The Essential HIV
Treatment Fact Book

"THE ESSENTIAL HIV TREATMENT FACT BOOK is even more than its title implies. It is an amazingly complete medical guide to all aspects of HIV infection. While a thorough tool kit for individual patients who wish to take charge of their health, it is also an exceptional reference book for health care providers working in the field. Patients, doctors, nurses, physician assistants, psychologists, and case workers would have a hard time finding a more comprehensive and up-to-date guide to the subject. It is one of those rare books which seems to anticipate just about every question a reader might ask. Highly recommended."

> —Martin Delaney,
> Executive Director and Co-Founder, Project Inform

"Pinsky and Douglas have done the impossible—they've written an 'AIDS Bible.' THE ESSENTIAL HIV TREATMENT FACT BOOK is an invaluable resource for those who are HIV+ and their loved ones."

> —Derek Hodel,
> Executive Director, People With AIDS Health Group

"This is a comprehensive up-to-date guide for the newly diagnosed person with HIV infection who wishes to be empowered to confront the illness with a solid knowledge base."

> —Gabriel Torres, M.D.,
> Medical Director, St. Vincent's Hospital Infectious Disease Clinic;
> Medical Consultant, GMHC *Treatment Issues*

Most Pocket Books are available at special quantity discounts for bulk purchases for sales promotions, premiums or fund raising. Special books or book excerpts can also be created to fit specific needs.

For details write the office of the Vice President of Special Markets, Pocket Books, 1230 Avenue of the Americas, New York, New York 10020.

The
Essential
HIV
Treatment Fact Book

by Laura Pinsky
and Paul Harding Douglas
with Craig Metroka, M.D., Ph.D.

POCKET BOOKS

New York   London   Toronto   Sydney   Tokyo   Singapore

For those we love as family,
both by blood and by choice

And for Charles Barber

An *Original* publication of Pocket Books

POCKET BOOKS, a division of Simon & Schuster Inc.
1230 Avenue of the Americas, New York, NY 10020

Pinsky, Laura.
    The essential HIV treatment fact book / by Laura Pinsky
and Paul Harding Douglas, with Craig Metroka.
        p.   cm.
    Includes bibliographical references and index.
    ISBN: 0-671-72528-9 : $14.00
    1. AIDS (Diseases)—Treatment.   I. Pinsky, Laura.   II. Metroka,
Craig.   III. Title.
    [DNLM: 1. HIV Infections—therapy—popular works.   WD 308 D735ea]
RC607.A26D69   1992
616.97'9206—dc20
DNLM/DLC
for Library of Congress   92-1716
                                                                              CIP

First Pocket Books trade paperback printing November 1992

10 9 8 7 6 5 4 3 2 1

Acknowledgments

The following people generously gave their time to review some or all of the manuscript:

Kevin Armington
Charles Barber
Richard Carlson, M.D.
Douglas Crimp
Jack DeHovitz, M.D.
Martin Delaney
Carolyn Douglas, M.D.
Richard Flaste
Garance Franke-Ruta
Douglas Goldschmidt, Ph.D.

Thaddeus Grimes-Gruczka
Samuel Grubman, M.D.
Derek Hodel
Gerard Ilaria, C.S.W.
Richard Isay, M.D.
Jonathan Jacobs, M.D.
Donald Kaplan, Ph.D.
Robert Kertzner, M.D.

Robert LaFosse
Jeffrey Laurence, M.D.
David Petersen
Judith Rabkin, Ph.D.
Charles Schable
Jeffrey Schmalz
Gabriel Torres, M.D.
Simon Watney
Daniel William, M.D.
Ron Winchel, M.D.

Any errors that may remain are the responsibility of the authors.

We would also like to thank the following people who have supported this work in diverse ways:

Dina Bisagna
Black Dot Graphics
Jonathon Brodman
Gina Centrello
the volunteers of the
  Columbia Gay
  Health Advocacy
  Project
the staff of the
  Columbia Health
  Service
the staff of the
  Columbia Mental
  Health Division
Tina Dobsevage, M.D.
Dorothy Fanning, R.N.
Bruce Francis
Peter Ginsberg

Richard Glendon, M.D.
Milton Horowitz, M.D.
Rose Inman, N.P.
Dan Kaney
Leslie Kantor
David Klotz
Donald Kotler, M.D.
Gary Ledet
Elena Levine, M.D.
Billie Lindsay
William Lloyd, M.D.
Irva Mandelbaum
the Monday and
  Wednesday Night
  Support Groups

Elizabeth Murray, R.N.
Cade Fields Newman, M.S., R.D.
Elaine Pfefferblit
Florence Pinsky
Juliette Pinsky
Michel Radomisli, Ph.D.
Ian Tattenbaum
Jess Taylor
Anita Tierney
Diane Watkin
Robert Withers
Jerry Wolbert, N.P.

Acknowledgments

We remember the lives of:

Allen Barnett
Robert Cohen
Roy Lynn Crawford
Larry Deccle
Frank Fedornick
Mark Fotopoulos
Robert Freedman
Stuart Garcia

Barry Gingell, M.D.
Tom Hannan
Craig Harris
Chris Hill
Dan Hirsch, Ph.D
Michael Hirsch
Dan Krumholz
Sal Licata, Ph.D.

Jay Lipner
Tyler Mackintosh
Kevin Mahoney
Michael Mitchell
Jean-Paul Mustone
Ray Navarro
Vito Russo
Joseph Stonehouse

Contents

Part One
Early Intervention

Part Two
Managing Complications

Part Three
Understanding the Science

Contents

Part Four
Practical Matters

Introduction

HIV DISEASE AND AIDS

In 1981 physicians around the nation began to report clusters of young homosexual men who had developed a then-rare pneumonia caused by the organism *Pneumocystis carinii*. These patients went on to develop numerous other rare complications, previously seen only in those with severely damaged immune systems. A pattern began to emerge as physicians reported more and more cases.

To track this new epidemic, the Centers for Disease Control (CDC) named it *acquired immunodeficiency syndrome* and defined it with a formal set of symptom-based criteria. To be defined as having AIDS a patient had to have one or more of a specific list of diseases and have no other reason to be immune deficient. (For more on this, consult Chapter 16: Immunology, Pathogenesis, and Etiology in Part 3: Understanding the Science.)

In 1983–84, researchers identified a virus as the probable cause of AIDS. The virus had various names initially (LAV, HTLV-III). The virus's official name is now the *human immunodeficiency virus,* or HIV.

When the HIV antibody test became widely available, the CDC changed the definition of AIDS to include a positive HIV antibody test (see Chapter 1: HIV Antibody Testing). Still later, the CDC widened the definition to include HIV-infected people who had lost substantial amounts of lean body mass *(wasting syndrome)* or who had certain cognitive deficits *(AIDS dementia complex).* In 1992, the CDC will change the definition of AIDS yet again: all HIV-infected people with certain blood-test values indicating immune deficiency (T4 lymphocyte count below 200 cells per mm^3; see Chapter 3: Monitoring the Immune System) will then fit the official criteria for a diagnosis of AIDS.

AIDS activists pay attention to the formal definition of AIDS for several reasons. Before the inclusion of people with wasting or dementia, a number of people with HIV disease were sick, unable to work, and yet not eligible for benefits because they did not fit the formal CDC definition of AIDS. In addition, government agencies based policy decisions and the allocation of resources on the official CDC statistics. These statistics in turn relied on narrower definitions of AIDS that understated the extent of the epidemic. However, epidemiologists who traced the course of the disease were reluctant to alter the definition because it determined their case figures: it is much harder to interpret trends in figures for a disease whose definition is constantly changing.

Researchers found it hard to perform accurate epidemiologic analysis on a moving target.

The word *syndrome* is part of the acronym AIDS because the cause was unknown when the term AIDS was coined. AIDS refers to an advanced stage of a viral illness. HIV *disease,* on the other hand, refers to the full range of illness caused by infection with this virus. HIV is necessary to cause AIDS: the full syndrome does not occur in the absence of HIV infection. HIV may be sufficient to cause AIDS by itself. However, HIV-infected people develop AIDS at such different rates that many researchers have suspected the existence of a *co-factor* (such as co-infection with another organism) that accelerates the appearence of AIDS.

IMPORTANT NEWS ABOUT TREATMENT

Most people think the AIDS epidemic consists solely of the approximately 200,000 Americans diagnosed with any of the life-threatening complications of HIV infection. You may be reading this book because you or someone you care about has a formal diagnosis of AIDS. This book directly addresses your situation.

However, there are another estimated *one* to *two million* HIV-infected Americans who have not yet developed any serious symptoms. If you are one of these people, you can now get medical care before you get sick—care that may prevent you from getting sick. Officials estimate that only one in ten HIV-infected Americans has been tested for the virus. The message of our book is that—since HIV infection has become treatable—you need to take action to protect your health *now.*

Early intervention refers to HIV-infected people acting to control the virus and fight symptoms while they are still healthy. Early intervention prevents or at least delays the onset of illness, lengthens the time patients remain healthy, and increases life span. This strategy is not hypothetical; it is currently a proven part of the clinical practice of physicians expert in treating HIV disease.

Sixty percent of the deaths from AIDS have been due to a single illness: *Pneumocystis carinii* pneumonia, or PCP. Some people survive multiple episodes of PCP, but fully 25 percent of those who get it die during their first bout. **PCP is now *preventable* with antibiotic drugs.** Given enough warning of decline in the immune system, an HIV-infected person can begin taking medication to forestall (perhaps permanently) the onset of this deadly pneumonia.

HIV disease typically causes few noticeable symptoms over the ten years (on average) from infection to development of serious complications. The immune system gradually weakens until infections and cancers appear, often without any warning signs obvious to the patient. Physicians can use blood tests to determine the condition of the immune system: these tests can tell when an HIV-infected person needs to begin medication to avoid life-threatening complications. Currently, very few HIV-infected people are aware of the need for regular blood tests to monitor the immune system.

Many infected people who might be able to get PCP prevention and other therapies are falling ill and dying needlessly. People need to know that early intervention is necessary and available. They also need to know how to overcome practical, psychological, and social barriers to get effective treatment. You may have been told that AIDS is untreatable and inevitably fatal and therefore believe that there is nothing you can do to protect yourself. We intend this book to reveal that this is a potentially life-threatening misconception. We hope to move you to take prompt action.

INFORMATION PRESENTED WITH INSIGHT

Most people go to the doctor only *after* illness appears, rather than before. Those with HIV cannot afford to wait until they are sick to get help. Even people who see a physician regularly are not going to hear about early intervention from their doctors. *The New England Journal of Medicine* states that very few physicians are aware of proper care for AIDS, and fewer still know anything about early intervention. According to the federal government, in 1992 and 1993 hundreds of thousands of previously healthy people will learn they have HIV disease by getting sick, and still more will need care without realizing it. HIV-infected people need to learn about developments in treatment. This will not be easy—unfamiliarity, fear, and the disease's link with stigmatized people and activities block education about HIV.

It may be difficult for you to take the first steps toward getting care for your HIV infection because it requires you to acknowledge the possibility that you might become dangerously ill. Acknowledging this reality is emotionally painful but necessary if you are to get proper care. We will describe this pain realistically and suggest ways in which you can counter the difficulty of this situation. Early intervention *is* possible if you address the emotional barriers and break down the practical task into small, manageable steps.

Two components are crucial to successful delivery of this message: usable information and psychological insight.

New attitudes toward medical care are developing in the context of the AIDS epidemic. Patients are now demanding more information and seeking to make better-informed choices. In our work counseling HIV-infected people, we have found that people *can* absorb and effectively use sophisticated medical information, if we present the material correctly. People frequently underestimate their ability to understand medical information. The medical establishment bears some responsibility for its historical failure to teach patients about their illnesses. The motivated individual can understand all the necessary information, if it is demystified and properly explained. **Usable information can help you replace passivity with action.**

Writers frequently offer scientific information about this disease as an unorganized collection of isolated facts. Technical information should be conveyed with both power and simplicity; you need enough information to make decisions that affect your care, but not so much that you are paralyzed with irrelevancies. Some facts about HIV are simply more *useful* than others—in particular information relevant to those decisions that you yourself can make. We advocate courses of action based on proven clinical studies, consensus among expert physicians and researchers, and our own experience in working with HIV-infected people. We describe those instances in which experts disagree substantially. This book treats practical, medical, psychological, and emotional issues as part of a coherent and comprehensive survival strategy.

This book attempts to set down current knowledge of the treatment of HIV disease according to established medical authorities. Although we sometimes describe unproved and controversial treatments, we emphasize the consensus of HIV-expert physicians regarding diagnosis and treatment. We believe that this viewpoint represents the present best hope for people who are HIV infected. This book does not discuss holistic, alternative, or non-Western strategies for treating HIV disease. We suggest that interested readers pursue further reading.

No book can give you back complete control of your life. However, this book may at least provide a clear picture of the choices you face and help you manage your illness rationally and competently.

Information alone may not be enough. Emotional conflicts can make information difficult to *understand,* no matter how clearly presented. You may associate information about HIV and AIDS with pain, stigma, loss of control, and thoughts of death. This book takes into account the conflicts you may experience about being sick, becoming a patient, taking medication, going to the doctor, or being hospitalized.

Other emotional barriers may keep you from *acting* upon information, even if you have thoroughly assimilated and understood that information. Even well-informed HIV-infected people may have difficulty acting on their knowledge. For example, you may have seen friends and lovers get sick and die relatively early in the epidemic, before many of the treatments that are now saving lives became standard. This painful experience may have influenced your idea of treatment for HIV. Memories of terrifying and futile treatment keep people from learning about more recent advances and discourage them from believing in the very possibility of effective treatment. In addition, those who associate treatment entirely with the most debilitating terminal phases of AIDS may be hostile to early intervention because they may wrongly interpret it as prolonging a painful end rather than adding years of healthy productive life.

Introduction

Our strategy to help you overcome psychological resistance to medical care will be to:

- Alert you to possible problems by acknowledging and explicitly describing emotional barriers
- Remind you that emotions in response to serious illness vary from person to person and over time, and that anxiety, numbness, anger, or sadness are to be expected.
- Explain how social factors such as discrimination may worsen your psychological distress
- Encourage you to analyze feelings and thoughts that may keep you from acting in your best interest medically
- Encourage you to talk with friends or counselors
- Urge you to fight isolation by joining together with other infected people for information, strategies, and support
- Break down tasks that may initially seem overwhelming into smaller, more manageable steps
- Provide a structure within which you can monitor whether you are following through with your health-care plans

Other people in your situation have been able to get the right kind of medical treatment and benefit from it. Our culture stigmatizes this disease, and, as a result, you may not feel comfortable discussing your situation with others. Exposure to an informed and sympathetic consensus about early intervention will help you confront your need for medical care.

HIV brings worries and grief: give yourself permission to be anxious, to mourn, to feel sad. Once you express these strong emotions, you may be able to take productive action toward resolving the practical questions surrounding medical care.

If you explore and challenge obstacles to understanding and action you may be able to overcome reluctance to find and use effective medical care. Listen to your emotions as well as your physical symptoms and you may improve your understanding, increase your cooperation with medical care, and reduce your psychological distress. You bring your own character and conflicts to the experience of HIV disease. Other aspects of your life and experience influence your feelings about HIV. These psychological reactions affect your ability to understand and use medical care.

How to Use This Book

Read different sections of this book depending on your particular medical, social, and psychological needs. There is absolutely no need to read this book from cover to cover.

The book addresses people with varying degrees of illness. We expect that some readers have no current medical symptoms and are leading active lives unimpeded by physical disability. We also expect that some readers have life-threatening symptoms that therefore motivate discussions of serious disease, hospitalization, and the physical and emotional aspects of disability.

The situation of an asymptomatic HIV-positive person is both similar to and very different from that of those living with advanced AIDS. If you have few symptoms it may be frightening to identify yourself with people who are more seriously ill. If you are a veteran of this disease, the worries of asymptomatic HIV-infected people may seem trivial. One insight remains true for all: you can derive strength, knowledge, and support from other people who are HIV infected or who have AIDS.

Because of the variability of the course of the disease, to some extent you will have to take things one day at a time. At any one time, only some of the information in this book will be relevant to you.

Everyone should read the material presented in Part One: Early Intervention.

Part Two: Managing Complications, contains detailed specific material on a vast range of infections and cancers, only some of which will ever be relevant to any particular individual. It may be anxiety-provoking to read descriptions of complications that may never affect you. Balance your curiosity against your anxiety.

If you are interested in understanding the scientific issues connected with HIV disease, more technical topics have been presented in Part Three: Understanding the Science. You do not need to read this material to understand your medical care. However, some people like to know more of the medical and scientific background.

Everyone should read Part Four: Practical Matters on insurance, benefits, discrimination, and wills. The Appendices contain listings of telephone numbers and other contact information for AIDS service organizations and other groups that may be helpful to you.

We would like to acknowledge here that this book will be less useful to those who have had less access to education or to those whose economic situation is such that they are profoundly disadvantaged in terms of access to health care.

How to Use This Book

A CAUTION TO THE READER

At the end of the book, we have listed those sources that may be most helpful to readers who want more information on specific topics. However, we have attempted to capture a snapshot of current medical practice, which necessarily runs in advance of the published literature. Much of the material presented is still under debate. Much that is accepted practice among expert clinicians may never receive full proof in the form of controlled clinical trials. In the text we have indicated the status of evidence when evidence is available. We have also tried to incorporate consensus opinions among clinicians and researchers, or to mark controversy among experts where it persists. This is not a medical textbook. **Take no action that might affect your health without obtaining the advice of a physician expert in the management of HIV disease.**

Authors' Note

Laura Pinsky and Paul Harding Douglas have based this book on seven years' work with the Gay Health Advocacy Project at Columbia University (which we serve as director and co-director) and also with the Gay Men's Health Crisis in New York City. Laura Pinsky is also a psychotherapist in private practice in New York City. In addition, she runs support groups for HIV-infected people. Paul Douglas, trained as an artist and computer scientist, now divides his time between AIDS work and the graphic arts. They have also written *The Essential AIDS Fact Book,* basic information on AIDS for a general audience, now in its fourth printing.

Craig Metroka received his M.D. and Ph.D. from New York University. He is trained in the fields of internal medicine, hematology, and medical oncology. Dr. Metroka is an associate editor of *AIDS Targeted Information Newsletter,* a contributing editor of the *AIDS/HIV Treatment Directory* of the American Foundation for AIDS Research (AmFAR), and a former contributing editor of *AIDS Clinical Care.* He is a member of the scientific advisory committee of AmFAR and of the Community-Based Clinical Trials (run by AmFAR). He is a member of the Oncology Core Committee of the AIDS Clinical Trials Group of the National Institute of Allergies and Infectious Disease. He is the author of numerous articles in the field of HIV disease. Dr. Metroka is an attending physician at St. Luke's/Roosevelt Hospital Center in New York City and assistant professor of medicine at Columbia University College of Physicians and Surgeons.

Writers should have empathy with their readers, but with AIDS, it has seldom been forthcoming. Articles in the press about HIV disease are often written as if no readers were themselves at risk or infected. Medical books usually assume the point of view of the researcher, which may make the HIV-infected reader feel like a laboratory animal. Our goal has been to speak to you, the infected reader, directly.

This book has been shaped by our own experience of the disease, by that of our lovers and friends and colleagues, as well as by our professional work with HIV-infected people. We have met and lost remarkable people. It has been difficult, heartbreaking work, frustrating but fascinating and worthwhile; providing small triumphs in the face of great tragedy. We appeal to you: first, work to stay healthy; then, join the thousands of people of every description who call themselves AIDS activists.

Part One
Early Intervention

This part of the book provides information you need to understand and obtain early effective medical treatment for HIV infection.

Some people reading this book may not yet know whether they are HIV infected, so we begin with a chapter on the HIV antibody test. This chapter may also be useful for those who have already tested positive and want a clear description of the implications of the test results and help in coping with emotional reactions to the test.

Your work together with an expert physician crucially determines your chances for continued health. Chapter 2: You and Your Doctor discusses how you can locate a physician with the necessary expertise. The chapter also suggests ways you can work compatibly and productively with your physician. (Part 4 contains some useful general information about health insurance and other ways to pay for medical care.)

The third chapter, Monitoring the Immune System, describes how you can keep track of the damage that the virus has caused to your immune system. This information will give you the opportunity to intervene against the virus and its secondary complications at the appropriate moment.

The next chapter is largely concerned with AZT and other antiviral drugs. We discuss antivirals first because, for most people, antivirals will be the first medical intervention used against the virus. The chapter discusses how HIV grows, and what can be done to stop its growth. HIV-infected people starting antivirals may worry about these powerful drugs.

Once you know the status of your immune system, you can act to prevent the onset of opportunistic infections. Chapter 5: Preventing PCP and Other Complications, describes treatments and strategies that have already greatly improved the survival of people with HIV.

Chapter 6 covers a great range of issues surrounding general health care. It includes discussions of when to get medical help for your symptoms, what immunizations to get, and other great and small matters from nutrition to travel to pets.

Chapter 7 is titled Your State of Mind. This chapter has two sections. The first describes the range of psychological reactions that we have seen in

1

people with HIV disease, and talks about how to manage emotional problems that may arise. The second part describes more purely medical (or psychiatric) factors that affect your state of mind. This part also explains how treatment can help you lessen problems with anxiety, depression, low energy, sleep disturbances, and pain.

The first part ends with a chapter devoted to special issues for women, children, and members of racial and ethnic minorities, and finally a brief chapter describing ways that you can educate yourself further about unproven treatments.

Chapter 1
HIV Antibody Testing

Many people are now struggling with HIV antibody testing issues: whether to be tested, whether the test is accurate, how to go about being tested. Since HIV antibody testing is the first step toward getting adequate medical care, people need help to understand how they can benefit from testing and how they can overcome their fear and reluctance. This chapter describes the test in detail, considers the various economic, social, and psychological obstacles you face in using testing to get medical care, and offers some suggestions as to how you may be able to overcome these obstacles. This chapter will lead you through the medical, legal, and psychological aspects of HIV antibody testing. You will learn how to assess your risk for being HIV infected; how to be tested accurately and anonymously; when to be retested; and how to get the best possible psychological support.

Until early intervention became a practical reality, many people saw no persuasive medical reason to be tested, as long as they practiced *risk reduction* (used condoms for sexual intercourse and did not share needles). The consensus against testing and for safer sex was a cornerstone of successful community-based self-help and advocacy efforts. However, the very success of this agenda (which was correct and appropriate in the past) now interferes with the acceptance of testing for the purpose of early intervention.

OLD LINE: DON'T GET TESTED

Soon after the introduction of the HIV antibody test, many AIDS service providers decided that antibody testing was not generally productive for people who actually had significant risk for having been infected who were already practicing risk reduction. There were several reasons for this.

People thought to have AIDS or HIV have sometimes suffered injurious discrimination or harassment. People with AIDS have sometimes lost jobs, housing, or the support of friends or family. Association with this illness carries with it a profound stigma. Early on, the media frequently discussed the possibility of mass coercive screening with the HIV antibody test. This terrified people who felt they might be infected, who justifiably feared loss of civil liberties, quarantine, or even violence. Initially, provisions for confidentiality of the testing process and test results were few and inadequate, a situation that persists in many areas of the country.

Testing can be very distressing. If the result is positive, then you have to face the fact that you have a real risk of getting seriously ill. Awareness of the stigma mentioned above further increases the stress of testing positive. Stress alone can cause illness, and in the presence of HIV it was feared it might actually precipitate a medical crisis.

When the test first became available, technique and interpretive standards varied from lab to lab. Some labs did not confirm reactive results from the initial sensitive screening test with more specific tests, which raised the possibility that some people might falsely be told that they were HIV infected (*false positives*), causing terrible and unnecessary distress. In addition to false positives, it was not then known whether false negatives might also be a problem: cases in which infected people might fail to be detected by a test based on screening for antibodies.

Finally the prognostic significance of testing was not immediately clear. Perhaps only a minority of HIV-infected people might get ill, in which case it was irresponsible to throw the majority into a panic for no benefit. No one knew how long HIV-infected people remained healthy before developing serious symptoms.

Since **no treatment for asymptomatic infection was widely available until relatively recently,** it seemed that there was no medical benefit to being tested.

The argument popularly advanced in support of testing was that people who might be infected had a duty to determine this fact and take steps to ensure that they did not transmit the virus to any sexual partners. **However, people at significant risk for infection are encouraged to commence or continue risk reduction in any case,** so no extra benefit is derived from testing in terms of restricting the spread of the virus.

NEW LINE: GET TESTED TO GET TREATMENT

In recent years some of these considerations have changed significantly. There are now compelling reasons for people at risk to be tested.

Discrimination continues to be a major aggravating problem in this epidemic. The increasing tendency of state and federal legislatures and courts to protect people against HIV-related discrimination has not significantly deterred widespread discrimination and harassment of those perceived as "having AIDS" or "spreading AIDS."

Testing continues to cause great psychological stress. Testing is now more frequently accompanied by at least some counseling, but the majority of those testing positive can still expect to experience substantial depression for a period of weeks to months.

Researchers have provided more information supporting confidence in the accuracy of the whole testing procedure.

The problem of false positives has virtually been eliminated through the

4

use of confirmatory tests for all those whose initial result is reactive. If performed properly, the odds of a positive result being false are very small. One estimate of the false-positive rate when screening a low-risk population is 1 in 135,000.

Given that enough time has elapsed between the last possible exposure to HIV and the time blood is drawn for the test, **a negative result is also very reliable.** (See p. 6, "Window Period" for a more complete description of this reasoning.)

What really convinced AIDS service providers to begin recommending testing to their clients who were at significant risk was the advent of **medical treatment proven useful** *before* **the appearance of noticeable symptoms.** Testing became the first step toward getting medical care that was potentially life saving. Medical breakthroughs outweighed considerations of psychological stress and potential discrimination.

Recent information has strengthened the case for (near-) universal adoption of safer sex practices. It is clear that infected people should protect themselves against infection with other (possibly more virulent) strains of HIV as well as against infection with sexually transmitted disease that may accelerate the progression of HIV disease.

PSYCHOLOGICAL RESISTANCE TO BEING TESTED

You may be reluctant to be HIV antibody tested. It may seem easier to avoid thinking about HIV altogether. You may feel that the stress of knowing that you were infected would be unbearable. These are understandable deterrents to testing.

In this book we hope to demonstrate the benefit of early medical intervention against HIV infection. We believe that the prospect of extra healthy and productive years provides a strong incentive to be tested and to face the consequent psychological stress.

The stress is real: living with HIV is often upsetting. However, in a few weeks to a few months most people recover from the stress of testing positive, regain their psychological equilibrium, and get on with their lives. Given preparation and support, testing and early intervention offer you the best chance for the best quality of life.

DETECTING ANTIBODIES VERSUS DETECTING VIRUS

There are several possible ways to determine whether you are infected with HIV. The most common method is to test for the presence of *antibodies* to HIV, rather than to test for the virus itself. The antibody test is typically used because it is cheaper, technologically simpler to perform and interpret, standardized, and widely available. Other tests attempt to detect the virus itself directly and can sometimes be useful in addition to the antibody test. We will discuss these other tests later.

NORMAL ANTIBODY FUNCTION

Your immune system normally responds to infection by manufacturing proteins called *antibodies*. The production of measurable levels of antibodies usually occurs within a few days to a few weeks of the time of infection (though it may take somewhat longer in the case of HIV infection, as we will see). Each infectious organism stimulates the production of antibodies specific to certain of the organism's component molecules. These component molecules that trigger an antibody response are called *antigens*. Each antibody matches one specific antigen and is drawn from a genetically determined repertoire of hundreds of millions of possible antibodies. This repertoire has evolved over time to provide protection against many of the infectious organisms that the average person encounters. An antibody functions by binding to its specific antigen, effectively marking the organism containing that antigen for destruction by other parts of the body's immune system.

The presence of antibodies specific to a particular infectious organism is in general a good sign. Antibodies help the body resist the proliferation of that organism. The presence of circulating antibodies to an organism helps (in some cases) to provide *immunity* against future infections by that organism. However, the antibodies produced against HIV—while helpful—are not completely effective in controlling the growth of this virus. The presence of antibodies to HIV thus indicates infection but not immunity or total protection from the virus's ability to cause disease.

WINDOW PERIOD

Most infections will stimulate the production of a detectable level of antibodies within a fairly short period—days to weeks. Antibodies to HIV may not be detectable for a longer period. Debate over the length of the time between infection and the production of detectable levels of HIV antibodies has now been resolved (refer to Part 3: Understanding the Science, for more information on the debate over *long latency).* The Centers for Disease Control observes that most subjects in whom the date of infection is known have tested antibody positive within three months of their infection. It is conceivable that some may take longer to develop antibodies in response to HIV infection. In order to leave a margin for error, the CDC now recommends that you interpret a negative antibody test result as indicating that you were uninfected as of six months prior to the time blood was drawn for testing. If you have not shared needles or had intercourse without a condom in the six months prior to a negative test, you may consider yourself to be uninfected.

INITIAL AND CONFIRMING TESTS

When performed on humans, the HIV antibody test is really a sequence of several different tests. The initial test used (called the *ELISA* test) may be repeated several times, and may also ultimately be checked against any one of several confirming tests (variously the *Western blot, IFA,* or *RIPA).*

ELISA stands for "enzyme-linked immunosorbent assay" and is pronounced like the name Eliza. This test was developed to screen donated blood so as to eliminate HIV-infected blood from the blood supply. Only later was it used for detecting HIV infection in humans. A negative (nonreactive) result from the ELISA very accurately demonstrates that the blood sample contains no HIV antibodies. However, a reactive result from the ELISA may sometimes be false. Donated blood with a reactive ELISA result is simply discarded or set aside for reasons of economy, though it might be a false positive. When testing people for HIV infection, an initially reactive ELISA should not immediately be accepted as a true positive. A reactive ELISA should be repeated twice. Consistently reactive ELISAs are then subjected to confirmation with another laboratory test that is even more specific for HIV antibody and so has fewer false positives.

The ELISA reacts to various anti-HIV antibodies without providing any information on which of the different types of HIV antibodies are specifically present in the sample. **The Western blot test,** on the other hand, indicates which specific antibodies are present. This additional information can help distinguish samples that are true positives from those that are falsely positive on the ELISA.

We usually think of antibodies to an infectious organism as all being of one type. In fact, there may be many different antibodies directed against different antigens that form the parts of a single infectious organism. In the case of HIV, humans form antibodies against at least nine different molecular components of the virus. A test result that implies the presence of certain of these antibodies is a more definite indication of HIV infection than a result indicating the presence of other antibodies.

The ELISA test does not distinguish between the various different antibodies against HIV: the test reacts if any one of the HIV antibodies is present. But a reactive ELISA may not indicate HIV infection, because other non-HIV antibodies may cross-react and mimic an HIV antibody. The Western blot is designed to detect whether each of the possible HIV antibodies is present. The pattern of antibodies that is found can determine whether HIV infection has indeed occurred.

Some laboratories confirm ELISA-positive results with tests other than the Western blot. Alternatives include the *immunofluorescence assay* **(IFA)**, and the *radio-immunoprecipitative assay* **(RIPA)**. These tests provide confirmation as accurate as that of the Western blot.

7

ACCURACY OF RESULTS

The rate of false positives after confirmatory testing is extremely low. If you receive a confirmed positive result despite low risk for HIV infection, seek further lab investigations. Generally this will involve repeating the entire testing sequence on a fresh sample of the subject's blood, but, if available, more sophisticated testing (e.g., polymerase chain reaction, PCR) may provide a conclusive result more quickly (see discussion of PCR in Part Three: Understanding the Science, p. 324).

If enough time has elapsed since the last possible exposure to HIV, the ELISA–Western blot antibody test sequence is extremely accurate in both the negatives and positives. Positive results in people with significant risk for HIV infection are very likely to be true positives, and repeat testing is probably not necessary to confirm the result. Positive results in subjects with low risk are likely to be false positives, and testing therefore should be repeated.

Occasionally, a Western blot or other confirmatory test will have an indeterminate result. An indeterminate result should occasion a new cycle of testing with a fresh sample of blood. Indeterminate results can occur if the subject is in the process of *seroconverting*—changing from negative to positive. This type of indeterminate will eventually resolve into a positive result if testing is repeated at a later date. But indeterminates on Western blot can also resolve as negative results, for reasons not completely understood. Subjects with low risk for HIV infection who persistently receive indeterminate results on Western blot are unlikely to be HIV infected. Their serostatus may be determined by DNA amplification testing such as PCR. Have your physician contact the Laboratory Investigation Branch of the Centers for Disease Control in Atlanta for further information on how to resolve persistently indeterminate Western blot results. Again, indeterminate results are rare; testing should be repeated after a few weeks' wait.

HIV-2 is a variant of HIV that is prevalent in western Africa and very rare in the United States. HIV-2 is transmitted through the same routes as HIV-1 and, like HIV-1, can cause AIDS. The HIV antibody test commonly available in the United States is a test for antibodies to HIV-1 and does not always detect infection with HIV-2. Few cases of HIV-2 infection have been reported in the United States. Most identified HIV-2–infected U.S. residents have been immigrants from western Africa. Beginning in 1992 blood centers in the United States test donated blood for HIV-2 as well as HIV-1.

If any portion of your risk for HIV infection (from transfusion, needle sharing, or unprotected sexual contact) occurred in, or through a person coming from, a western African nation (including Guinea Bissau, Ivory Coast, Senegal, Burkina Faso, Cape Verde Island), you should be tested not only for antibodies to HIV-1 but also for antibodies to HIV-2. See the appendices for more information.

SIGNIFICANCE OF RESULTS

What is the significance of the results obtained from HIV antibody testing?

A **negative HIV antibody test result** is usually good news. A negative means that antibodies to HIV were not detected in the sample of blood supplied. If six months or more has elapsed since the last episode of unprotected vaginal or rectal intercourse, the last episode of needle sharing, or the last instance of other risk, then it is extremely probable that the absence of antibodies to HIV means no infection with HIV has occurred. Without infection, disease due to HIV is impossible. A negative result also implies that transmission to others through blood, semen, or vaginal or cervical secretions is impossible. However, despite a negative result, infection with HIV is still possible in the future. Therefore, even those people with a negative result should avoid sharing needles and should use condoms for intercourse, with narrow exceptions.

Nobody likes to get a **positive HIV antibody test result.** However, a positive result can provide early notice of the opportunity to start medical action to control the virus and prevent illness. A positive result means that antibodies to HIV were found in the blood sample you provided. Therefore, you are infected with HIV. Infection with this virus must at present be considered lifelong. A positive result implies that you may be able to transmit the virus if your blood, semen, or vaginal or cervical secretions come into contact with the wet internal linings (*mucous membranes*) of another person's vagina, rectum, or urethra (the tube through which urine passes). You may also be able to transmit HIV infection by sharing needles for intravenous drug use, or if another person's bloodstream is directly exposed to your blood, as via transfusion. If you are an HIV-positive woman, your pregnancy has a 25 to 30 percent chance of resulting in an HIV-infected newborn.

What does a positive result imply in terms of your chances of getting sick? Even without treatment, this virus is very slow to cause any serious symptoms. Most HIV-infected adults stay relatively healthy for eight to twelve years following infection. A minority of infected people fall seriously ill sooner than eight years after infection. A recent study showed that one in five infected people remained healthy after eleven years.

The message of this book is that you do not have to let the virus run its course without opposition. The decade-long period of relatively good health following infection with HIV may be extended to an unknown degree by medical treatment. In later chapters we will describe how existing treatments have been proven to slow the progress of HIV disease. Early intervention with these treatments buys you healthy, productive years during which researchers may develop even more effective treatments.

OTHER TESTING

There are other tests that can determine whether you are HIV-infected: viral culture, DNA amplification, and p24 antigen assays. For various reasons, these tests are not generally used to detect HIV infection. These tests are described below for the curious; others may skip this section without missing anything vital.

Researchers use the term *viral culture* to describe a test-tube attempt to grow the virus in blood or tissue samples. Since viruses cannot reproduce on their own, host white blood cells from non-HIV-infected donors must be provided. These cells are stimulated with a chemical called PHA (*phytohemagglutinin*) to make them more receptive to HIV infection. Stimulated host cells are then exposed to sample cells from the patient, and the whole system is then incubated for days or weeks. The system can be assayed at various points and in various ways for evidence of HIV.

Viral culture is technically difficult. Initially, culturing HIV was so difficult that it was not possible to find virus even in many patients with frank AIDS. As culture techniques have improved and laboratory experience has grown, the success of viral culture has also improved. At this point a good lab can culture virus from the vast majority of people with AIDS. However, the technique remains difficult—so difficult that it is not suitable for mass application. In addition, the sensitivity of the ELISA-Western blot sequence remains higher than that of viral culture techniques. That means that testing for HIV via viral culture alone will result in some false negatives. Because of the difficulty and the lack of sensitivity, viral culture is not a good general method for the detection of HIV infection.

DNA amplification by the DNA polymerase chain reaction, or PCR, is a novel laboratory technique that allows the detection of very small amounts of specific sequences of nucleic acid (such as the genetic material of HIV as integrated into the cellular chromosomes) that may be contained within much larger sequences (such as the entire complement of DNA in the chromosomes inside a human cell).

In PCR, a selected target region of DNA is located and replicated, while the larger host DNA is not replicated. This process is repeated, with the amount of target DNA doubling after each cycle. After a number of cycles, an amount of the target DNA will be generated that is detectable by conventional assays.

A problem in using PCR is that it is very easy to get false-positive results if the lab technique used isn't perfect. The slightest contamination of the sample with HIV DNA from previous tests will cause a false positive, since this technique is so sensitive. This is why PCR is not the best test for mass screening for HIV. It is useful for the detection of HIV nucleic acid in circumstances where HIV antibody testing cannot

10

provide a reliable result, such as in newborn infants of HIV-positive mothers (where maternal antibodies will render the infant seropositive whether or not the child is actually HIV infected); and in the case of people whose Western blot is indeterminate.

Part of an inner shell of the virus is composed of a protein called *p24 antigen.* This antigen is sometimes detectable in the blood of HIV-infected people. The p24 antigen test is not currently used for the purpose of determining whether an individual is HIV infected. It may have certain uses in the evaluation of new drugs and possibly in decisions about treatment in later stages of HIV infection (these will be discussed in Chapter 3: Monitoring the Immune System).

PSYCHOLOGICAL PREPARATION FOR TESTING

Prepare before getting tested: it will make things easier for you. Assess realistically your risk of being infected. Risk assessment may help you decide about HIV antibody testing and further medical evaluation. Contemplating the possibility that you may be positive is unpleasant, but you will have had more time to adjust if you actually get back a positive test.

If the odds are that you will be positive, it is a good idea to do as much planning as possible beforehand so that you will not have to cope with a number of things when you will undoubtedly be upset. This applies to practical issues (checking out your insurance, finding a doctor) and emotional issues such as deciding whom you will tell in the short run and what kind of support you want and can get when you are feeling bad. You may be able to anticipate difficult areas and make arrangements to lessen difficulties. For example, you may want to plan to get your test results back at a time when you are not going to be under a great deal of other stress.

Counseling before and after testing will help you understand the test process and the significance of the results.

You should spend some time thinking about what your reaction is likely to be if you are HIV positive. Although you cannot always anticipate how you will feel, having explored the possibilities will make things less confusing and overwhelming if you find out that you are infected. You should think about how you have reacted to bad news in the past. Do you tend to do self-destructive things impulsively when you are upset? Being conscious of your behavior in the past can help you avoid some mistakes. Plan how to take care of yourself by thinking about what has been helpful in past times of stress.

The single most crucial issue to think about in advance is how to arrange the best possible emotional support to help you face a positive test result. What this boils down to is finding people who will help you. At the very minimum, someone you trust should know that you are going to be tested. If possible, talk with this person (before getting back your test results) about your thoughts and feelings about possibly being HIV infected. Many people feel better if they bring someone with them when they go to get back the test results. Make arrangements in advance to be with someone if you get back a positive result. It is almost always a bad idea to be alone when you first get bad news.

RISK SELF-ASSESSMENT

If you have not yet been HIV antibody tested you need to estimate the odds that you might be infected so that you can prepare for the likely result. Ideally, you should consult with a trained HIV counselor who can review your sexual and drug-use history and help you assess your risk for having been HIV infected. This section provides guidelines that you may use to assess your risk if professional counseling is not available.

Remember, this type of risk self-assessment is not useful for determining what risk-reduction behavior is appropriate for your situation. If you or a sexual partner has not yet been reliably tested negative, you need to use condoms for intercourse. A self-assessment of low risk for you and your sexual partners is not a substitute for safer sex. Similarly, all needle-drug users must avoid sharing needles, or at least must effectively clean shared needles before and after use. A self-assessment of low risk for you and your needle-sharing partners is not a substitute for safer injection practices.

Risk self-assessment is usually the first step toward testing, but do not substitute risk-assessment for reliable antibody testing.

The method of risk assessment described below will assign you one of three levels of risk: significant risk, low risk, or no risk. We have chosen three levels of risk rather than a point-based or other scoring system because there are three recommended courses of action that you should take, depending on your level of risk. Any further refinement of the estimate serves only to heighten anxiety prematurely or create a false sense of security.

RISK CATEGORIES AND TESTING

Risk Category	Risk Reduction Recommended	Testing Recommended	Primary Purpose of Testing
No Risk	Yes, if risk activity is contemplated	Only for anxiety or if otherwise desired	Reduce inappropriate anxiety
Low Risk	Yes	Yes	Reduce inappropriate anxiety; discourage risk behavior
Significant Risk	Yes	Yes	Motivate testing and early intervention

The risk-assessment method used here depends on three factors: the concrete information available to you; the varying risk of transmission associated with various past actions; and the risk of the partners with whom these past actions were performed.

A person's **information about his or her risk** for infection may be *incomplete* if the person may have performed actions of which he or she has no conscious knowledge, as when drunk or drugged or unconscious.

The **risk associated with various activities** is fairly well characterized. Sharing needles and unprotected rectal or vaginal intercourse confer significant risk, while all other sexual activities confer less-than-significant risk.

The **risk of partners** is in general hard to determine with accuracy. This is because most people have limited information regarding the risk history of partners and *their* past partners. A characterization of a partner's risk based solely on membership in a population not defined by specific behavior may be inaccurate in three ways: the characterization depends on the accuracy of the *perception;* it may be inaccurate if the reference population is chosen incorrectly (e.g., some men consider themselves "straight" despite having unprotected intercourse with other men); and finally because assumptions about the prevalence of infection in the reference population may be wrong.

Determine the risk of your partners in exactly the same way as you determine your own risk. Assign each partner one of the three levels of risk: no risk, low risk, or significant risk. The portion of your risk attributable to your contact with each partner will then depend on the partner's risk and the riskiest activity you performed with that partner.

The rule of thumb that most people use is to decide whether any sexual partners were men who have had unprotected intercourse with other men or were people who shared needles. Such partners do have a greater statistical chance of having been HIV infected. However, we are at a transition point: we must begin to consider all people who have intercourse without condoms as at significant risk for HIV infection.

Have you ever been tested for HIV antibody? **If you have ever tested positive, you are HIV infected.** If your most recent test result was negative, then you must assess the risk of your activity since six months prior to the time blood was drawn for that test.

If you received certain blood or blood products for medical purposes at any time before March 1985, you are at risk for having been HIV infected. Blood products known to have transmitted HIV are: whole blood, blood cellular components, plasma, and clotting factors. Blood products that are not known to have ever transmitted HIV are: immunoglobulin, albumin, plasma protein fraction, and hepatitis B vaccine.

If you have shared needles or other equipment *(works, gimmicks, sets, points, cookers)* for drug use since 1977 you have significant risk for having been HIV infected, unless your needle-sharing partners are explicitly known to have tested HIV negative. Shared needles may transmit HIV not only during injection into a vein (intravenous, IV), but also during injection into a muscle (intramuscular, IM), or during injection of drugs just under the skin (subcutaneous injection, sometimes called *skin-popping).*

If you have had **unprotected intercourse** since 1977, your risk depends on the risk of your partners. Unprotected intercourse is defined as vaginal or rectal intercourse without a condom (however briefly), or intercourse with a condom that broke while the penis was inside the partner's body. The risk of unprotected vaginal or rectal intercourse is significant whether you were the *insertive* or the *receptive* partner. (The insertive partner puts his penis inside the receptive partner's vagina or rectum.) In the United States, the receptive partner is probably at greater risk. Ejaculation in the body during unprotected intercourse increases the risk of transmission to the receptive partner.

Oral sex has not been a significant risk for HIV transmission unless semen or blood enters the mouth. Oral-genital sex includes *fellatio* (the stimulation of a man's penis with the mouth, also called "blow jobs," or "going down" on a man) and *cunnilingus* (the stimulation of a woman's vulva and clitoris with lips and tongue, also called "going down" on a woman). While we recommend that you avoid getting blood or semen in your mouth, very few cases of AIDS have been traced to transmission via the mouth. Oral-anal contact (stimulation of the anus with the lips and tongue, also called "rimming") is not a likely route of HIV transmission, but may transmit intestinal parasites that can produce serious medical problems and possibly exacerbate an existing HIV infection. The use of latex barriers in oral-genital and oral-anal sex further reduces the risk of transmission of HIV or other organisms.

Kissing, including tongue kissing or wet kissing, poses no significant risk for HIV transmission. For a more detailed discussion of sexual risk reduction, please refer to Part 4: Practical Matters.

ARRANGING FOR TESTING

To find a reliable source of HIV antibody testing, call the nearest AIDS service organization or department of health. Some are listed in the appendices. Ask for the location of the testing site, the procedure, time you must wait until you get your results, the availability of counseling, provisions for anonymity, and availability of referrals to medical and psychological services. Make sure that positive ELISA testing is confirmed by more specific tests such as Western blot or IFA.

ANONYMITY PROTECTS AGAINST DISCRIMINATION

Anonymity is your first line of defense against discrimination. Some legal protections exist but they rely on the prospect of enforcement to deter discrimination. Statistics show that the incidence of discrimination has not been reduced by the passage of protective legislation. In most cases this legislation provides recourse but not protection beforehand. Confidentiality laws are helpful in certain situations.

The clearest way to protect yourself from possible discrimination is to be tested anonymously. HIV antibody testing is anonymous only if those doing the testing never know your real name, address, or any other identifying information. In anonymous testing you are assigned a code that identifies your blood specimen without revealing your identity.

All states provide HIV antibody testing at alternate test sites (ATS's) funded by the Federal Centers for Disease Control. ATS's provide some type of anonymous testing in forty-one states, Puerto Rico, and the District of Columbia. ATS's record names of all those being tested in: Alaska, Alabama, Colorado, Idaho, Minnesota, North Dakota, South Dakota, South Carolina, and Virginia. If you live in one of these nine states, you may want to travel to another state to obtain anonymous HIV antibody testing. Locations and telephone numbers of some anonymous testing sites are listed in the appendices. If you decide to be tested, go to one of these sites, or call your local AIDS service organization for advice. Some people without access to a test site that offers anonymity have used false names to protect their privacy.

You may choose to be tested through a physician's office. If so, be aware that such testing is at best confidential, not anonymous. Testing through a physician should be done only with a trustworthy doctor who is expert in treating HIV disease.

If you are HIV antibody tested, whether positive or negative, be careful to whom you tell your test results. Since HIV infection cannot be transmitted by casual contact, there is no medical need for you to tell co-workers or acquaintances. Avoid leaving any written record of any risk you may have for HIV infection. Avoid leaving any written record of the fact that you have been HIV antibody tested, even if test results have been negative. Medical records are a problem area for protecting your confidentiality. If you test positive and seek treatment for your HIV infection, claims to health insurers will ultimately reveal your HIV infection. The solution is to arrange your insurance in an airtight fashion before submitting claims that would compromise your health insurance.

REACTION TO TESTING POSITIVE

What will happen if you get back a positive test result? How are you likely to react? What should you do to help yourself emotionally? What kind of decisions do you need to make? What practical steps should you take and how fast should you take them?

People react in a wide variety of ways to finding out that they are HIV infected. You will probably feel very upset. **You have a right to be upset;** there is nothing weak or babyish or neurotic about responding to bad news with strong emotions. You may find that you are crying a lot or feeling scared. You may have difficulty sleeping, eating, concentrating, or working. You may feel that nothing is much fun, that you're not interested in sex, or that you are grouchy and irritable.

Intense negative reactions are usually temporary. You will probably have a lot of strong reactions for a few weeks to a few months and then, as time goes on, get back on a more even keel. The emotional difficulties of being HIV infected should not be underestimated; the knowledge of your infection will be a factor in your emotional life from now on. On the other hand, it is very unlikely that you will remain in a state of permanent crisis.

Take good care of yourself during the period of crisis. This means something different for everyone. There is no right or wrong way to react. Some people best cope with crises by continuing their normal routine. For example, you may find that involving yourself in work or other projects that have nothing to do with HIV will take your mind off your worries. Other people find that they cannot concentrate and need to take time off and avoid some daily tasks and responsibilities for a while. Every person has a different style of adaptation and a different rhythm of dealing with difficulties. The point is to try to think realistically about what works to make you feel better and to use trial and error to figure this out.

You may get some unhelpful advice in this area. Someone might tell you that if you are trying to distract yourself you are "denying" and that you should "let your feelings out." Or, if you are thinking a lot about HIV and needing to talk about it and cry, you may be told that you are "wallowing in it" and you should get your mind off HIV. These suggestions are bad advice. As long as you are doing the things necessary to take care of your health and not doing anything grossly self-destructive, you are doing what you as an individual need to do.

Danger signs to watch out for during this period are suicidal ideas, ignoring responsibilities and commitments in a way that is irreversible, drinking or using other drugs too much, or isolating yourself entirely. There is a big difference between taking a vacation and walking out on your job without notice. There is a difference between treating yourself to some new clothes and impulsively spending your entire life savings. You need not make any major life decisions during the first few weeks or months of learning that you are HIV-infected. This includes major changes in work, living situation, and love relationships. Because you are under a good deal of stress, your judgment may not be as clear as it will be later on. You will probably find that things will feel different to you in a few months. Also, major changes are likely to add to your anxiety.

You deserve emotional support. Professional help and/or peer support may be very helpful for you. You may want to enter psychotherapy, at least for a time. AIDS organizations may be able to suggest therapists (either privately or through a clinic) who are experienced in this area. If you have been in satisfying psychotherapy in the past, this may be a good time to see your former therapist for a period of time. Involvement in a group with others who are HIV infected is extremely helpful for many people. Again, check with the major AIDS organizations in your area for suggestions.

Some people find that getting involved in the political issues that surround HIV disease is actually helpful in coping as well as being socially useful. Volunteer work with local AIDS service organizations or political organizations such as ACT UP (see appendices) is a good way to meet other people who are HIV positive and knowledgeable about the disease. Although you may not want to add any new responsibilities to your life, some people find it a relief to get involved early on in these groups and to feel that they are doing something active to fight for better treatment.

For most people, the best comfort is friends. There are many social and psychological factors involved in deciding whom to tell. Some people are in a situation where telling could lead to discrimination. Some people find that if they tell a lot of people immediately they are overwhelmed by too much talk on the topic. What is clear is that you need some people to talk with and to understand your situation. Do not deal with the situation alone. If you feel that there is no one in your life with whom you can discuss your situation, it is crucial for you to seek an organized support group or professional counseling.

Chapter 2
You and Your Doctor

Once you know you are HIV infected, your first and most important task is to find a physician who can help you. This may not be easy; the medical system is large and complex, and many doctors do not currently have sufficient knowledge of HIV disease to provide state-of-the-art treatment. You may also have a limited choice of doctors because of financial or geographical limitations. This chapter will describe strategies for locating the best medical care available. You will learn what happens during an initial visit to the doctor and how to make the best use of the medical care available. The chapter will also help you to assemble past medical information, and learn how to improve the chances of getting adequate care when options are limited.

BECOMING A PATIENT

HIV-infected people have to think seriously about medical care and make regular visits to the doctor. If you are young and relatively healthy, this may be a new and disturbing experience for you. Probably, like many healthy young people, you have seen a doctor only periodically and only for routine matters or occasional emergencies. If you are HIV infected you will have to see your doctor more frequently and give much more serious attention to medical matters.

You do not have to adjust to this all at once. If you have no symptoms and your immune system is functioning well, your main task will be to see your doctor three or four times a year. You do not have to make all decisions—or even many decisions—about your medical care in the first few days, weeks, or months of finding out that you are HIV-infected. You do not have to stay forever with the first doctor you see.

Although it is, in general, a good idea to know as much as possible about the disease that affects you, you do not have to become an instant AIDS expert. Some things take time to learn. Anxiety may interfere with your understanding of scientific material relevant to HIV disease. You may find it easier to learn things a few months down the road, when you are calmer. As long as you have been evaluated by a competent and knowledgeable physician and had your HIV infection treated, there is no need to memorize every page of this book. Give yourself a break.

It is a very good strategy to involve another person (in addition to your doctor) in helping you deal with medical matters and decisions. It feels better not to have to think about these things alone. Another person familiar with your medical situation may be able to help you with practical matters such as finding a doctor, keeping up with current information, making good medical decisions, and even helping in talking to your doctor. Having a medical confidant will make you feel less alone. Obviously, you have to choose such a person carefully. Look for someone who is discreet, smart, calm, and not afraid to learn about medical issues. Pick someone close to you: this is a serious responsibility. A lover or family member may or may not be a good choice. Sometimes a person very close to you may be too upset to provide you with good support or your relationship may already be too complicated without adding more issues.

You have three initial tasks. First, check out your medical insurance; this will play a major role in determining what kind of medical care you can afford. For more information, refer to Chapter 20: Medical Insurance. Second, find a doctor, and third, plan for your initial visit to the doctor. We will describe these last two steps in detail here.

FIND DECENT MEDICAL CARE

If you find out that you are HIV infected, you should see a physician promptly. Ideally, find an appropriate doctor before you find out that you are infected. Once you know you are infected you may be anxious to see a physician; your anxiety may make the job of finding a doctor harder, and any confusion or delay may make your anxiety worse.

If you aren't sick now, you are not likely to have a serious medical problem in the next few days or weeks. However, a physician can tell you whether you need medical intervention. It will also be reassuring for you to know that you have begun to act to control the virus, and that you have someone to call in case of questions or emergencies.

"Choosing a doctor" is an option only for some people who are HIV infected. It will be possible for you to choose if you have insurance that allows you to pick your own physician and if you live in a geographical area where there are many doctors who are HIV knowledgeable. We will first discuss an approach to choosing a physician for people who are in this situation. Later, we will discuss strategies for people who are not as free to choose due to limitations of insurance (Medicaid or health maintenance organization, HMO) or geographical location.

▲ Expertise

It is highly preferable to see a physician who is expert in HIV disease and has treated many HIV-infected patients. HIV care has in some ways become a medical specialty of its own. Information is fast changing and complex. A physician who has not been seeing HIV patients will not be adequately informed despite being otherwise an excellent doctor. A recent survey indicated that one-quarter of United States physicians have

19

never treated an HIV patient and that most of the rest have treated only one HIV patient. Physicians with large HIV practices form an informal network and keep one another up-to-date on recent developments. They also know more about experimental treatments. There are a number of factors that will play a part in your choice of doctor. HIV expertise is not the only variable, but it is a crucial variable.

How do you find doctors who are HIV knowledgeable? The best place to start is by contacting organizations that work in the field. Major AIDS service organizations such as the San Franciso AIDS Foundation, AIDS Project L.A., or Gay Men's Health Crisis (GMHC) in New York City all maintain referral lists of doctors.

If there is no active AIDS organization in your area, contact a highly respected hospital, particularly one that is affiliated with a medical school. Ideally, contact a hospital that is known for caring for HIV patients. A hospital that participates in the official tests of new drugs for HIV disease is called an AIDS Clinical Trial Unit (ACTU). An ACTU hospital will be a good source of referrals.

Call and ask to speak to someone in the infectious disease or immunology department. You will have to be somewhat persistent and inventive in getting information from a hospital. It can be difficult to get to the person you want in a hospital; even getting through to the hospital switchboard may take time. You may have to call many times, leave repeated messages, and be prepared to stay on hold.

Contact more than one source of referrals, if you have the energy. A physician on multiple referral lists is more likely to be reliable. For example, a physician suggested both by your local AIDS organization and by a teaching hospital is likely to be a good choice.

Friends who are HIV infected themselves are a source of information about possible doctors. Take into account the judgment of the friend you ask: Is this a sensible person who has become well informed about HIV disease? Remember also that many factors influence people's opinions of their doctors. A doctor who is just right for your friend may not be right for you.

Many HIV physicians have practices that are full and will not accept new patients. However, you can call their offices and ask for referrals. They are in a position to judge who is competent and will often know of younger doctors who are starting practices and have openings for new patients. A younger doctor, one who has just finished a residency in internal medicine or a specialization in infectious disease or immunology, is often a good choice. If the doctor has trained in a hospital with a large case load of AIDS patients, he or she will be experienced in treating HIV disease.

You may be in a situation in which you already have a trusted doctor whom you like and respect. Should you continue with a doctor who is not an HIV expert? A good answer to this question is to continue to see this doctor in addition to seeing an HIV expert. Check with both doctors to make sure they are willing to collaborate with each other. The HIV specialist can make necessary treatment decisions and you can continue to see your regular physician if this contact is reassuring and helpful.

Some doctors who are well known for treating HIV have medical opinions that differ dramatically from those of most HIV experts. For example, there are physicians who never use AZT or who are trying a radically different unproven treatment. If you are seeing a doctor who is in disagreement with the consensus of AIDS experts, be sure that you understand the difference. Choosing such a doctor should be a carefully thought-out decision and one you should make only if your own level of information about the disease is excellent. Sometimes unconventional physicians have been right in their opinions; more often they have been wrong. If you are betting against the odds you need to do so carefully and with the knowledge that you are taking a risk.

▲ Hospital Affiliation

What are some of the factors besides HIV expertise that may play a role in your choice of doctors? One factor should be the hospital with which a physician is associated. Hospitals choose which doctors can admit patients to their facilities; this is known as "admitting privileges." Some doctors have admitting privileges to more than one hospital. Ask the hospital affiliation of doctors recommended to you. Then consider whether this is where you would want to be hospitalized if it becomes necessary. Again, reputation for quality and experience in treating patients with HIV disease are the most important factors. Hospitals with special AIDS units often provide the best care. They are the most experienced and will have nursing staff who have chosen to work with HIV patients. You may also want to consider the geographical location of the hospital and its physical characteristics.

In addition, a few hospitals may have special programs that could be useful. Some hospitals have areas for patients who need more intensive care than is available at home but do not need full hospitalization. For example, a patient undergoing extensive diagnostic tests may find this kind of service appropriate. It may be much more pleasant to be treated in such a facility where you will not be confined to bed and will have more independence, more privacy, more pleasant physical circumstances, and more flexible visiting hours.

▲ Compatibility

There are other issues that will play a role in your experience with a physician. HIV disease is a serious illness that requires close collaboration with a doctor. You need someone whom you can work with as well as whose medical abilities you trust. The balance between these two issues is hard to strike. No matter how much you like your doctor, you will not get adequate care if he or she is not medically competent. On the other hand, the most brilliant physician cannot help you if you dislike her or him so much that you put off necessary appointments.

What makes a patient and a doctor compatible? Some of the factors may be easy to define. Do you have preferences regarding the age, gender, or sexual orientation of your physician? If you live in an area with a wide choice of AIDS physicians you may be able to act on your preference. Other factors are more intangible. Some people prefer physicians who provide them with full information and a large role in making a choice about treatment options. Other people find that this is too anxiety-provoking and prefer more guidance from their doctors. Although everyone should learn enough about her or his disease to make informed decisions, this preference is a matter of personal psychology and not a moral right or wrong. Some people like physicians who are chatty and informal; others feel a more distant and formal relationship is more comfortable.

It is very difficult to figure out before you see someone whether your styles will be compatible. This is not the kind of information you can get from an AIDS organization or a hospital. Friends who can describe their experiences may be more helpful. Think back on past experiences with doctors and what qualities in them you found helpful.

When you are choosing a doctor to see initially, remember that you don't have to find the perfect doctor right away. You only need to see someone who is competent to start to monitor your immune system. Seeing more than one doctor initially is usually burdensome both emotionally and financially. Instead, pick a doctor who sounds like a good candidate. Give the relationship a chance. You can always switch later on. If you really don't get along with the physician from the start, try another doctor.

One thing to remember is that no matter how long you look, you are unlikely to find a physician who seems ideal to you all the time. For example, almost all AIDS doctors are terribly busy. Seeing an expert will require more time in the waiting room and a longer wait for returned calls than you would like. This is an unfortunate reality of the system that you will have to accept.

Does this description of choosing a doctor seem like a lot of work? It is difficult but you can probably go through all the steps outlined above in a couple of hours. The investment of time and energy will be worth it in the long run. Enlisting a helper is a great idea. If you have a friend who is thoughtful and willing, you could have this person make most of the phone calls. You may be anxious if you have just found out that you are HIV positive, and this is a good time to have someone help you with projects that are likely to make you more anxious.

▲ Finding a Doctor If Your Choice Is Limited

Many people with HIV disease will not have the best alternatives among which to choose. This is usually due to either financial or geographical reasons. Without private health insurance it is not easy to get good or even passable medical care in the United States. A very large number of Americans do not have access to decent medical care; 34 million American citizens have no health insurance; 62 percent of these people work full-time and another 24 percent work part-time. There will be no real solutions for HIV disease and other serious health problems until the health care system is radically overhauled. Nonetheless, as an HIV-infected individual it is worthwhile to struggle to get the best health care possible. If you are willing to strategize, put up with some problems, and fight back, you can get medical care that could be crucial to your health and survival. Don't give up. Careful planning and persistence can help you find the best possible medical care even when your options are limited.

Medicaid (or MediCal in California) is the federally sponsored health insurance that provides payment for a portion of people who live in poverty. (It actually covers only 36 percent of uninsured Americans.) It is an inadequate program that pays unrealistically low fees to physicians and hospitals and that often involves users and providers in a mess of red tape.

The majority of private doctors will not accept new Medicaid patients due to the relatively low fees and the huge amount of paperwork required of doctors. However, if you have been seeing a private doctor and have been forced to switch to Medicaid due to loss of insurance, generally the private doctor will continue to see you. If you are on Medicaid and do not already have a private doctor, the best option is to go to a clinic affiliated with a major teaching hospital, particularly one that is an AIDS Clinical Trial Unit.

There are some definite problems connected to this. You may end up seeing different doctors at each visit, rather than being followed by one doctor over time. In many clinics, if you have an emergency you will have to be seen in the emergency room of the affiliated hospital rather than be able to get a timely appointment with your own doctor. However, the picture is not entirely bleak. Many hospital-affiliated HIV clinics are staffed by excellent and dedicated physicians. Although they may still be completing their training, they will have experience with the disease and supervision from a senior physician. In addition, at some of the better clinics you can get important additional services such as psychiatric and psychological care, nutritional counseling, and social services.

Medicaid pays for hospitalization and should pay for all tests and other services that you receive while hospitalized. It also pays for most prescription drugs. Most but not all drugs commonly used for treating HIV disease are covered by Medicaid.

If you rely on Medicaid clinics for your care you may face inconvenience and impolite treatment. There is really no way to make this less painful. Try to remember that the problems with getting good health care are caused by an inequitable system, and not by something you did wrong.

If you are HIV infected and uninsured, investigate the possibility of obtaining Medicaid or of buying private insurance. If your income is too high for Medicaid and too low to afford private insurance, you will need to look for a clinic in your area that accepts patients on a *sliding scale* of payment (fees are adjusted according to income). Sliding-scale clinics have many of the problems that apply to Medicaid clinics; nevertheless, some provide very good care.

Some people have insurance through plans known as **pre-paid insurance or health maintenance organizations (HMO's).** HMO's provide comprehensive services for a fixed, pre-paid amount that is independent of the number of services actually used. If you belong to an HMO, you are only covered for treatment by those doctors who work for the HMO. The advantage of HMO's is that they pay for 100 percent of medical expenses and are often a good bargain financially. The (very significant) disadvantages are that there may be no doctors expert in treatment of HIV-related illnesses affiliated with your HMO, you will have a limited choice of hospitals to which you can be admitted, and there may be long waits for appointments.

If you belong to an HMO, you should check about the possibility of switching to a plan where you can choose your own doctor. If you have to stay on the HMO—temporarily or permanently—you should obtain the list of physicians available to you and check out whether any of the providers are HIV specialists. Again, you can call your local or nearby AIDS organizations for help with this. You may also want to consider— if you can afford it—occasional visits to an HIV expert whom you pay privately to supplement your care from an HMO.

Geographical factors must be taken into account. It is easiest to find good HIV medical care in New York, San Francisco, Los Angeles, or other large urban areas. Most medium and small cities at this point have at least some physicians available who have experience in treating HIV disease. Call the nearest AIDS organization and ask for a referral. If they have no names in your area, call someone they recommend in the next closest city and ask for a referral closer to you. Again, be persistent and invest some initial time in the detective work necessary to find an appropriate doctor; it will pay off in the long run.

If you live in a rural area where there are no physicians available with expertise in HIV, your best bet (if you can afford it) is to try to arrange a combination of care. See an AIDS expert in the nearest large city periodically and arrange for her or him to collaborate with a good local physician. Obviously, this plan requires sufficient funds and insurance for multiple doctors' visits and occasional travel.

▲ Educating Yourself

Educate yourself about treatments for HIV disease, especially if your sources of medical care may not be reliable. Chapter 9: Learning About Experimental Treatments lists newsletters written to inform HIV-infected people of the latest developments. Reading such newsletters is reassuring for some people and anxiety-provoking for others. However, if you are not certain that you are getting up-to-date medical advice, you need some independent source of current information. Again, consider the possibility of trying to find a friend to help you with this project.

▲ Physicians Are Not the Only Health Care Providers

Throughout this discussion we have talked about physicians. Actually, many people get expert HIV care from nurse practitioners or physicians' assistants. These are health care providers who are not doctors but who have sophisticated training. They generally work in tandem with a private doctor or in clinics and refer to doctors as necessary. If they have had extensive HIV experience they can provide excellent care. They have the additional advantage of often having more time to spend with you and greater sophistication about psychological issues than do many doctors.

INITIAL VISIT TO THE DOCTOR

You will get more benefit out of your first visit to the doctor if you do some advance preparation. This has two aspects: organizing information that will be helpful to your doctor and figuring out what questions you want answered by your doctor.

▲ Information for Your Doctor

Your doctor needs good information to provide good medical care.

Because of discrimination, information about HIV-infected status is sensitive. Discuss with your doctor what information needs to be written on the chart and what information will be sent to insurance companies.

Your new doctor will want to know your medical history. Make a list of the following information before your initial visit:

- Any current physical problems or changes in your body or functioning. Try to think of a clear way of describing these things. Write down when they started, any pattern you have noticed about when symptoms come and go, when they have been better and worse, and whether anything seems to trigger them. Include both specific physical symptoms and changes in functioning.
- History of past illnesses, injuries, and hospitalizations. Don't include minor problems such as unremarkable colds. A history of childhood illnesses is useful if you can get this information from a

25

family member. As much as possible, make a list of dates and treatments received for each problem. Include all sexually transmitted diseases. Include major psychological problems and any psychiatric hospitalizations.

• Current and past medications. Include, if possible, dosage, duration of medication, effectiveness in treating the illness, and side effects or allergies to the drugs. In your current-medication list record everything you are taking, including vitamin supplements, frequent use of over-the-counter medications (aspirin, other pain killers, cold medicines, etc.), herbal remedies, non-traditional therapies or so-called "blackmarket" or "underground" drugs. Even apparently benign drugs might sometimes affect you adversely or interact with other medication. Include psychiatric medications such as tranquilizers and antidepressants.

• In addition to drug allergies, be sure to mention any allergies to foods, pets, plants, or other substances.

• Vaccinations. These are the shots you got as a child to prevent measles, mumps, etc., as well as ones you might have gotten later on for travel. Tell your doctor whether you have been vaccinated against hepatitis B.

▲ Workbook for Initial Visit

You may want to organize your medical information for a new doctor in a workbook form before the first visit. Some possible things to mention might include:

Current Physical Symptoms	Changes in Functioning
Rashes, sores, or growths on skin or in mouth	Appetite
Fevers, night sweats, weight loss	Sleep
Cough, shortness of breath, pain on inhalation	Concentration
Diarrhea, constipation, abdominal pain	Memory
Headaches, changes in vision	Energy level
Weakness, aches, and pains	Menstrual cycle
Abnormal bleeding, rectal bleeding, or vaginal bleeding outside of menstruation	Sexual functioning

Refer to the section later in this chapter for more on keeping a medical logbook.

▲ Other Information Your Doctor May Ask

Certain infectious organisms are more common in people from a particular **geographical area.** For example, the parasite *Histoplasma capsulatum* is more commonly seen in patients from the central United States (Indiana, Ohio, Mississippi, Missouri, and Tennessee). For this reason, your doctor may ask you questions about where you have lived or traveled.

26

Your physician may ask you questions about your **sexual history.** He or she will be concerned about whether you are now using condoms for intercourse, and about possible current or past exposure to other sexually transmitted diseases. By asking about your history of intercourse without condoms, your physician may get an idea of when you were infected.

Ideally, a physician should be able to ask you questions and provide information about sexual matters in a fashion that is helpful, fully informed, and not judgmental. In fact, doctors, like most other people, tend to be anxious about sex and this can be reflected in the way they talk about sex. Doctors, like other people, may be homophobic, have negative attitudes about sex, and be moralistic about issues such as the number of sexual partners. If you feel that your doctor is homophobic or judgmental, it would be best to find a physician who is not. However, you may be in a situation in which you cannot choose another doctor. The best you can do in this situation is to remember that your doctor has medical expertise but may be uninformed about many other things. The widespread prejudices about sexuality and especially homosexuality in our culture may influence her or him. If your doctor tells you something about safer sex that seems overly restrictive, ask questions about the scientific rationale for the advice.

Your doctor also may ask you questions about present or past **use of recreational drugs.** As with questions about sex, this is not idle curiosity. This information is relevant for a number of reasons. A history of intravenous drug use is associated with multiple medical problems such as staphyloccocal disease, endocarditis (a heart infection), abscesses caused by needles, and hepatitis. If you are currently using alcohol or other recreational drugs in a way that is damaging to you physically or psychologically, this information is relevant to your medical care. Your physician may be a good source of support or referral in dealing with drug problems. However, many physicians are uninformed about drug use and it is possible that your physician will be critical and prejudiced rather than helpful. Again, if this is the case and if it is upsetting to you, try to switch doctors if possible. Remember that you are seeing your physician for certain specific purposes and that another source may be more helpful regarding substance abuse problems.

Some doctors may ask you questions about current and past **emotional, vocational, and social functioning.** If your doctor is sensitive, psychologically minded, and supportive, this could be helpful to you and improve the quality of your medical care by taking into account psychological factors. Some doctors are not equipped by training or personality to deal with these issues; you can't expect everything from your doctor. You should also feel free not to answer these questions if you feel that discussion with your doctor may not be useful. However, it may be worth overcoming initial discomfort about talking to obtain emotional support. Physicians are ethically obligated to inquire about any ideas you may have about suicide.

▲ Physical Exam

The physical examination your doctor will perform at your first HIV appointment will be essentially the same as physicals you may have had before. The physical examination is likely to include the following items:

- Doctors use the term **vital signs** to include internal body temperature, pulse rate, blood pressure, and body weight. Abnormalities in vital signs are initial indicators of many medical problems.
- Because HIV infection often manifests itself early on as **skin problems,** your doctor will inspect your skin carefully. Point out any unusual lumps, bumps, or discolorations you may have noticed.
- Your physician is likely to feel for **swollen lymph nodes** behind the neck and under the arms. Lymph nodes, part of the lymphatic system, are located throughout the body (see pp. 327–35 in Chapter 16: Immunology, Pathogenesis, and Etiology for a description of the lymphatic system). Important clusters of lymph nodes occur in the back of the neck below the ears, deep under the armpits, and in the groin. Lymph nodes (sometimes called *lymph glands)* swell when an infection is present nearby. Swollen glands are an expectable part of many illnesses; they are not a cause for alarm. Sometimes people with HIV disease develop chronic swollen glands *(generalized lymphadenopathy);* although this is due to HIV infection, it is not a sign that the disease is progressing and is not a bad prognostic sign. HIV-infected people with chronic swollen lymph nodes do just as well as those whose nodes are not chronically swollen.
- Your doctor will examine your **eyes** by looking at them with a small hand-held instrument called an *ophthalmoscope.* This provides some information about both your eyes and your nervous system.
- Your doctor should visually examine your **mouth and throat.** The doctor will be looking for indications of herpes simplex, candidiasis, hairy leukoplakia, or (rarely) lymphoma, or Kaposi's sarcoma. In early HIV disease, herpes, candidiasis, and hairy leukoplakia are not serious problems; they are either treatable or go away on their own.
- Your doctor will examine your **chest** by listening to it with a stethoscope, tapping your back and chest, and determining your rate of breathing. Lung problems, particularly *Pneumocystis carinii* pneumonia (see Chapter 5: Preventing PCP and Other Complications), are common in HIV disease, but it is extremely unlikely that your physician will diagnose any serious problems with your lungs if you have not had any symptoms. Tell your doctor about any persistent coughing or shortness of breath.
- In addition to recording your blood pressure and pulse rate, your

doctor obtains information about your **heart and circulation** by listening to your heart with a stethoscope.

- Your doctor will examine your **abdomen** by pressing on it to check for the possible presence of any masses and to establish the baseline size of the spleen and liver so that any changes in the future that might mark illness can be noted.
- The doctor will examine the **testicles and penis** for any signs of tumors or for sores that might indicate a sexually transmitted disease, such as gonorrhea, chlamydia, or condyloma. If there is a discharge from the opening of the penis (the urethra) a sample of this will be collected to look at microscopically for diagnostic purposes.
- A **gynecological exam** should include visual inspection of the external genitalia, a Pap smear, a manual exam (by inserting lubricated gloved fingers into the vagina while pressing on the abdomen), and possibly a magnified exam of the cervix (colposcopy). For more complete information, refer to Chapter 8: Sex, Age, Race, and Ethnicity, pp. 161–64. Your physician will be looking for signs of sexually transmitted diseases such as gonorrhea, chlamydia, or condyloma; for candida (yeast infection); and for signs of any disorders of the cervix.
- Your physician will look at the external area of your **anus** and then examine your **rectum** digitally (by inserting a lubricated gloved finger into the rectum). A small sample of stool will be examined for signs of blood, which could indicate gastrointestinal problems.
- Your doctor will examine your **muscles and joints** for signs of soreness, swelling, or weakness. These are general symptoms that can be caused by a number of different medical problems.

▲ Tests

In Chapter 3: Monitoring the Immune System, we will cover the specialized laboratory tests that you and your physician will use to determine the status of your immune system and the progression of HIV disease. These are primarily blood tests.

Your physician is also likely to perform the following other tests: a set of standard blood tests; tests to see whether you have been infected with the organisms that cause tuberculosis, syphilis, hepatitis B, or toxoplasmosis (described in Chapter 11: Infections); and a chest X ray. Some physicians perform a group of skin tests called an *anergy panel* that indicates whether your immune system is able to react properly to previously seen infections.

These tests are described in detail in Chapter 13: Procedures and Tests.

▲ Questions to Ask Your Doctor in the First Few Visits

You should think carefully about the questions that you want to ask your doctor. Write them down and bring them with you. Most people get nervous when they see a doctor and forget the questions they want to ask unless they have a list. You may want to take notes about what the doctor tells you. Your questions may include:

- What is the general state of my health?
- Do I have any specific medical problems other than HIV infection?
- What kinds of blood tests or other tests do I need at the present time?
- How often do I need to see you?
- Are there any specialists I should see now?
- Do I need to take any medication?
- Do I need to make any changes in my daily habits?
- What symptoms or changes should I report to you?
- When is the best time to call with questions?
- What should I do in an emergency?

To answer these questions your doctor needs information about you, such as blood-test results that may not be available until your second visit.

COLLABORATING WITH YOUR DOCTOR

In an ideal world many things would be different about medical care. Good care would be available to all. You could be certain that the doctor who treated you was expert. There would be plenty of time to talk with your doctor. Health education and discussion of preventive issues would be part of routine care. Your doctor would be sensitive to your psychological needs and cultural issues relevant to you. You would be able to reach your doctor easily in cases of emergency and would have a convenient way to ask the doctor questions between appointments.

Realistically, you must assess what medical care is available to you and strategize to use that medical care in the most productive way possible. Realize that you cannot always get what you want and need from your physician.

Squeeze the most out of visits to your doctor. Make decisions about whether to switch to a different physician based on the real possibilities for better medical care and not on some wished-for but unattainable goal.

It is useful to recognize that you are often right to feel frustrated and angry at the care you receive. Medical care is complicated and there are many possibilities of mistakes. There really are major faults in the system and you are not being unreasonable to be bothered by them. At the same time, your physician and other health care providers are also constrained by the system in which they work. Every problem that comes up in your medical care is not necessarily the fault of your doctor. Some problems your doctor cannot remedy.

▲ Time

Long waits in **the waiting room** are inevitable. The wait may vary from doctor to doctor. It will depend on your geographical location and the nature of your doctor's practice. If your doctor always keeps you waiting for very extended periods of time, you may consider looking for a physician whose practice is less busy. However, since there are a limited number of expert HIV doctors, since they mostly have very busy and demanding practices, and since they frequently deal with emergencies, it is unlikely that you will find a doctor who does not keep you waiting at least some of the time.

Try to schedule your appointments so that if you are kept waiting you do not miss something that is important to you. Call ahead to see if your doctor is running behind. Bring something to read or something else to do while you are in the waiting room. Consider asking a friend to come with you if you will be anxious while waiting.

Similarly, there will probably be **times that you feel rushed while talking to your doctor.** This is inevitable some of the time, but if you *always* feel that your doctor does not have time to listen and explain, you should consider trying another doctor. You can help by organizing in advance what you want to know (see below) and by being clear with your doctor about things that you don't understand or times when you need further explanation or attention.

Many people who are generally organized and clear thinking find that they feel confused and even "stupid" when talking to their doctor. The cause of this difficulty is anxiety. Most people feel anxious about seeing their doctor, especially if they anticipate problems. Anxiety causes difficulty in concentration and slows down the ability to learn new material. You can lessen these problems by planning in advance what you want to ask and writing it down. If you find that your mind really goes blank while you are talking with your physician, consider having a friend come into the office for the discussion part of your visit.

Schedule regular visits with your doctor. See your physician at least three times a year if you are asymptomatic—more often if you have symptoms. Regular office visits allow appropriate monitoring, timely diagnosis, and a chance to develop a working relationship. Ask at the end of *every* visit when to schedule the next appointment. Your doctor may easily forget to tell you when to come back to have something checked or to get lab tests. You should make it your business to ask.

Do not wait to contact your doctor until a symptom has gone on for an extended time or becomes an emergency. It hurts your chance to get the best treatment; also, your doctor may be rushed and unable to give you adequate attention and time for discussion.

Be considerate of your doctor's schedule, too. Don't postpone necessary action until Friday afternoon at five. Ask as many questions as you need, but be organized. If your doctor gives you something to read regarding your medical situation, read it.

▲ Organize the Visit

Plan to make the best use of your time when you see your physician.

It is important to tell your doctor about all the medical problems that are bothering you and the physical changes since your last visit. Sit down and make a list. Then consider in what order to present your complaints. **Start with the problem that seems most serious to you.** Think about how to describe problems concretely and clearly. Note when symptoms started or stopped and what else was going on at the time.

Make a written list of questions you want to ask. Ask the most important question first. Make the questions as understandable and specific as you can.

Do not expect simple answers to complex questions. However, if your doctor uses medical language that you don't understand, ask for a translation into ordinary language.

If you are dealing with a new illness or starting a new medication, you should be given information about what to expect.

Following is basic information you should get about any new illness.

- Name of the illness
- Cause of the illness
- Possible course and prognosis
- Further diagnostic procedures needed
- Treatment
- Side effects of treatment
- How fast treatment should work
- How to prevent recurrence
- When to schedule next visit
- Possible consultation with a specialist
- What emergencies might arise

However, do not expect your doctor to be able to predict the future. Your doctor may not be able to give you specific information about the course of the disease or how well you will respond to medication. Often, the best that the doctor can do is to indicate several likely possibilities.

Here is a scenario to use as a model when you are seeing your doctor about a new symptom(s). Let us say, for example, that you have developed a cough. Here's what you should report to the doctor:

"I have a cough. It started about two weeks ago and has gotten worse over time. By 'worse' I mean more frequent and more painful. I cough up a lot of greenish stuff. I've also had a fever of about 101 degrees for the last two days and feel very tired."

Your doctor will probably ask you more questions and then examine you. When you talk afterwards your doctor may say something like this:

"The most likely possibility is that you have bronchitis. I think it will get better. I want you to take antibiotics. If they don't help, we'll do more tests."

This does not give you enough information. You might also want to ask:

- What is bronchitis?
- How long can I expect it to last?
- Are there any other symptoms that might appear? Are there symptoms I should report to you immediately?
- How fast will the antibiotics help? How long should I wait to contact you if the symptoms do not get better?
- What are the antibiotics? Do they have any side effects? If so, what? Are they incompatible with any other medication that I am taking?
- Is there anything else I can do to lessen discomfort?
- Is there anything else that I should do to help get better? Can I go to work? Should I stay in bed (change my diet, make other changes in daily routine)? Am I contagious to others?
- If it is not bronchitis, what are some of the other likely possibilities? If I do not get better from the antibiotics, what is the next step?

Whether to ask the last question on this list (What comes next?) depends on you. Some people like to know about what diagnostic and treatment options the physician is considering and feel more secure when they understand the various possibilities. You have a right to this information. However, other people feel overwhelmed when they have to consider too many possibilities and like to take one step at a time. Remember also that in terms of diagnosis your physician needs to follow an orderly process. Many of your questions cannot be answered on the basis of preliminary information and if you want to know every single diagnostic possibility you have to be prepared to hear something broad and confusing and possibly more frightening than necessary.

Write notes on information that your doctor gives you. If a complicated procedure or a medication with many side effects is being explained, ask your doctor if printed information on the topic is available. Some doctors have nurse practitioners, physician's assistants, nurses, or other health care personnel working in the office who may be able to answer questions at greater length.

Your physician should know something about **your mental state and most pressing concerns.** At a minimum, tell your doctor about any medication you are taking that affects the mind (for example, anti-anxiety drugs or antidepressants), and any current or past serious problems with depression or anxiety. If your physician seems sensitive to emotional issues, it can be helpful to discuss your personal life, history, and attitudes toward HIV disease. For example, if your physician is going to make treatment plans with you after a hospitalization, talk about what kind of support and help is available to you after discharge. If you are particularly frightened of a certain disease or treatment, tell your physician in advance.

People have **different attitudes toward treatment** of HIV disease. One person may prefer aggressive treatment, even at the cost of discomfort and side effects. Another person may prefer a wait-and-see attitude even at the cost of delay in important treatment. Your attitude may change over time. Your physician cannot read your mind: express your preferences as clearly as possible.

During the treatment of HIV disease, you may have **diagnostic or therapeutic procedures that cause pain.** Give your doctor feedback: describe the location, extent, and duration of the pain. People vary in sensitivity to pain both in general and during any particular procedure. Some people prefer to take more pain medication. Others prefer using less pain medication because it makes them feel sleepy or "out of it." Make your preferences known. Pain medication is discussed in detail in the latter part of Chapter 7: Your State of Mind.

In general it is very important to **give your physician feedback.** This is easier said than done. Of course you do not want to complain all the time and it can be difficult to criticize someone whom you depend upon. Nonetheless, if something is happening on a repeated basis with your doctor that you do not like, it is important to raise the issue. You have to give your physician the benefit of the doubt; your physician may not be aware of the problem if you have not said anything. If you do bring up problems, your doctor has a chance to make changes, or at least to explain her or his point of view in a way that makes a difference.

▲ Contacting Your Doctor Outside of Visits

Ask your doctor how you can make contact between visits. Is the physician available on the phone? What time of day will the doctor return phone calls? If you feel that an urgent situation may be developing, can you make unscheduled office visits?

Leave clear telephone messages with your doctor's office staff. If the situation is urgent, tell this to the person taking the message. Be sure to leave your name, the reason for your call, and telephone numbers and times so that the doctor can return your call. Consider in advance whether you want your doctor to leave a message containing explicit medical information at these numbers. If you want a full message from your doctor, mention this to the staff.

Your doctor may not return telephone calls promptly. If the situation is not an emergency, it is reasonable for your doctor to not to call you back immediately. Some doctors set aside a specific time at the end of the day for answering nonemergency phone calls. If your call is important, call again. It is a serious problem if your doctor never returns repeated or urgent calls.

You should always have medical care available to you in case of an emergency. If your physician is not available, another physician should be "covering" and able to deal with emergencies. **Find out whom to call when your doctor is away or on vacation.**

▲ Your Doctor Is Human

If you are HIV infected, much depends upon your doctor. He or she tends to become a very important person in your life. **Every doctor has limitations you must accept.** At times you may wish to have your doctor fill needs that no doctor can reasonably fill on a consistent basis. A physician often plays some nurturing and supportive role in the process of caretaking. Your doctor may or may not seem warm and supportive. Some physicians who are in fact compassionate may not convey this to patients.

Some physicians develop friendly relationships and even friendships with some patients. This is a matter of personality on the part of both the doctor and the patient. Either one may have preferences about the formality of the relationship. Your physician has to have a say in this; people can't change their personalities on demand. Friendship between patient and doctor is complicated, and some people feel that it interferes with the necessary objectivity on the part of the physician.

Some doctors are psychologically-minded and sensitive to emotional issues. They may have been in psychotherapy themselves. Other doctors are neither knowledgeable nor comfortable with psychological issues. Your doctor may be a good person for you to talk to, but you cannot expect her or him to fill the role of the psychotherapist. Your doctor may not have the aptitude for this type of work and is unlikely to have the time on a steady basis.

Both you and your doctor will have **personal feelings** about your care. You have the right to make the final decisions in your treatment. Nonetheless, your doctor is not a machine and also has a right to have opinions and feelings about your treatment. For example, if you are refusing a treatment that your doctor feels is crucial and has limited side effects, you should expect your doctor to argue vigorously in favor of the medication. It is neither reasonable nor desirable to think that your doctor should passively comply with all your wishes, just as it is unreasonable for your doctor to expect you to be totally compliant and without preferences.

Of course you know that your doctor is "just human." However, it is easy to wish that a person who has so much influence on your well-being were more than human. From time to time, you may have to step back and **get some perspective on your doctor's attitudes, personality, and limitations.**

It is unrealistic to expect doctors to be perfectly consistent. They have good and bad days, strengths and blind spots. Evaluate what these strengths and weaknesses are and decide if they match what you need.

For example, you may have a physician who is competent, kind, and available, but terrible at explaining things or giving you information. If explanations are important to you and you do not have another source, this may not be the right doctor for you. To use another example, your doctor may give you excellent care but have nonscientific biases about safer sex. In this case, you might want to stick to your doctor but get safer-sex advice elsewhere. Again, you may feel that your doctor is a brilliant clinician but cold or psychologically insensitive. You may decide to continue with this doctor (since good medical care is the central issue) and get your psychological help from a therapist or friends. On the other hand, if you feel so uncomfortable with the doctor that you are missing visits or miscommunicating in major ways, it may be better to switch to another physician if this is possible.

Facing the fact that your physician has limitations will make this process easier. It is in your interest to try to understand your doctor, to some extent, in order to develop a good working relationship.

HOW TO KEEP YOUR OWN MEDICAL LOG BOOK

Writing down information in an organized fashion will improve your understanding of your treatment and will probably help your doctor provide you with medical care. If things are written down, they can be more complete and exact. You do not have to try to reconstruct history when you are feeling sick and under stress. You will be able to give all the relevant information to any new doctor you see.

Here is a suggested system for keeping track of medical information. It is designed for people who are organized and good at keeping records. If you don't fit this description, at least keep an up-to-date record of your current medications. You will need a notebook divided into seven sections.

HOW TO READ A PRESCRIPTION

It can be useful to understand the drug prescriptions that you are given. Prescriptions are written using simple abbreviations. Unfortunately, the abbreviations are of Latin words! Nonetheless, you can easily decode your prescriptions by referring to the following examples and table of abbreviations.

MEDICAL LOG BOOK

Section	Description
Physician Information	Name, address, and phone number of your primary doctor and other medical specialists you consult.
Insurance	Name of insurance company. Social security number. Policy and group number. Telephone number(s) to call for information or if your policy requires advance notification for hospitalization.
Medication	Medication allergies or other serious allergies.
	Current medication. Include prescription drugs, over-the-counter drugs, vitamins, herbal remedies, and "underground" drugs. Include name of medication, dosage, and the dates you start and stop taking it. Keep this list up-to-date by crossing out medications no longer used and adding new medications.
Medical History	Past medical history including:
	Past hospitalizations (reason, name of hospital, doctor, treatment, duration, outcome). Include any surgery done in hospital or out-patient surgery (reason, name of doctor, outcome).
	Past injuries (type, treatment required).
	Major illnesses not included in hospitalization (nature of illness, treatment, outcome). Include Hepatitis A and B.
	Childhood illnesses (measles, mumps, chicken pox, whooping cough).
	Immunizations (childhood and adult).
	History of sexually transmitted diseases (nature, treatment, outcome). Include syphilis, gonorrhea, chlamydia, condyloma, herpes.
	History of intestinal parasites (nature, treatment, outcome).
	Psychiatric history. Include hospitalization(s) and medication(s).
	For women: Gynecological and obstetric information, menstrual cycle, birth control method (if relevant), history of childbirth(s), miscarriages and abortions (if relevant).
Laboratory Markers	HIV laboratory markers. Include T4 counts, p24 antigen, beta-2 microglobulin, neopterin. (See Chapter 3: Monitoring the Immune System.)
Symptom Diary	Describe any illnesses. Record by date. List symptoms, diagnosis, treatment, outcome.
Current Questions	Current information and questions for your doctor. Record any current symptoms you should report to your doctor. List questions you want to ask at your next visit.

Examples of Prescriptions

Your doctor prescribes AZT (brand name: Retrovir). Each pill contains 100 mg of drug.

Take one pill every four hours by mouth.

The pharmacist is instructed to give you 240 pills and to refill this prescription four times.

TELEPHONE 999 765-4321

JANE Q. DOE, M.D.

123 MAIN STREET

DEA NO. AM 12345678ZZ
LIC. NO. 123456

ANYTOWN, OK

NAME *Bill Smith*   AGE *28*

ADDRESS *987 Oak Drive*   DATE *5/26/92*

℞

Retrovir 100mg

Sig † (one) q4h p.o.

Disp 240

Jane Doe, M.D.

☐ REFILL *4* TIMES

THIS PRESCRIPTION WILL BE FILLED GENERICALLY
UNLESS PRESCRIBER WRITES 'd a w' IN THE BOX BELOW

Dispense As Written

TELEPHONE 999 765-4321

JANE Q. DOE, M.D.

DEA NO. AM 12345678ZZ
LIC. NO. 123456

ANYTOWN, OK

123 MAIN STREET

NAME *Rita Mendez*   AGE *44*

ADDRESS *789 Shady Lane*   DATE *3/23/91*

℞

Prozac 20mg

Sig †† (two) qd p.o.

Disp 100

Jane Doe, M.D.

☐ REFILL ____ TIMES

THIS PRESCRIPTION WILL BE FILLED GENERICALLY
UNLESS PRESCRIBER WRITES 'd a w' IN THE BOX BELOW

Dispense As Written

Your psychiatrist has prescribed the antidepressant fluoxetine (brand name: Prozac). Each capsule should contain 20mg of drug.

Take two pills, once each day, by mouth.

The pharmacist is instructed to give you 100 pills.

CODES AND SYMBOLS ON PRESCRIPTIONS

Abbr.	Latin	English Explanation
Sig	*signa*	take Directions for use
Rx		prescription Starts prescription
Disp		dispense Doctors usually write the total number of pills or capsules (i.e., disp 260)
q	*quaque*	every
d	*die*	day
qd	*quaque die*	once a day, every day
q3d	*quaque 3 die*	every three days
bid	*bis in die*	twice a day
tid	*ter in die*	three times a day
qid	*quater in die*	four times a day
qh	*quaque hora*	every hour
q4h	*quaque 4 hora*	every four hours (six times a day)
qw	*quaque* week	once a week, every week
tiw	*ter in* week	three days a week Your doctor should write which days (e.g., Mon., Wed., Fri.)
prn	*pro re nata*	take as needed Often "prn sleep" (take as needed for sleep), or "prn anxiety" (take as needed for anxiety)
po	*per os*	by mouth, orally
pc	*post cibos*	after meals
hs	*hora somni*	at the hour of sleep, bedtime
†		one
† †		two
† † †		three
daw		dispense as written

Adapted with permission from "It's all Greek to me, or how to read a prescription," by Garance Franke-Ruta, in *Notes from the Underground*, issue 11, PWA Health Group, New York, Sept./Oct. 1991.

Chapter 3
Monitoring the Immune System

For several years after exposure to HIV, an infected person will typically have either no symptoms or only minor ones such as chronic swollen glands. However, despite the absence of noticeable symptoms, the virus is silently causing damage. HIV infects and kills certain white blood cells called *T4 lymphocytes,* reducing their number. The number of T4 cells in the body gradually declines in an HIV-infected person.

T4 cells act as the On switch for part of the immune system, so as the number of T4 cells drops, damage to the immune system progresses. Over time, individuals become increasingly susceptible to diseases caused by organisms that are usually kept in control by people whose immune systems are healthy. Several years after infection many HIV-infected people—because their immune systems are partially impaired—may develop symptoms such as night sweats, chronic diarrhea, fatigue, fever, and various skin problems. These symptoms vary in severity and persistence. In studies of HIV-infected gay men, typically three to eight years passed between the time of infection and the development of these types of non-life-threatening symptoms. (These symptoms may of course also accompany later stages of disease.) If the individual receives no treatment and further immune impairment occurs, the body frequently becomes susceptible to more dangerous life-threatening complications. Typically, this occurs only after eight to twelve years of infection.

This chapter discusses how you and your doctor can determine what preventive treatment is needed and when it should begin. It will explain the various laboratory tests that are now used to help make these decisions, including tests for T4 lymphocyte count, beta-2 micro-globulin, p24 antigen, and routine blood tests. Research into these predictive tests (called *prognostic markers*) is an area of intense interest, and significant breakthroughs are anticipated.

No one test can by itself determine a course of treatment, but the T4 lymphocyte count is currently the single best indicator as to when preventive treatment should begin. T4 counts are usually performed once every three months. If the numbers on this test come back relatively high, serious illness is unlikely in the near future. If the numbers come back low, the consensus of doctors and researchers is that you should begin treatment with drugs to protect against illness and to slow the progress of the infection. No single T4 count can be considered definitive: only the trend over time is truly significant.

Monitoring the Immune System

Regular monitoring with T4 cell counts or other tests raises many of the same psychological problems as HIV antibody testing. However, you will need to monitor your immune system repeatedly, usually every three months. You may well be anxious every time you get your T4 cells counted. Most people adapt to it over time and have diminished anxiety.

For a more technical discussion of the immune system and of the immune deficiency caused by HIV, please refer ahead to Chapter 16: Immunology, Pathogenesis, and Etiology in Part 3: Understanding the Science. This information may help you to understand what it is that prognostic markers measure and how these markers may best be interpreted. Some people like to know more detail about these mechanisms— it may provide a feeling of increased control or power over the disease. If this type of detail discourages you, skip it. You won't need it to understand how you and your physician can use T4 cell counts and other tests to warn you of illness and guide your medical care.

MONITORING STRATEGIES AND PSYCHOLOGIES

Laboratory tests can measure the status of the immune deficiency caused by HIV. These tests, or *prognostic markers,* play a crucial role in deciding the course of prevention and treatment in HIV disease. The underlying benefit of early intervention motivates monitoring the immune system with prognostic markers, just as it motivates HIV antibody testing. Monitoring and early intervention can buy healthy years during which research into more effective treatment can progress. Results of prognostic markers may provide reassurance by demonstrating that disease is unlikely in the near term. On the other hand, prognostic markers will raise anxiety if they warn that disease is imminent: however, timely warning makes early action and prevention possible.

Some argue that they would prefer to wait until they feel sick before taking action, and that therefore monitoring is unnecessary. Unfortunately, immune suppression can occur without any warning: you may be at risk for PCP, for example, and still feel perfectly healthy. Your subjective sense of your health does not tell the whole story and cannot substitute for laboratory testing.

T LYMPHOCYTE COUNTS AND THE COURSE OF ILLNESS

Several different measures can be obtained from a set of blood tests called *lymphocyte subset studies:* absolute T4 cell count, absolute T8 cell count, T4:T8 ratio, and the T4 cell percent (that is, the percent of all lymphocytes that are T4 cells). The absolute number of T4 lymphocytes per unit volume of blood is the prognostic marker most commonly used to measure the immune deficiency of HIV disease.

▲ T4 Lymphocyte Count

Many people refer to this number as the *T4 count,* or simply as *T4's.*

Normal values for T4 count vary widely. Different laboratories may have different ranges of T4 count that they consider normal, because of slight variations in the way the test is performed. Normal values for an individual vary depending on age, health history, genetic predisposition, and even geographical location.

The T4 count is a volatile changing measure, analogous to your pulse rate. Just as exercise can raise your pulse and resting can slow it down, the degree of challenge to your immune system can change your T4 count very rapidly in either direction. Counts performed on two blood samples drawn from the same person twelve hours apart may differ widely, occasionally by as much as several hundred points. The overall trend over months of time is therefore much more significant than any single number.

With these caveats, a reasonable normal reference range for T4 count is from 600 to 1400 cells per mm^3 of blood (mm^3 = cubic millimeter, a standard unit of volume—for convenience we will in future omit the units when referring to T4 cell count).

After HIV infection the T4 cell count typically drops below 800. Individual measurements of T4 count may vary considerably. However, the trend of the T4 count over several consecutive measurements will typically be smoothly and steadily downward over the course of un-treated asymptomatic HIV disease, averaging a drop of about 40 to 80 per year. As immune deficiency worsens, this downward trend may accelerate. Consequently more frequent monitoring is necessary as T4 count declines.

Early intervention has been documented to slow the decline of T4 counts. As long-term experience with antiviral drugs accumulates, we will have more information about how intervention alters the course of the disease and the profile of T4 counts over time.

In the weeks immediately after infection, HIV reproduces in the body. The immune system has not yet begun to make sufficient antibodies. The load of virus in the body increases, and the T4 count decreases well below normal. As the level of antibodies against HIV rises, the reproduction of the virus is suppressed and consequently the viral load decreases. T4 counts rebound at this point, usually stabilizing at a level somewhere below 800.

A **plateau phase** of several years then typically commences, with T4 trends relatively stable or decreasing at a low, even rate. Again, individual T4 counts may vary considerably, but the trend is likely to be fairly predictable. A minority of HIV-infected people have a more rapid and unstable course, with T4 counts declining in only a few years to the point of serious immune suppression.

Lymphadenopathy means swollen glands (lymph nodes). It may occur

42

at any level of T4 cell counts. The swollen lymph glands may be noticeable in the back of the neck, under the jaw line, or in the armpits. Swollen nodes may be tender or painless. Earlier in the course of HIV disease they may wax and wane without clinical significance. When T4 count drops below 250, swollen lymph nodes may shrink just before the onset of an opportunistic infection, and so should be reported to your physician.

Certain **minor symptoms** may occur during the plateau phase (T4 count below 800) but do not necessarily indicate serious immune suppression. Minor symptoms include occasional low-grade fevers, mild limited diarrhea, night sweats, and transient skin problems. Such symptoms may well trigger anxiety, but they are not out of the ordinary.

Given the state of evidence from clinical trials as of late 1991, most **expert physicians recommend that HIV-infected patients begin antiviral medication only when the T4 trend drops below 500.** Many believe that in future, as information accumulates, physicians may recommend medication even earlier.

There is little risk of life-threatening illness when the T4 trend remains between 500 and 250. An exception is that tuberculosis (TB) has been reported at relatively high T4 counts. Tuberculosis manages to cause illness when the immune system is still relatively intact because it is more virulent than other opportunistic infections. In HIV-infected people TB has usually responded well to treatment. Some drug-resistant TB has recently been reported—this may cause serious problems if resistant strains spread.

Kaposi's sarcoma may appear at any T4 count but is rarely serious until more serious immune suppression sets in (T4 below 250). Thrush, or oral candidiasis, is also seen in patients with T4 below 500.

The possibility of serious life-threatening opportunistic infection begins when T4 trends drop below 250. Different infections appear at different levels of immune deficiency. Preventive therapy for these infections therefore becomes appropriate at different times. Refer to Part 1, Chapter 5 for a detailed discussion of the current preventive options.

Preliminary studies and extensive clinical experience point to the following stratification of risks and therapeutic opportunities:

- T4 count above 500—opportunistic disease rare
- T4 count below 500—possibility of oral candidiasis, tuberculosis, shingles (herpes zoster), Kaposi's sarcoma, or lymphoma. Antiviral therapy recommended. Prophylaxis against TB is recommended for those who may have been exposed, independent of T4 count.
- T4 count below 250—possibility of *Pneumocystis carinii* pneumonia, cryptosporidiosis, severe herpes simplex ulcerations, tox-

oplasmosis, cryptococcosis, and esophageal candidiasis. PCP prophylaxis is recommended.

- T4 count below 50—possibility of *Mycobacterium avium* complex (MAC), and cytomegalovirus (CMV) disease. Prophylaxis against CMV is unproven but common. Prophylaxis against MAC is not yet routine.

These are very rough guidelines as to what risks you face at various T4 counts. Keep in mind that some people do get opportunistic infections with a high T4 count, and some people with very low T4 counts (below 50) remain healthy for a long time.

Strategies for use of T4 counts vary somewhat. The fundamental principle is to **obtain T4 counts often** enough that you can anticipate the emergence of opportunistic disease and prevent it if possible. The frequency of T4 testing depends on the current T4 level and on the rate of decline of the T4 trend. T4 counts are most commonly done every three months. Some physicians feel that testing every four months is adequate while the T4 trend remains above 500.

Physicians previously did not recommend continued T4 testing after the trend dropped below 250, feeling that no treatment decisions depended on the measure at that point, and that repeated testing simply increased anxiety. Opinion is moving toward **continuing T4 testing below the 250 level** as more clinicians experiment with prophylaxis.

T4 counts must be interpreted differently in young children. T4 counts are typically much higher in HIV-infected children than in HIV-infected adults. However, HIV-infected children demonstrate serious immune suppression at much higher thresholds than do adults. The figures listed above as T4 thresholds at which the risk of various opportunistic infections becomes significant must not be used to decide the treatment of young children. Refer to Chapter 8: Sex, Age, Race, and Ethnicity for a brief treatment of pediatric HIV disease.

Unusual or unexpected individual T4 count results must be interpreted carefully. The final number provided as T4 count is the product of three separate measurements performed on the blood sample. Many variables may act together to produce a value that does not truly reflect the underlying state of the immune system. Also, laboratory errors do happen. If you get a result that is very far from the value predicted by your overall T4 trend over time, have the T4 count repeated.

▲ T4:T8 Ratio

T8 cells come in two varieties. One kind, *suppressor T8 cells,* balances the activation of T4 helper cells to help to turn off the immune reaction to a specific antigen. The other type, *killer T8 cells,* works to destroy body cells transformed by disease. (See Chapter 16: Immunology, Pathogenesis, and Etiology.) The absolute number of T8 lymphocytes per unit volume of blood is not by itself a useful measure of immune competence or immune deficiency. T8 lymphocytes typically rise early in the disease and remain high, providing little information during the later stages of disease when treatment decisions are more often made. This measure was most often used in combination with the T4 count. The T4:T8 ratio is obtained by dividing the T4 count by the T8 count.

Normal values range from 1.0 to 4.0—that is, from a situation in which there are equal numbers of T4 and T8 cells to a situation in which there are four times more T4 cells than T8 cells. In HIV-infected people the T4:T8 ratio is typically 0.5 or lower—that is, there are fewer than half as many T4 cells as T8 cells. As the disease progresses the T4:T8 ratio declines further. A low T4:T8 ratio may be due either to a low T4 count or to a high T8 count.

▲ T4 Cell Percent

The T4 cell percent is a useful addition to the absolute T4 count. In some cases the T4 count alone may be misleading. Immune suppression may be present despite a high T4 count if the total lymphocyte count is also high. In effect, the T4 cells may be out-voted even if there are many of them.

A T4 cell percent under 20 percent indicates serious immune deficiency, even if T4 count is high. Begin prophylaxis against PCP if T4 cell percent drops below 20 percent, even if T4 count is above 250.

SUPPLEMENTARY PROGNOSTIC MARKERS

In addition to T4 count, T4:T8 ratio, and the T4 cell percent, a number of other laboratory measurements are sometimes helpful in making decisions about when to start treatment. We will briefly mention beta-2 microglobulin, serum neopterin, p24 antigen, and p24 antibody. These tests are not necessarily available from all laboratories. These additional prognostic markers are not in wide use yet, but if available, one or more of these markers may provide some useful information to supplement T lymphocyte testing.

▲ Beta-2 Microglobulin (B2M)

Beta-2 microglobulin (B2M) is a protein that appears on the surface of any cell that possesses a nucleus. (It forms part of the *class I major histocompatibility complex,* described in Chapter 16: Immunology, Pathogenesis, and Etiology.) The quantity of B2M found in blood increases whenever lymphocyte activation or destruction increases. B2M levels may be higher in certain populations with a background of immune-system stimulation, such as people who have shared needles for intravenous drug use.

B2M levels above 5.0 milligrams per liter indicate an increased chance of disease progression. Of all the supplementary prognostic markers, testing for B2M is the most available and predictive, and therefore the most often used.

BETA-2 MICROGLOBULIN PREDICTS PROGRESSION OF UNTREATED DISEASE

(Moss and Bacchetti)

Beta-2 Microglobulin Level (mg/L)	3-yr. Progression to AIDS
< 3.0	12%
3.0–5.0	33%
> 5.0	69%

▲ Neopterin

Neopterin is a low-weight protein molecule whose imposing chemical formula is 6-D-*erythro*-trihydroxypropylpterin. Macrophages (a type of white blood cell) activated by stimulated T lymphocytes release large amounts of neopterin. Increased neopterin levels in serum (the liquid part of blood) are not specific for HIV disease since neopterin will increase as a result of any activation of macrophages.

Neopterin levels are normally below 2.0 nanograms per milliliter of serum. Neopterin levels above 15.0 nanograms per milliliter indicate disease progression.

NEOPTERIN PREDICTS STAGE OF UNTREATED DISEASE

(Reddy and Grieco)

Neopterin Level (ng/mL, ± SD)	Stage of disease
1.19 ± 0.12	Uninfected controls
1.76 ± 0.14	HIV-negative homosexuals
3.05 ± 0.20	HIV-positive asymptomatic homosexuals
18.60 ± 2.10	People with AIDS

SD = Standard deviation

▲ p24 Antigen and p24 Antibody

As was mentioned in Chapter 1: HIV Antibody Testing, p24 antigen is a protein that forms part of an inner shell of the virus. The p24 antigen test has often been used in the evaluation of new drugs, but until recently had limited clinical applications.

The amount of p24 antigen in the body increases as viral activity increases. However, the immune system makes antibodies to p24 that bind to the antigen, forming an *immune complex.* Antibodies "mop up" p24 antigen, effectively hiding the antigen from testing. Until recently, serum p24 antigen was often detectable only when the amount of antigen was greater than the amount of antibodies. This doesn't necessarily happen even in people with advanced AIDS. In the previous uses of the p24 antigen test, a positive result definitely indicated progression, but a negative result provided no information, since you could be quite ill and still be p24-antigen negative.

Recent developments have shown that the immune complexes formed when p24 antibody and antigen bind may be at least partly dissolved by pretreatment with acid before testing for p24 antigen. This is called an *acid-hydrolysed* p24 antigen assay, and is not yet generally available. Experience is still limited with this test: it may extend the utility of p24 antigen assays as a prognostic marker.

Antibody to p24 is usually detectable in inverse relation to the amount of p24 antigen. If there is little p24 antigen in the blood, p24 antibody will be high; if lots of p24 antigen is present, the antibody will bind to the antigen forming immune complex, and so the measurable p24 antibody will be low.

Both acid-hydrolysed p24 antigen and p24 antibody are measured as a *titer,* which is a measure of the relative concentration of a substance in a solution. The original sample is tested. If the sample is negative for the substance, that is reported directly. If the sample is positive, the sample is diluted by a factor of 10 and retested. Dilution continues as long as the sample remains positive. The final titer is the dilution of the original sample that was necessary before the substance became undetectable.

Thus a 1:10,000 titer of p24 antigen means that the sample was initially positive for p24 antigen, and had to be diluted by a factor of 10,000 before p24 antigen became undetectable. A *low titer* means there was a low concentration of the substance; a *high titer* means a high concentration. A titer of 1:10 is *lower* than a titer of 1:10,000.

Unfortunately, these measures have not yet been standardized in any way that allows comparison of results across different laboratories.

Chapter 4
AZT, ddI, and ddC

We now turn to the topic of medical treatment that is currently available to help slow the progress of HIV disease. This chapter describes antiviral drugs used to control the damage caused directly by the virus itself—the foundation of long-term treatment for HIV disease. The next chapter will discuss the prevention of the secondary or opportunistic illnesses that arise as a result of HIV-induced immune suppression. Then we will discuss general health care issues relevant to HIV-infected people, some issues specific to populations other than white male adults, and conclude the first part of the book with suggestions on how to keep abreast of developments in treatment.

The bulk of this chapter covers one family of antiretroviral drugs called *nucleoside-analog reverse-transcriptase inhibitors* (often simply called nucleoside analogs). These drugs inhibit the activity of an enzyme called *reverse transcriptase,* which HIV requires to copy its genetic material. (For more, consult pp. 342–47 in Part 3: Understanding the Science.)

There are many different nucleoside analogs that have been studied for use as reverse transcriptase (RT) inhibitors. They have different profiles of safety and efficacy both in the test tube and in human patients. Comparison of these drugs is complicated and will become more so as ever more candidate drugs enter human trials. We will discuss in depth the three nucleoside analogs for which substantial data are available:

ANTIRETROVIRAL DRUGS IN COMMON USE

Common Name	Brand Name	Chemical Name	Structural Name	Manufacturer & Status
AZT (azido-thymidine)	Retrovir	Zidovudine (ZDV)	3'-azido-3'-deoxythymidine	Burroughs-Wellcome FDA approved in 1987
ddI	Videx	Didanosine	2',3'-dideoxyinosine	Bristol-Myers FDA approved in 1991
ddC	Hivid	Zalcitabine	2',3'-dideoxycytidine	Hoffman-LaRoche FDA conditionally approved in 1992

AZT, ddI, and ddC. We will present the evidence that AZT offers healthier patients demonstrable benefit with few side effects. The issues that surround AZT therapy in general will be thoroughly treated, including side effects and data on the safety and efficacy of lower doses of the drug.

AZIDOTHYMIDINE (AZT)

Azidothymidine (AZT) is an anti-HIV medication taken by mouth in capsule form. AZT was the first drug approved for use against HIV by the Food and Drug Administration (FDA). AZT was the only anti-HIV drug approved by the FDA from February 1987 until October 1991. Other scientific names for AZT are zidovudine (ZDV), or 3'-azido-3'-deoxythymidine. AZT is sold by the Burroughs-Wellcome company under the brand name Retrovir.

The current recommended dosage of AZT is 500 to 600 mg per day (five to six capsules per day). Most AIDS experts recommend starting AZT if your T4 cell count drops below 500. Treatment with AZT now costs about $3,000 to $4,000 per year. It is paid for by Medicaid and some other government programs and is reimbursable under any insurance policy that pays for medication.

Clinical trials of experimental drugs can be difficult to interpret (see Chapter 19: Understanding Clinical Trials). Most experts agree that AZT delays progression of HIV disease; the drug may also prolong the disease-free survival period. If you are asymptomatic or have only minor symptoms, AZT will delay progression to AIDS. AZT delays the decline of T4 cells and (in higher doses) is helpful in treating neurological symptoms and a blood-clotting complication of HIV called ITP *(idiopathic thrombocytopenia purpura)*. It has no effect on the course of Kaposi's sarcoma itself, but will help those with KS from developing infectious complications.

A study done over two and a half years, published in 1992 (Hamilton), compared patients who began to use AZT early in the course of illness (T4 count between 200 and 500) with patients who began later (T4 count below 200). Although there was no difference in total survival time, there was significant difference in the amount of healthy time. Patients who started AZT earlier had a longer time before the development of opportunistic infection; AZT delayed the rate of progression to AIDS by nearly 50 percent.

AZT is not an ideal drug. It is not a cure for AIDS. It seems to stop working after a period of time (years in those who are asymptomatic), perhaps due to a phenomenon called *resistance*. Side effects of the standard dose are almost always minor and transient in those who are asymptomatic or have only a few symptoms. However, in some patients AZT has serious but reversible side effects and must be discontinued. No one knows whether AZT may have adverse long-term side effects. AZT is expensive if not covered by health insurance.

We need much better drugs for treating AIDS and we need them as soon as possible. The reason to use AZT now is that it is the most reliable and best understood anti-HIV drug now available. Newer anti-virals such as ddI may prove to work better (at least for some people) but are less well documented and have their own disadvantages. The idea is to survive long enough to benefit from newer drugs. The use of antiviral medications buys you time during which research continues. Think of AZT not as "Mr. Right," but as "Mr. Right Now."

NEGATIVE FEELINGS ABOUT AZT

AZT has been the focus of some bad feeling among some people with HIV disease, particularly on the east coast of the United States. However, after six years of experimental trials and clinical experience, it has become clear that AZT significantly benefits many HIV-infected people. The drug probably has more benefit when used earlier in the course of HIV disease. For this reason, it is important to sort out the current facts about AZT from concerns that date from the past.

AZT was the first drug approved against HIV. In 1986–87 **people were bitterly disappointed that AZT did not prove to be a cure.** Unfortunately, many infected people saw sick friends die despite taking the drug and were intensely disillusioned and angry.

We now know that **the original recommended dose of AZT was too high.** At the time the drug was approved by the FDA, patients were given 1,200 to 1,500 mg per day—twice as high as the current recommended dose. The drug was given only to people who had already been diagnosed with AIDS or those who had T4 cell counts below 200. At this higher dosage and in this population of sicker patients, AZT frequently caused side effects.

The worst of the side effects was anemia, which left some people feeling exhausted and very weak. This meant that some people who began to take AZT felt worse rather than better after starting the drug and needed regular transfusions. Some people with serious anemia from AZT had to stop taking the only antiviral then available, which left them feeling terribly vulnerable. Serious side effects from the current standard dose of AZT are rare.

Though HIV-related research on AZT was done by federal agencies and with federal funds, the patent was granted to the pharmaceutical company, Burroughs-Wellcome, that had originally developed the drug. **The manufacturer was seen as a profiteer,** setting an initial price that meant that AZT cost $10,000 to $12,000 per year. Burroughs-Wellcome justified this price as necessary to recover its development costs. Following standard pharmaceutical-industry practice, the drug company declined to publish details about its cost of research and development.

Since that time, in response to pressure from AIDS activists, Burroughs-Wellcome has reduced its price for AZT by 20 percent. In addition, the lower dose now being used reduces the yearly cost by another two-thirds. There has been a legal challenge made to Burroughs-Wellcome's exclusive right to sell AZT. If this challenge holds up in court and other companies can manufacture the drug, the price should go down further.

Remember, if you lack insurance to pay for medication, don't give up. There may be ways to get drugs you need but cannot afford: Medicaid, insurance, special government programs such as the AIDS Drug Assistance Program (ADAP), or by enrolling as a research subject. Call an AIDS service organization for advice.

AZT was first developed in the 1960s as an anti-cancer drug. It was not particularly successful and was not used for treatment. In the mid-1980s, many existing drugs were screened to see if they inhibited reverse transcriptase in the test tube. AZT showed considerable promise for this purpose and so became a prime candidate for development as an anti-HIV drug.

When the drug was tested on humans, subjects receiving AZT did so much better than those not receiving the drug that trials were stopped early or modified so that all subjects got the drug. AZT was eventually licensed in February 1987 for use in HIV-infected people with a diagnosis of AIDS or with T4 cell counts below 200.

The methodology of the first of these early trials was criticized, with some justice. However, the results from the early trials have since been confirmed and strengthened in many separate trials conducted by many different researchers on different continents. A summary of a few of the most significant trials is included later.

CRITERIA FOR STARTING AZT

Low-dose AZT is the first recommendation for HIV-positive people with **T4 cell counts below 500.** This includes those with T4 cell counts below 200 and those who have been diagnosed with AIDS.

Many expert physicians also recommend low-dose AZT for people with T4 cell counts above 500 who have significant **constitutional symptoms** (fever, night sweats, weight loss, diarrhea).

People with Kaposi's sarcoma (KS) who have T4 cell counts below 500 should also take AZT or another antiviral. **Although AZT does not affect the course of KS, it will help slow the progression of HIV disease.** Like other HIV-infected people, those with KS are vulnerable to opportunistic infections once their T4 cell count drops below 200.

DOSAGE

The recommended standard (lower) dose of AZT is now 500 to 600 mg per day: five to six 100-mg capsules per day, taken one every four hours (skipping the 4:00 AM dose). Larger doses may be prescribed to treat central nervous system symptoms. If side effects develop your physician may recommend that you take a lower dose; 300 mg per day seems to have antiviral action, although it is not clear whether this dose is as effective as 500 mg per day.

ADMINISTRATION

There has been some debate as to the timing of the doses. Is it better to divide the standard dosage up evenly during waking hours, or to take the medicine in two or three doses per day? There is no need to wake up in the middle of the night to take AZT. Although there are no hard data, expert physicians suggest that the most important consideration is to take the full amount of the medication each day. If you find it too difficult to take AZT five times a day, it is probably better to take several pills at once than to miss medication.

It seems that AZT may reach peak concentration in the blood better (and therefore act more effectively) when it is taken alone rather than with a meal, particularly a high-fat meal. However, some people feel nauseated when they take AZT without food. Experiment with this. **If you can take the drug on an empty stomach, do so.** If this makes you feel sick, take AZT with your meals.

Take your AZT with plenty of water or other liquid while sitting up. There have been a few reports that people who habitually took AZT without water while lying down developed esophageal ulcers that may have been caused by the drug staying in the esophagus for a long time before reaching the stomach.

BENEFITS

In repeated clinical trials it has been demonstrated that AZT:

- Increases T4 cell counts. A major study of AZT in asymptomatic HIV-infected people showed an increase of T4 cell counts of 26 percent to 39 percent in AZT subjects versus a 16 percent decrease in subjects not taking AZT.
- Decreases frequency and severity of opportunistic infections. The same study showed half as many episodes of opportunistic infections among those taking AZT.
- Delays progression to AIDS.
- Leads to weight gain in those who have been involuntarily losing weight.

- Improves daily functioning as measured by a standardized test called *Karnofsky scores.*
- Improves neurological status and cognitive functioning. In patients with dementia, AZT was associated with improvement sustained up to eighteen months. AZT was less helpful with certain other neurological conditions (peripheral neuropathy and myelopathy).
- Increases response to *anergy panels,* a skin test of the ability to mount an allergic response. Increased response on anergy panels implies improved cellular immunity.
- Decreases levels of p24 antigen in blood and cerebrospinal fluid. This is a sign of decreased viral activity in the body.
- Increases platelet count. Platelets are *formed elements* in the blood that play a major role in the coagulation (clotting) of blood. Some patients with HIV disease have a low platelet count, a condition known as *HIV-induced (or idiopathic) thrombocytopenia purpura.* Thrombocytopenia can occur at any stage of HIV disease. AZT helps patients with HIV-induced thrombocytopenia purpura develop an adequate platelet count.

PROBLEMS

In people with T4 cell counts above 200, side effects are very rare. In people with T4 cell counts below 200, AZT may occasionally produce anemia and neutropenia (decrease in a type of white blood cell needed to fight bacterial infections). Serious anemia may require transfusion, drugs to counteract anemia, or the cessation of AZT.

Transient minor side effects may appear in the first to fourth weeks after starting AZT. They occur in only a minority of patients and usually subside on their own after a few weeks. Although they may be uncomfortable, none are dangerous or require treatment. These side effects include:

- Headache
- Fatigue and malaise
- Abdominal discomfort
- Nausea or vomiting

Some people taking AZT develop a **harmless discoloration of the fingernails and toenails.** The discoloration consists of longitudinal streaks in shades from blue to brown-black on the nails. This side effect does not occur until AZT has been used for at least six months. It does not have any adverse effects other than cosmetic.

Low-dose AZT rarely causes serious anemia or neutropenia. Myopathy (muscle disease) and myalgia (muscle pain) may occur but are also less common than with high-dose AZT. These side effects are all reversible by stopping the drug.

Anemia is a reduction of the level of red blood cells below normal. Anemia occurs in some patients after taking AZT for one to three months. It rarely occurs in patients who have T4 cell counts above 200. HIV itself, diseases associated with HIV, and various medications can all interfere with a process known as *erythropoiesis,* the formation of red blood cells in the bone marrow. Reverse transcriptase inhibitors such as AZT may interfere with blood-cell formation because some of these drugs may also inhibit human DNA polymerase, an enzyme particularly needed by fast-dividing cells like the bone marrow (for more information, refer to Chapter 18: Blood and Blood Cells).

Ordinary blood tests can easily detect anemia as one of three abnormal results: a low *hematocrit* value, low *hemoglobin* level, or a low *total red blood cell count.* For an explanation of these tests, refer to Chapter 13: Procedures and Tests.

There are three strategies for dealing with anemia while continuing on AZT. First, reducing the dose may solve the problem. Periodic blood transfusion is a second option. Over the period when the higher dose of AZT was prescribed, about one-third of patients with advanced AIDS required transfusions to continue AZT. These statistics will probably improve radically now that the lower dose is standard. The third option is to use a synthetic hormone to increase the production of red blood cells.

This hormone is called recombinant human *erythropoietin* (EPO, Epogen). Erythropoietin is a natural hormone secreted by the kidneys that acts on the bone marrow to stimulate production of red blood cells. Recombinant EPO is a synthetic version of this hormone. In a clinical study of patients with AIDS, use of synthetic EPO in patients with low natural EPO levels significantly reduced both the number of patients who needed transfusions and the number of transfusions for those who needed them. Patients who are anemic despite normal levels of natural EPO are not helped by receiving synthetic EPO. The drug appears to have very few side effects but may occasionally cause *thrombosis* (unwanted blood clotting). EPO is very expensive and must be injected.

Neutropenia is a reduction of neutrophils (a type of white blood cell) below normal levels. Among patients with T4 cells below 200 who were taking the old higher dose of AZT, neutropenia occurred in about 50 percent of patients and was usually the reason patients had to stop AZT. The rate is much lower with lower dose AZT. Neutropenia is rare among patients with greater than 200 T4 cells. Neutropenia appears from one to six months after starting AZT, most frequently at about three months. Neutropenia is detected on a routine blood test called a *neutrophil count.* Generally, physicians will diagnose neutropenia if your neutrophil count falls below 500 to 750 cells per mm^3 of blood.

Other medications may also sometimes induce neutropenia. These include the anti-CMV drugs ganciclovir (DHPG), Bactrim, acyclovir, and some drugs used as chemotherapy against cancer. To avoid neutropenia it may be necessary to decrease the dose of AZT taken in combination with these medications.

Neutropenia may be treated with *granulocyte colony-stimulating factor* (G-CSF), an expensive but effective injected medication.

Myopathy means "disease of the muscles." Some people who are HIV infected may at times develop pain or weakness of muscles, particularly in the legs. Both AZT and HIV themselves may cause myopathy. If it is caused by AZT it can usually be treated by temporarily lowering the dosage. See also the discussion of **myalgia** (muscle pain) under neurological disorders on pp. 207–08 in Chapter 10: Organ System Complications.

Not enough people have taken AZT long enough to determine whether the drug has long-term adverse side effects. So far there is no evidence of increased rates of cancer among people taking AZT for HIV disease. Burroughs-Wellcome has performed some laboratory studies on mice and rats that concluded that AZT could be cancer-causing in extremely high doses.

Some people have worried that increased appearance of cancers of lymphatic tissue (*lymphomas*) might be due to AZT use. Current opinion is that lymphomas are due to profound immune suppression. Lymphomas are more common simply because people with advanced AIDS are now living longer with immune suppression.

As we have mentioned, AZT is a stop-gap, to be used to buy time until better drugs can be developed. No one is likely to take a ten-year course of AZT. **For now, expert physicians feel that the danger of leaving HIV untreated is greater than the unknown long-term side effects of AZT.**

MONITORING FOR SIDE EFFECTS

While taking AZT you need to see your physician regularly to have blood tests performed. This will guard against the development of possibly dangerous side effects such as anemia. The necessary tests are a complete blood count (CBC) with differential, CPK (*creatinine phosphokinase,* an enzyme that increases with muscle damage), and renal and liver function tests. (See Chapter 13: Procedures and Tests for more information.) Have a complete blood count done before beginning AZT. The CBC should be repeated every four to six weeks.

INTERACTIONS WITH OTHER MEDICATION

AZT has no interactions with other medications except as noted above in the description of neutropenia. It was initially believed that using Tylenol (acetaminophen) in combination with AZT might lead to increased bone-marrow toxicity. Further research has contradicted this: it is safe to take Tylenol and AZT in combination. Probenecid, a drug often taken in combination with penicillin, makes AZT remain in the body longer, effectively causing an increase in dosage which increases the chance of side effects. AZT and the antiviral drug ribavirin have been shown to lose efficacy when used together in the test tube.

RESISTANCE

Extended use of any medication to control an infection brings with it the risk that the target organisms will evolve resistance to the medication.

Most people initially respond to AZT with increased or stabilized T4 cell counts, or perhaps with a decrease in or disappearance of symptoms. After some period of time these gains may begin to fade, perhaps because the drug's effect on the virus may have waned. **AZT may work for only a limited time**—from six months to a few years depending on the stage of illness when the drug is started. The reason why this occurs is imperfectly understood, but many experts believe that HIV develops resistance to the drug.

An HIV-infected individual has a population of many HIV particles or copies of HIV genetic material (*provirus*) in the body at any one time, representing many different strains of HIV with different properties. Just as a population of animals evolves when natural selection operates on random mutations, the population of HIV in the body also evolves. Because HIV reproduces and mutates at a rapid rate, evolution progresses much faster than in animals.

The addition of AZT to the body simply adds an artificial selection pressure to the system. Most strains of HIV have been sensitive to AZT and are referred to as "wild-type" HIV. When wild-type HIV is exposed to AZT, reverse transcriptase is successfully inhibited: this prevents AZT-sensitive virus from replicating. Mutants of HIV that are less sensitive to the drug are better able to replicate and pass on their resistant genes. Eventually, **AZT-resistant strains of HIV** come to dominate the viral population in the body.

The degree of resistance to AZT of a strain of HIV can be measured in research laboratories. Virus isolated from people taking AZT has been studied in this way for resistance. Experiments show that AZT-resistant strains of virus can develop in people with late-stage HIV disease as soon as six months after AZT therapy begins.

If AZT is discontinued, the population reverts to the AZT-sensitive wild type. This would argue for a regimen that alternated antivirals, except for the fact that AZT-resistant strains reappear quickly as soon as the drug is reintroduced.

Resistance develops more slowly and at a lower rate in patients who are

at an earlier stage of HIV disease, as indicated by higher T4 cell counts and fewer symptoms. This is logical because there is simply more virus in later stages of HIV disease: more virus means more viral replication, which speeds the evolution of resistance.

Some have argued that AZT should not be used early in the course of HIV disease because the drug's limited period of effectiveness should be hoarded until life-threatening complications loom close. Patients who start AZT with T4 count below 100 tend to develop resistance within one year. However, studies indicate that patients with early HIV disease (T4 cell count over 400) require three years of AZT therapy to develop resistant strains of virus. This slower development of resistance in healthier patients provides theoretical support for the use of AZT early in the course of HIV disease.

Resistance as measured in the test tube does not develop more rapidly at lower doses of AZT, regardless of the stage of the disease. Thus, there is no hidden resistance penalty for using the safer lower doses that are now standard.

A piece of good news is that AZT-resistant strains of HIV in general remain sensitive to other antiviral drugs—that is, **there is little *cross-resistance* between AZT and other drugs.**

We have said that resistance to a drug (call it Ralph) develops as Ralph-sensitive organisms exposed to the drug are unable to pass on their genes, leaving the field open to Ralph-resistant mutants. If the Ralph-resistant mutant is (by virtue of the mutation) able to replicate despite the presence of another drug (call it Alice) to which the organism has never been exposed, then the organism is said to be *cross-resistant* to drugs Ralph and Alice.

Cross-resistance develops between AZT and other nucleoside analog drugs only if the other drug contains a piece of the AZT molecule called the *3'-azido portion,* as does the antiviral called AZDU. The other nucleoside analogs currently in use—ddI and ddC—lack the 3'-azido portion. Consequently, people who have taken AZT for an extended period need not worry that this has caused them to develop strains of HIV resistant to ddI or ddC (a considerable relief).

Combination therapy may combat resistance. If AZT-resistant virus is not cross-resistant to another drug—ddC, for example—then using both AZT and ddC at the same time puts considerable pressure on the evolution of the organism. Mutants that are both AZT-resistant and ddC-resistant may be extremely rare, with the consequence that double resistance may take a much longer time to appear. This may considerably extend the duration of the effectiveness of both drugs. So combination therapy is attractive partly as a strategy for reducing the impact of resistance.

The connection between resistance to AZT (as shown in the test tube) and its effect on clinical outcome in people is not yet clear. Patients who develop AZT-resistant virus do not show increased levels of viral activity as measured by the p24 antigen test (Larder). At least one study (Singer) showed increased progression of the disease in those with resistant virus. Clinical benefit of AZT for patients who start with T4 cell counts below 200 seems to last only six to eighteen months. Clinical benefit lasts longer (perhaps three years or more) for patients who start AZT at a higher level of T4 cells.

It is theoretically possible that unsafe sex could transmit AZT-resistant strains of HIV to a person infected with strains of the virus that are not resistant to AZT. **Thus, resistance provides an additional reason why HIV-infected sexual partners should continue to use condoms for intercourse.**

THE EXPERIENCE OF STARTING AZT

If you are HIV infected with T4 cell counts below 500, it is likely that you will be starting on AZT or possibly another antiviral medication. This is often a psychologically significant event.

Emotional reactions vary. Some people feel a sense of relief at starting medication because they are finally taking action against the virus. Some people feel upset because starting medication makes the illness seem more threatening to them, even if they have no symptoms. Most people have a complicated mixture of these and other reactions. If your mood or behavior changes at this time, it may be that you are reacting psychologically to the stress of beginning the medication.

For many people, starting AZT feels like reaching a new stage in HIV disease. Since initially only people with a formal diagnosis of AIDS took AZT, you may associate starting medication with the onset of advanced disease. This association may make you feel as if you are sicker than you really are. Taking AZT may be your first significant protracted action to fight the virus. Some people feel that taking medication is a constant reminder of their HIV infection and, for a period of time, worry more about getting sick.

Many people find themselves feeling angry when they begin to take AZT. It is burdensome to remember medication, to visit the doctor, to pay for pills, and to fill out insurance forms. You may feel it is very unfair that you have to worry and make sacrifices to protect your health when other people do not. Taking medication may also make you feel isolated or different from other people.

If you have no previous experience with chronic illness you may never have taken medication on a regular basis for more than a few weeks. **Remembering to adhere to a schedule of medication multiple times each day may be difficult at first.** This is partly a matter of habit; any chore like this needs to become part of your daily routine. Sometimes negative feelings about taking AZT may unconsciously lead you to forget to take it. It is understandable that people push out of their mind reminders of a frightening situation. Some people prefer to use a watch beeper or a special pill box with a beeper attached to help remind themselves to take AZT. Others feel that this makes their use of AZT too noticeable to others. If you cannot remember to take your AZT five times a day, take the medication in two or three doses. This is better than taking fewer than the prescribed number of capsules per day.

Privacy versus support is often an issue. In general, taking AZT may raise further questions of how "public" you want to be about your HIV status. If you are taking AZT three to five times a day, going to the pharmacy to pick up medication, and taking pills with you when you travel, it may be hard not to have others see that you are on medication.

Decide consciously whom you want to know about your medication and organize your pill-taking accordingly. It is a good idea to have at least one person you can talk with about your physical and emotional reactions to starting AZT. In fact, it is useful at this time to belong to an HIV-positive support group. Other people who have started AZT have had very similar reactions. Talking with people who understand what you are going through will probably reduce your anxiety, increase your ability to take the medication correctly, and make you feel less alienated.

Most people have no side effects when starting the current standard dose of AZT. However, some people do have some minor side effects for a few days to a few weeks. The most common side effects are nausea and an uncomfortable feeling in your stomach. It is extremely likely that these side effects will go away as your system adjusts to the medication.

Minor initial side effects are almost always manageable. You may decide to stick it out, knowing that the side effects will probably fade in a while. On the other hand, if you feel really uncomfortable, don't let yourself or your doctor dismiss your discomfort as trivial. You may need to take the drug on a full stomach to reduce nausea. Sometimes it may help to start with a low dose and slowly increase to the standard dose. You may also be able to take medication to reduce uncomfortable side effects.

Anxiety about starting AZT may contribute to your symptoms. It does not really matter in this instance whether your symptoms have a known physiological cause or are anxiety-related. It is probably not possible to tease apart these issues. The goal should be reduction of distress by all reasonable means. If thinking and talking about the emotional issues connected to AZT is helpful, be sure to do so. If taking antacids helps, do this too. Psychological and physical relief are in no way contradictory in this situation.

The negative psychological reaction to starting AZT often fades within a few weeks as taking AZT becomes part of your daily routine and therefore less noticeable. It may be easier for you to manage the first few weeks if you remember that the physical and emotional reactions to taking AZT are both probably temporary.

RESULTS OF CLINICAL TRIALS OF AZT

Our discussion of AZT concludes with a review of the major studies done on AZT. Readers who want details of the evidence that AZT is effective should read this section: others may skip it. (For explanation of how clinical trials of experimental drugs are conducted and of terminology used below, please refer to Chapter 19: Understanding Clinical Trials.) It is always difficult to interpret the results of drug trials on human subjects. Many aspects of studies differ: subjects, duration of the trial, other medications allowed, dosage used, and method of analysis applied. As an example, most subjects in studies of AZT have been middle-class gay white male adults. It is conceivable—though unlikely—that results could be significantly different in women, people of color, or intravenous drug users. All studies done so far bear out the utility of AZT in most HIV-infected people. The bottom line is that almost all HIV experts agree that AZT is useful in treating HIV disease and that its benefits outweigh its costs for many people.

The first clinical trial of AZT that suggested efficacy was completed in 1986 (Yarchoan). This phase I trial tested safety and dosage. The study followed 19 patients with AIDS for six weeks on AZT. There were few side effects during this brief period. Because the study showed possible positive clinical and immunologic effects, large-scale, double-blind, randomized trials were started to determine efficacy.

In 1987 a larger trial provided data that persuaded the FDA to approve AZT for certain patients. This trial was done in a number of medical centers working together as the AZT Collaborative Working Group (Fischl, Richman, Hirsch). The study followed 282 patients with AIDS (recently recovered from PCP) or with T4 counts below 200. Half of the subjects took 1,500 mg per day of AZT and half took placebo. The study was terminated before the majority of patients had been followed for the planned twenty-four weeks because data showed dramatic benefit to the group taking AZT.

Some criticism has been raised of this study. Particularly, it was charged that the study may not have been truly double-blind and that patients and doctors might often have known who was on AZT and who was on placebo. The same degree of difference in survival rates has not been duplicated in subsequent studies, but other results have been duplicated repeatedly.

As a result of this study, AZT was licensed in February 1987 for use only in those with an AIDS diagnosis or T4 cell counts below 200.

This same group of patients was eventually followed on AZT for a mean of twenty-one months. This longer term follow-up continued to show benefit of reduced opportunistic infections and longer survival. Those in the group who delayed more than six months in starting AZT had the worst survival rate. The only new side effect that developed was some myopathy (muscle disease).

RESULTS OF 1987 PHASE II AZT STUDY (N = 282 subjects)

Result	AZT Group (1500 mg/d)	Placebo Group
New opportunistic infections	24	45
Deaths (after 9 month follow-up)	6.2%	39.3%
T4 counts	Increased	Decreased
Viral activity (p24 antigen)	Decreased	No decrease
Body weight	Weight gain	Weight loss
Functional ability (Karnofsky score)	Improved	No improvement
Neutropenia	16%	2%
Anemia	24% (some subjects required transfusion)	4%
Other side effects	Headache, nausea, muscle ache, insomnia	—

Other reports observed this reduction in opportunistic infections and improvement of clinical markers with the use of AZT. See, for example, a study of 700 homosexual men followed in Vancouver (Schecter) and a study of the efficacy of AZT in reducing viral activity (Jackson). A statistical review of national AIDS incidence (Rosenberg) indicated the likelihood that taking AZT was a factor contributing to the delay in onset of AIDS recently seen in patients with HIV disease.

Another review (Graham) indicated that despite these hopeful results, 42 percent of patients being followed as part of the Multicenter AIDS Cohort Study with T4 cells below 200 were not taking AZT as late as 1989. The proportion using AZT in the general HIV-infected population is likely to be even lower. This means that failure to use a currently available drug is leading to illness and death that could be stopped or at least postponed.

In 1990, ACTG Trial 016 showed little toxicity in those with T4 counts above 200. This placebo-controlled trial of AZT followed 711 subjects. Patients had T4 cell counts between 200 and 800 and one symptom of

HIV disease (oral candidiasis, oral hairy leukoplakia, herpes zoster, or unintended weight loss of more than 10 percent of body mass, dermatitis, diarrhea, chronic fatigue). The subjects were divided into two groups. One had T4 cell counts from 200 to 500, the other T4 cell counts over 500. Subjects were followed for a mean of eleven months.

The study showed the following results:

- AZT (1,200 mg per day) inhibits progression to advanced symptoms or AIDS in patients with T4 counts of 200 to 500.
- Twice as many patients in the placebo group progressed to AIDS.
- Patients in the AZT group had fewer and less serious opportunistic infections.
- Patients in the AZT group showed a decline in viral activity as measured by reduction of p24 antigen.

The study showed the following side effects:

- The incidence of serious side effects among patients with T4 cell counts between 200 and 500 was dramatically lower—only 5 percent as compared to 50 percent in patients with more advanced HIV disease. Only 3 percent of patients on AZT required blood transfusions.

For the group with T4 cell counts between 200 to 500, the benefits of AZT on T4 cell count in this study was similar to past studies. T4 cells increased significantly as compared to the placebo group for six months and did not decline below baseline for a year.

For the group of patients with T4 cells over 500, the results were inconclusive, because very few subjects in either group had any symptoms. Those on AZT did no worse than those on placebo. This study was stopped early because of evidence of clear benefit to the group taking AZT. A group of 145 subjects from this study were followed for 22 months and showed no significant increase in the rate of disease progression, indicating continuing benefit from the drug.

In 1990, ACTG Trial 019 showed the superiority of low-dose AZT and safety and efficacy for those with T4 counts below 500. This placebo-controlled AZT trial followed 1,338 patients for a mean of 55 weeks. Of these patients 92 percent were male, about 90 percent white and non-Hispanic, and 70 percent homosexual. Patients were stratified into groups by T4 cell counts: below 200, between 200 and 500, and above 500. Each group was then divided into three parts: patients taking placebo medication, patients taking 500 mg per day of AZT, and patients taking 1,500 mg per day of AZT.

The study showed benefit for all patients who were asymptomatic and had below 500 T4 cells. For those patients with T4 counts below 200, the benefit was similar to that demonstrated in earlier studies. The study was inconclusive for those patients who started with T4 counts greater than 500. So few patients with high T4 counts advanced to opportunistic infections and AIDS that it was difficult to compare the AZT and the placebo group. Dramatically, the study also demonstrated that patients who took 500 mg of AZT had as much benefit as those who took 1,500 mg while having significantly fewer side effects.

RESULTS OF ACTG TRIAL 019 OF AZT

(Results shown for those subjects with 200 < T4 < 500)

Result	High-dose AZT (1500 mg/d)	Low-dose AZT (500 mg/d)	Placebo Group
Progression to AIDS	14	11	33
Time-adjusted progression	—	2.3%	6.6%
T4 counts	Significant increase +26/yr	Significant increase +39/yr	Decrease −16/yr
Viral activity (p24 antigen)	Decline	Decline	No decline
Anemia and neutropenia	12.6%	2.9%, no transfusions	1.8%

Analysis of trials 016 and 019 retrospectively showed that benefit was independent of ethnic background. African-Americans and Latinos showed the same benefits and side effects as whites.

Possible ethnic differences in AZT efficacy have been a subject of controversy. Relatively few people of color have been subjects in the clinical trials of AZT. The Veterans Administration did a study beginning in 1987 regarding use of AZT. This study apparently showed that people of color did less well on AZT. However, on more careful analysis, this difference by race was probably a reflection of the poorer health care received by people of color, their entry into treatment later in the course of illness, and the use of a too-high dose of AZT. Although the numbers studied are small, women and intravenous drugs users (IVDUs) seemed to do as well on AZT as male non-IVDUs.

In 1990, ACTG Trial 002 confirmed the superiority of lower doses. This trial compared two doses of AZT, 1,500 mg per day and 600 mg per day (after a loading dose of 1,200 mg per day for the first thirty days). The study was conducted with 524 subjects who had had one previous episode of *Pneumocystis carinii* pneumonia, and no other infections or cancers other than minimal Kaposi's sarcoma on the skin. Both doses were equally effective in terms of time to development of opportunistic infections and effect on T4 cell counts. Those subjects on the lower dose showed increased survival benefits for two years. The low-dose group also had significantly fewer side effects (fewer hematologic problems, less severe toxicity). The rate of development of AZT-resistant virus seemed the same.

Several studies (Noore and Lemp, Graham 1992) **have indicated an increase in time of survival** for patients with AIDS over the course of the epidemic. Survival is increasing. Although it is difficult to sort out the contributing factors, data strongly suggest that AZT plays a large role. A large AZT study on safety and efficacy and resistance is being conducted in Europe. This is referred to as the Concorde 1 trial and is being conducted by MRC/INSERM. Data should be released by 1993.

Some people who challenged the efficacy of AZT initially asked whether the benefits observed in clinical trials of AZT could possibly have been due to the concurrent use of PCP prophylaxis. However, in patients from some early AZT studies who were followed over a longer period of time the benefits of AZT appear to be independent of PCP prophylaxis. A recent study done in the UK and Australia confirmed that those taking PCP prophylaxis and AZT had a slower rate of progression to AIDS than those taking PCP prophylaxis without antiviral medication.

WHAT TO DO IF AZT STOPS WORKING OR CAUSES INTOLERABLE SIDE EFFECTS

AZT is not a cure for HIV disease. Although the drug does keep many people from getting sicker, it has two glaring drawbacks: some people cannot tolerate AZT; and its benefits don't last forever. What should you do in these cases?

We have talked above about the side effects of AZT. Although serious side effects are much rarer now than they were among people taking higher doses of AZT, they do still sometimes occur. We described the various strategies physicians use to enable people with side effects to continue getting the benefits of AZT. Sometimes, however, the side effects outweigh the benefit, and it becomes time to stop taking AZT. Fortunately there are now alternatives to the drug.

One definition of **AZT intolerance** is any one of the following: anemia (decrease of hemoglobin of 2g per month), decrease in white blood count (a total neutrophil count of less than 750), nausea and vomiting, psychosis, severe muscle damage (myopathy) or inability to take AZT because of concurrent use of ganciclovir (Cytovene, DHPG) or chemotherapy for lymphoma.

The term **AZT failure** is commonly used to mean that the drug has ceased to provide clinical benefit. Broadly speaking, any decline in

AZT, ddI, and ddC

SUMMARY OF SELECTED CLINICAL TRIALS OF AZT

Trial	Patient type and number (N)	Dose, Duration	Benefits	Side effects
1986 Phase I Yarchoan et al., Lancet 1986, 1:575	AIDS/ARC N = 19	N/A 6 wks.	Suggestive	Few
1987 Phase II Fischl et al., New England Journal of Medicine, 1987, vol 317	AIDS (PCP) or T4<200 N = 282	1500 mg/d or palcebo <24 wks.	Dramatic: ↓ OI's ↓ Deaths ↑ T4 count ↓ p24 Ag ↑ Weight ↑ Function	Significant: ↑ Anemia ↑ Neutropenia Headache Nausea Insomnia
1990 ACTG 016 Fischl et al., Annals of Internal Medicine, 1990, vol 112	One symptom, 200<T4<800 N = 711	1200 mg/d or placebo ~ 44 wks.	In patients with 200<T4<500: ↓ AIDS ↓ OI's ↓ p24 Ag	Side effects ten times rarer in pts. with T4> 200 (5% vs. 50%)
1990 ACTG 019 Volberding et al., New England Journal of Medicine, 1990, vol. 322	Three groups: T4<200, 200<T4<500, 500<T4 N = 1338	1500 mg/d 500 mg/d or placebo ~ 55 wks.	For T4<500: low dose was just as effective For T4>500: inconclusive	Side effects rare when T4>200 Anemia and neutropenia: placebo group: 1.8% 500 mg. AZT: 2.9% 1500 AZT: 12.6%
1990 ACTG 002 Fischl et al., New England Journal of Medicine, 1990, vol. 323.	History of PCP N = 524	1200 mg/d 600 mg/d	Low dose was just as effective	Low dose group had fewer side effects
1992 MACS Graham et al., New England Journal of Medicine, 1992, vol. 326.	HIV infected N = 2,162	~ 24 mos.	Increased survival independently of PCP prophylaxis Slower progression to AIDS	—

Key: > = above, < = below, ↓ = decrease, ↑ = increase, ~ = about
mg = milligram, d = day, Ag = antigen, Ab = antibody, OI = opportunistic infection,
ACTG = AIDS Clinical Trial Group

immune parameters or increase in symptoms after use of at least 500 mg of AZT for greater than six months may indicate AZT failure. There is no universally-accepted strict definition of AZT failure. Expert physicians commonly base antiviral treatment decisions on some combination of the following criteria:

- New opportunistic infections or cancers
- T4 cell count decline
- Involuntary weight loss
- Increase of p24 antigen
- Neurological deterioration

Most people get noticeable benefit from AZT initially. Some remain stable on the drug while in others the benefit lasts months to years before the drug begins to fail. This initial benefit is marked by a rise or stabilizing of T4 cell counts. Some people, however, do not have even an initial benefit from the drug. If T4 counts continue to drop steadily over the first six months of AZT therapy without ever rising, then it is reasonable to consider alternatives to AZT as the sole anti-HIV drug therapy.

The **possible alternatives** are: to stop AZT as sole therapy in favor of one or more other antiviral drugs; to take AZT simultaneously with another antiviral; or to take AZT and another drug in alternation.

In October 1991 a second anti-HIV drug, ddI, was also approved by the FDA. Another antiviral, ddC, was approved conditionally in 1992 in combination with AZT. DDI alone might be more or less effective than AZT for some patients and have greater or fewer side effects. Conclusive data are not yet available. While ddC is probably not as good as AZT for sole antiviral therapy, it may be useful in combination with other antivirals.

Many AIDS experts think that the next important step in antiviral therapy will be the simultaneous use of combinations of antivirals. A combination of drugs could maximize antiviral benefit while reducing side effects and reducing the development of viral resistance. Various combinations of AZT, ddC, and ddI are being tried experimentally and in clinical practice. This is a rapidly evolving topic. You and your physician must keep up-to-date on new developments.

COMPARISON OF AZT, DDC, AND DDI AS SOLE ANTIVIRAL THERAPY

More information about AZT is currently available than about ddI or ddC. Most clinicians currently suggest:

- Starting anti-HIV drug therapy with AZT.
- If AZT stops working, consider adding ddC (or possibly ddI).

• If AZT causes intolerable side effects, discontinue AZT and use ddI instead. Recent evidence discourages the use of ddC as sole antiviral therapy.

There are no conclusive data at this point about the safety and effectiveness of combining AZT with ddC and/or ddI. More data on these drugs and their combinations should become available in 1993.

DIDEOXYINOSINE (DDI)

One anti-HIV drug in wide current use is dideoxyinosine (ddI). DDI was approved by the FDA in late 1991. DDI is an oral medication that belongs to the same class of drugs as AZT (nucleoside analogs) and like AZT works by inhibiting the viral enzyme reverse transcriptase. Other chemical names for ddI are 2',3'-dideoxyinosine or didanosine. DDI is manufactured by Bristol-Myers under the brand name Videx.

DDI has been approved by the FDA and is therefore **available by prescription**. Before approval—that is until very recently—ddI was available only in two ways: through clinical trials, or through an expanded access program run by the manufacturer.

Following promising phase I clinical trials, preliminary data from phase II trials, clinical observations from alternate access patients, and after political activity on the part of AIDS activists, the FDA allowed the use of ddI outside of clinical trials under limited circumstances. In this expanded access program ddI was made available free from its manufacturer. Patients paid only for the laboratory monitoring required by the company.

Patients had to meet the following criteria to receive ddI under the expanded access program:

• To avoid depriving the ddI trials of needed subjects, candidates for expanded access could only be people who for some reason would not have participated in a trial. So they had either to be ineligible for clinical trials of ddI or to live too far from any site of clinical trials.
• When it came out, ddI was the "new drug," and many people who could take AZT wanted ddI for that reason alone. Bristol-Myers intended the expanded access program to provide ddI only to those people for whom it was the drug of last resort. Therefore, the company required that candidates for expanded access be intolerant of AZT or not responding to AZT.

By the time the drug was approved, 22,000 patients had received ddI. Some data are available from about 7,000 of these patients. The side effects were the same as the ones in the clinical trial but appeared at a higher rate. Generally speaking, the response of patients of ddI through the expanded access program was less good than that of patients on clinical trials of ddI. This is because patients receiving the drug through expanded access were generally sicker than patients in trials. This does not argue against expanded access programs for ddI or other drugs.

The dosage currently used in adults ranges from 250 mg to 600 mg depending on body weight (see table below). Tablets are available in 25, 50, 100, and 150 mg dosages. The amount is usually divided into two doses, taken morning and evening. DDI is inactivated by gastric acid. For this reason, the tablets include a buffering agent to decrease acidity. Two tablets must be taken at a time; this allows the intake of sufficient buffering agent to allow the drug to work. DDI comes in tablet form which is chewed and then swallowed. It should be taken on an empty stomach, because taking it in combination with food reduces its concentration in the blood.

ADULT DOSAGE OF DDI BY WEIGHT (KAHN)

Weight	ddI Dosage
Above 75 kg (165 lbs.)	Two 150 mg tablets twice daily
50-74 kg (110-164 lbs.)	Two 100 mg tablets twice daily
35-49 kg (77-109 lbs.)	One 100 mg and one 25 mg tablet twice daily

The two drugs **ddI and dapsone** (used for PCP prevention) should perhaps not be taken together. The antacid used in the formulation of ddI may prevent dapsone from being absorbed, leaving you susceptible to PCP. Some people use ddI and dapsone in combination, but take them at least two hours apart to reduce the risk of a PCP breakthrough.

Studies have shown that **the benefits of ddI** are that it increases T4 counts and decreases viral activity as measured by levels of p24 antigen. Studies also show that ddI seems to slow the progression to opportunistic infections and cancers. Although some people develop serious side effects to ddI (particularly inflammation of the pancreas), most people seem to be able to tolerate the effective dose. DDI remains in cells for twelve hours after administration. In consequence ddI need be taken only twice a day.

Because ddI, AZT, and ddC are each somewhat different chemically, they have different **side effects.** The side effects of ddI are different from the side effects of AZT. DDI does not cause suppression of production of red or white blood cells. This means that some patients who are unable to tolerate AZT can take ddI.

The most serious side effects of ddI have occurred among patients receiving doses above 1.5 grams per day. There does not seem to be cumulative toxicity (over the period of use of the drug) as was once feared, but only toxicity to high doses of the drug.

The most serious side effect of ddI is **pancreatitis,** inflammation of the pancreas. This is a serious illness that in extreme cases can be fatal. The symptoms of pancreatitis are abdominal pain, nausea, and vomiting. If you are taking ddI it is crucial that you report any of these symptoms to your doctor promptly. Functioning of the pancreas is tested in the laboratory by measuring *lipase* and *amylase levels* in the blood. Even if you have no symptoms, you should discontinue ddI if your amylase level is five times greater than normal. Also discontinue ddI if *serum fasting triglyceride levels* are above 750.

It is probably best not to take ddI with other drugs that also can cause pancreatitis. DDI should be discontinued during treatment with intravenous pentamidine for PCP. Other drugs that may cause pancreatitis include sulfonamides, cimetidine, ranitidine, and azathioprine. You should avoid use of alcohol, which can contribute to pancreatitis. A history of pancreatitis or very high triglyceride levels usually means that you should avoid taking ddI.

Other side effects that have been reported are peripheral neuropathy (less frequently than with ddC), diarrhea, hepatitis, headaches, insomnia, increase in uric acid levels with no clinical signs or symptoms, and diabetes. The diarrhea may have been caused by the buffering agent used in the ddI; a different buffering agent is now used in the approved drug. If peripheral neuropathy develops, patients may stop the drug for four to six weeks and then restart ddI at a dose that is 25 percent to 50 percent less than that previously used.

Studies done so far have disagreed on whether some viral strains that are resistant to AZT have also developed **resistance to ddI.** Even if this is the case, it seems that not all AZT-resistant viral strains of HIV will be resistant to ddI. DDI-resistant strains of HIV seem to develop more slowly than AZT-resistant strains. It is not yet known how the growth of drug-resistant strains of the virus may affect your course of illness.

There have been a number of clinical trials of ddI alone. An overview of phase I trials was published in 1990 (Rozencweig). This information covered a total of 92 patients who had been seen in four sites. Studies were done by Yarchoan, Lambert, Cooley, and Valentine. In each of these studies, ddI was given intravenously for two weeks and thereafter was given orally. Doses varied, as did the number of times a day medication was given. Patients mostly had AIDS or ARC; about two-thirds had previously taken AZT. Generally, patients receiving higher doses of ddI did better. Major side effects were peripheral neuropathy, pancreatitis, abdominal pain, and diarrhea. The benefits observed are listed in the table following:

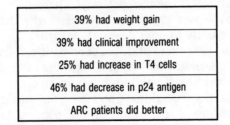

POOLED TRIAL DATA ON BENEFITS OF DDI (ROSENCZWEIG)

39% had weight gain
39% had clinical improvement
25% had increase in T4 cells
46% had decrease in p24 antigen
ARC patients did better

There are currently several different phase II–III trials of ddI going on that compare safety and efficacy of AZT and different doses of ddI. The major U.S. trials are ACTG 116, 117, and 118.

A number of trials are under way combining ddI with other antivirals. Preliminary information on the **efficacy of ddI in combination with AZT** is conflicting. Reports of good results from the combination (Collier) conflict with rumors that larger studies show antagonism between the two drugs that reduces efficacy below that of either drug alone.

DIDEOXYCYTIDINE (DDC)

In addition to AZT, an anti-HIV drug in current use is dideoxycytidine (ddC). DDC was conditionally approved by the FDA in 1992. DDC is an oral medication that belongs to the same class of drugs as AZT (nucleoside analogs) and like AZT works by inhibiting the viral enzyme reverse transcriptase. Other scientific names for ddC are zalcitabine and dideoxycytidine. DDC is manufactured by the Hoffman-LaRoche pharmaceutical company under the brand name Hivid.

Interpreting information about ddC is difficult, and **data are limited.** Although a number of studies have been done, they are small phase I and phase II studies. No large scale phase III studies have been completed. Early studies on the drug were halted when use of high doses of ddC led to many serious side effects. Only in the last few years has it become evident that lower doses of ddC can be used with much less frequent and less serious side effects; preliminary data are available from a number of studies.

Because some HIV-infected people have been using ddC for a few years, there is also a fairly extensive body of clinical information available. These data are important but do not substitute for formal drug trials.

As of June 1992, **ddC is available by prescription** and is reimbursable by insurance.

As of early 1992 the **most frequently used dose** currently is 2.25 mg per day (0.75 mg three times a day). (Notice that the weight of the recommended dose is smaller than the weight of the recommended dose of AZT mentioned above: about 2 mg per day of ddC versus 500 mg per day of AZT. This is simply due to the different properties of the two drugs.) Preliminary data suggest this dose of ddC may be effective while generally avoiding serious side effects. It is important to divide up doses and space them out evenly over the day in order to maintain adequate levels of ddC in the blood.

The best dosage for the combination of AZT and ddC has not been determined. Many experienced clinicians suggest combining the full standard doses of each drug: 2.25 mg per day of ddC and 500 mg per day of AZT.

A number of studies have shown that some **benefits of ddC** are that it decreases viral activity as measured by levels of p24 antigen and at least temporarily increases T4 counts. Studies have also indicated that ddC seems to slow the progression to opportunistic infections and cancers. Although some people develop serious side effects to ddC, most people seem to be able to tolerate an effective dose.

The common side effects of ddC are different from the most frequent side effects of AZT. **DDC rarely causes the anemia or suppression of white blood cells that are the major problem with AZT.**

Minor but potentially bothersome side effects of ddC are skin eruptions, canker sores in the mouth *(aphthous ulcers)*, general inflammation of the mouth *(stomatitis)*, nausea, and fever. These symptoms usually disappear after the first four weeks of using ddC. Local treatment can help symptoms that occur in the mouth.

A serious side effect of ddC that occasionally occurs is an inflammation of the nerves called *peripheral neuropathy*. Side effects of ddC depend on the dose used. The initial studies of ddC used what with hindsight is now seen as a very high dose. Some of the subjects taking high doses of ddC (up to 50 mg per day) developed extremely severe persistent peripheral neuropathy and related side effects. On the much lower dose now used (2.25 mg per day) **most ddC-induced neuropathies have been mild and reversible.** About a quarter of the patients taking low-dose ddC on expanded access still experience some peripheral neuropathy. However, less than 2 percent have had to stop taking the drug due to this side effect.

The symptoms of peripheral neuropathy are burning or numbing in the hands or, most often, the feet. Some people develop occasional shooting pains or cramps. The symptoms may start slowly. Some people develop only mild symptoms while others have to contend with serious pain that makes walking difficult.

In those taking low-dose ddC the symptoms of peripheral neuropathy usually stop when the drug is terminated. However, the symptoms may continue for a few weeks and even get worse before resolving. In the most severe cases, symptoms have persisted for six months after stopping the drug.

HIV itself can also cause peripheral neuropathy. A past history of peripheral neuropathy (due to use of the drug ddI or other causes) may predispose you to development of peripheral neuropathy on ddC.

If you develop tingling, numbness, and pain, you should discontinue the drug, at least for a period of time. It may be possible to resume ddC at a lower dose later.

Another possible serious side effect of ddC is pancreatitis, a potentially dangerous inflammation of the pancreas described in more detail previously in the discussion of the drug ddI. However, **pancreatitis seems to occur infrequently** and much less often than in patients taking ddI. Pancreatitis seems to occur in patients taking ddC who have a prior history of pancreatitis, for instance, as a consequence of intravenous pentamidine therapy for PCP. Because intravenous pentamidine therapy may increase the risk of pancreatitis, physicians commonly recommend that you interrupt ddC or ddI while on pentamidine. Avoid alcohol while taking ddC: alcohol can damage the pancreas.

Limited data suggest that **ddC has a synergistic effect with AZT.** This means that the therapeutic effect of the two drugs used together may be greater than the sum of the drugs' benefits when used alone. Each drug seems to make the other work better, without increasing the toxicity of the other drug.

Because ddC and AZT are somewhat different chemically, the two drugs have different side effects. DDC does not cause suppression of red or white blood cell production. Consequently, some patients who are unable to take AZT due to anemia or neutropenia can use ddC.

Studies done so far have disagreed on whether some viral strains that are resistant to AZT are also resistant to ddC. Even if this is the case, it seems that not all AZT-resistant viral strains of HIV will be resistant to ddC.

When **deciding between antiviral drugs,** probably the best strategy is to use AZT alone first. If AZT stops being effective, you may decide to take ddC together with AZT. If serious side effects develop from the use of AZT, you may decide to switch from AZT to ddI (or possibly ddC) alone.

As much positive information is known about ddC at this point as was known about AZT when it was licensed in 1987. However, as of early 1992 there is more extensive proof of the safety and efficacy of AZT than of ddC.

DDC as a sole antiviral therapy may not be as useful as AZT for treating neurological problems. The brain is protected from many toxins in blood by a mechanism called the *blood-brain barrier.* One drawback of ddC is that it does not penetrate the blood-brain barrier as well as AZT (Yarchoan).

Patients who are not doing well on AZT (presumably because they have developed AZT-resistant strains of HIV) may still respond to ddC. A combination or alternation of AZT and ddC, possibly with other antiviral drugs, may work better while reducing side effects. Trials combining or alternating the use of AZT, ddI, and ddC are currently under way and are of great interest.

Follow the development of data about the combined or alternative use of AZT and ddC. This combination is likely to become part of standard care for HIV disease. Many clinicians are using these drugs in combination even now.

The question is now more complicated than whether ddC slows progression of disease. Other questions that must be answered are how effective is ddC compared to AZT and are ddC and AZT more effective in combination or alternation than either drug alone. Studies compare ddC and AZT in different combinations and different doses, making it impossible to give simple, clear-cut answers about response to ddC as compared to AZT.

Interactions with other therapies: If you are starting radiation therapy, amphotericin B, pyrimethamine, sulfadiazine, intravenous Bactrim, ganciclovir, pentamidine, or acyclovir, you should discontinue ddC until you are stable on the other drug.

Several **clinical trials** initially indicated that ddC might have promise as sole antiviral therapy against HIV (Yarchoan 1987, Merigan 1989, Gottlieb 1989). However, a larger recent study suggests otherwise.

ACTG 114 is the largest clinical trial to date that compares AZT and ddC in people with no previous use of antiviral drugs. This study followed 320 patients on ddC and 315 on AZT for ten to twelve months. This study was halted because AZT appeared clearly superior to ddC as a single therapy. Thirty-three percent of ddC patients developed opportunistic infections or cancers as opposed to 28 percent of AZT patients.

DDC may be more useful in combination with other antiviral drugs.

Many experts think that the most promising use for ddC is in combination with AZT. A number of **trials of the AZT–ddC combination** have been undertaken and hopeful results of some of these were presented at the Seventh International AIDS Conference in 1991.

A study was conducted (Yarchoan) alternating AZT and ddC each for seven days at a time to see if side effects could be reduced. The alternation of drugs worked to reduce neuropathy; five times more ddC can be tolerated without neuropathy when it is used in this fashion. Nine patients continued on this regime for eighteen months and showed an increase in T4 counts and energy levels and less toxicity than would have been expected on either drug alone.

Trial ACTG 106 looked at 56 patients, 48 percent with AIDS and 52 percent with advanced ARC. The mean T4 counts of these patients was 60 to 70. The average length of time in the study was forty weeks. Five different combinations of AZT and ddC were used (0.015 mg per kg of ddC used in combination with either 150, 300, or 600 mg of AZT or 0.03 mg per kg of ddC in combination with 300 or 600 mg of AZT). One arm of the study was given AZT alone. None of the patients had been on previous antiviral therapy. The dose of AZT used alone (150 mg) was

Early Intervention

SELECTED CLINICAL TRIALS OF DDC

Trial	Type and No. of patients (N)	Dose, Duration	Benefits	Side effects
1988 Phase I High dose ddC Yarchoan et al., Lancet, 1988, Vol 1	AIDS or ARC N = 20 on ddC alone N = 6 on alternating ddC and AZT	High dose: 7-50 mg/d 6 wks.	Mildly positive: ↑ T4 (small) ↓ p24 Ag	Discouraging for ddC alone in these doses: Severe peripheral neuropathy Good results and fewer side effects in AZT ddC combination
1989 Phase I Low dose ddC Merigan et al. Annals of Internal Medicine, Vol. 110	AIDS/ARC N = 61	Lower dose: 0.03-0.06 mg/kg of body weight 3-6 months	Promising: ↑ T4 ↓ p24 Ag	Many fewer side effects
1989 Dose comparison Gottlieb et al. Vth International Conference, WB 327	T4 > 400 N = 21	0.03 mg/kg or 0.01 mg/kg t.i.d.	Lower dose more effective	Lower dose safer, no neuropathy
Ongoing ACTG 119 AZT vs. ddC	AIDS/ARC, > 1 yr. on AZT N = 102	AZT or ddC ~ 16 wks.	ddC slowed progression more than AZT	—
1989 AZT & ddC Yarchoan et al. Vth International Conference WBP 327 (preliminary data)	AIDS or advanced ARC N = 18	Alternate 7 days 1200 mg AZT and 7 days ddC in two different dosages 18 mos.	↑ T4 count ↑ Energy	Less toxicity than either drug alone
ACTG 114 AZT vs. ddC Ostreicher	AIDS/advanced ARC <3 mos. prior AZT use N = 635	—	AZT dramatically more effective than ddC	—

Key: > = above, < = below, ↓ = decrease, ↑ = increase, ~ = about
mg = milligram, d = day, Ag = antigen, Ab = antibody, OI = opportunistic infection,
ACTG = AIDS Clinical Trial Group

suboptimal; this limits the significance of the study. All arms of the study were very small. Questions about randomization have been raised; some groups started with higher T4 cell counts.

With the higher dose of ddC there was an increase of up to 120 T4 cells (higher than would have been expected from AZT alone) and most people maintained T4 levels above baseline for a year. P24 antigen levels declined. For patients with low T4 cell counts, the AZT/ddC combination provided the best results of any antiviral drug or drug combination tried so far. Patients on combination who were receiving at least 600 mg per day of AZT did the best in terms of sustained rise in T4 cells.

ACTG 155 is a fairly large clinical trial study (1,001 patients) testing the use of 0.03 mg per kg per day of ddC in combination with 600 mg per day of AZT. No results are yet available. Another study is looking at AZT plus acyclovir alternating with ddI and ddC. A third study is investigating whether it is better to discontinue AZT when declining T4 cell counts and progression to opportunistic infections occur or to add ddC (or ddI) to AZT. Results from these trials are expected by 1993.

Chapter 5
Preventing PCP and Other Complications

Opportunistic disease is the most frequent cause of death in people with AIDS, with *Pneumocystis carinii* pneumonia (PCP) responsible for over 60 percent of AIDS fatalities so far. The most dramatic example of the benefits of early intervention is that PCP is now largely preventable. If other opportunistic diseases could also be prevented, HIV-infected people might enjoy relatively normal life expectancies.

This chapter will describe medical treatment that is currently available to prevent the opportunistic complications of HIV disease. Preventive medications for many other infections common in HIV disease are in the process of being developed, tested, and used. Experts consider the development of further preventive treatments one of the brightest hopes for controlling HIV disease.

PROPHYLAXIS MEANS PREVENTION

The word *prophylaxis* is used interchangeably with the word *prevention;* medications (or other methods) to prevent the development of an illness are referred to as *prophylactic treatment.*

Prophylaxis is better than waiting to treat acute disease: drugs are more effective when used earlier, side effects are less severe, and the immune system is spared the strain of active illness.

Successful prophylaxis has two components: determining when particular opportunistic infections are likely to occur in an immune-suppressed person; and then using appropriate medication to block these infections.

Most opportunistic infections are the result of the growth and spread of microorganisms that have been in the body many years. **Monitoring** through the use of screening tests can sometimes indicate which people are infected with which organisms and therefore at risk for active infections.

The development of opportunistic infections is highly dependent on the degree of immune suppression. As was discussed in chapter 3, the most common measure used to monitor HIV-related immune deficiency is the T4 lymphocyte count. Opportunistic infections are rare in people with T4 cell count above 250 cells per mm^3. As the T4 cell count declines below 250, infections become more frequent.

Not every HIV-infected person should take all possible prophylactic medications simultaneously. The medications have side effects and interactions. T4 lymphocyte counts help determine when to start taking specific prophylaxes. Most physicians want to wait to start a particular medication until its utility is likely to outweigh its side effects.

There is no general agreement among physicians about when to begin prophylaxis for many infections. Preliminary studies and clinical experience suggest the following stratification of risks and opportunities for prophylaxis, based on T4 counts:

- T4 count above 500—opportunistic disease rare.
- T4 count below 500—possibility of oral candidiasis, tuberculosis (TB), shingles (herpes zoster), Kaposi's sarcoma, or lymphoma. Antiviral therapy recommended. Prophylaxis against TB is recommended for those who may have been exposed, independent of T4 count.
- T4 count below 250—possibility of *Pneumocystis carinii* pneumonia, cryptosporidiosis, severe herpes simplex ulcerations, toxoplasmosis, cryptococcosis, and esophageal candidiasis. PCP prophylaxis is recommended.
- T4 count below 50—possibility of *Mycobacterium avium* complex (MAC) and cytomegalovirus (CMV) disease. Prophylaxis against CMV is unproven but common. Prophylaxis against other infections is not yet routine.

Discuss the possibilities for prophylaxis with your physician. The physician's clinical experience is the best guide until more information becomes available from clinical trials.

The need for prophylaxis also depends on which opportunistic infections are common in the area in which the patient lives. PCP is common in North America, Europe, and Australia. Tuberculosis is common in Africa, Asia, the Caribbean, and South America, as well as in poverty-stricken areas of the United States. Histoplasmosis is common in the Ohio-Mississippi river valley of North America, the Caribbean (including Puerto Rico), and in Central and South America. Coccidiomycosis is found in the southwest United States and in Los Angeles. It is therefore useful to give your doctor a history of where you have lived and traveled.

A complete prophylactic strategy implies very long-term simultaneous use of multiple **medications:** antifungal, antiprotozoal, antiviral, and antibacterial. Some drugs can simultaneously prevent more than one opportunistic infection.

Prophylactic drugs should not produce dangerous or intolerably unpleasant short-term side effects. Specific side effects have to be balanced against the benefit of preventing particular opportunistic infections.

Long-term use of any drug may encourage the evolution of drug-resistant strains of microorganisms. Resistance is undesirable: it would reduce the effectiveness of both prophylactic and acute treatment. Long-term side effects and possible interactions with other drugs are also potential adverse consequences of prophylaxis.

Prophylaxis before a first episode of an acute illness is sometimes called *primary prophylaxis.* Prophylaxis against a relapse of an illness that has already appeared is called *secondary prophylaxis.* In general, we will use the term **prophylaxis** to mean prevention of the first episode of an illness, and will use the term **maintenance** to mean prevention of relapses or recurrence of illness. Current clinical practice recommends maintenance therapy starting after a first episode of most opportunistic infections, including PCP, candidiasis, toxoplasmosis, MAC, CMV, and cryptococcosis.

PNEUMOCYSTIS CARINII PNEUMONIA (PCP) IS PREVENTABLE

Pneumocystis carinii pneumonia (PCP) has been the major cause of sickness and death in the AIDS epidemic in the United States. Although almost everyone is infected with *Pneumocystis carinii* early in life, the organism is harmless unless people become immune compromised. In immune-compromised people the organism can cause a life-threatening pneumonia.

PCP has commonly been the first opportunistic infection that HIV-infected people suffer—43 percent of all AIDS patients received their AIDS diagnosis because they came down with PCP. Among all Americans who have been given a formal diagnosis of AIDS, 85 percent have had PCP at some point over the course of their illness.

In the last few years researchers have shown that PCP can in general be prevented. You can greatly reduce your chances of ever developing PCP if you receive the right kind of monitoring and treatment starting as soon as you know you are HIV infected. It is very important to prevent PCP: although treatment for episodes of active PCP has improved, 5 percent to 10 percent of people still die during their first episode.

In this chapter we will discuss prevention of PCP, and postpone discussion of treatment of acute PCP until Chapter 11: Infections.

▲ When to Start PCP Prophylaxis

If you are in immediate danger of developing active PCP you should start taking medication to prevent the growth of the organism. Multiple studies confirm that you are at increased risk of developing PCP in the near future if you are HIV infected and:

- You have had a prior episode of PCP. Forty percent of people with AIDS have a repeat episode of PCP within eighteen months if they do not receive PCP prevention.
- You have a T4 cell count below 250, or your T4 cells comprise less than 20 percent of your total lymphocytes. You are at high risk for PCP if your T4 cell count is below 250 and you have had a persistent fever over 100 degrees F (37.8 degrees C) or thrush (oral candidiasis).

In order to know when you are susceptible to PCP, you should have T4 cell counts done every three to four months. You may want to repeat your T4 cell counts sooner if your T4 cells are dropping rapidly or are between 300 and 200. Physicians will generally confirm a change in T4 trend before starting PCP prophylaxis. Once PCP prophylaxis has been started, physicians generally continue it even if T4 counts subsequently rise.

Although PCP is less common among people taking antiviral medication such as AZT, some people taking AZT still get PCP. Thus, if your T4 count is low, you need PCP prophylaxis as well as antivirals.

If you have active respiratory symptoms (such as shortness of breath or coughing), you should be evaluated before beginning PCP prophylaxis to see if you need treatment for some currently active illness (e.g., PCP, bacterial pneumonia, tuberculosis, cytomegalovirus). The medications and dosages used for prevention of PCP are not adequate to treat active PCP, and may not be effective at all if the symptoms are not caused by *Pneumocystis carinii.*

Several drugs have been shown in formal clinical trials to prevent PCP. There are also other medications that clinical experience suggests are effective in preventing PCP, although formal proof is as yet insufficient. We will discuss both the proven and the unproven drugs below. The principal drugs we will discuss are Bactrim, dapsone, and pentamidine (which is commonly administered as an inhaled aerosol for the purpose of PCP prevention).

▲ Bactrim

" Can not take "

Trimethoprim/sulfamethoxazole (TMP/SMX) is the chemical name for a commonly used compound of two antibiotics. This compound is sold under two different manufacturers' brand names: Bactrim and Septra. We will refer to this drug as Bactrim. Bactrim has been safely and effectively used for many years to treat common respiratory infections: for example, it is often prescribed to people who have sinusitis.

In the 1970s Hughes demonstrated that Bactrim effectively prevented PCP in children who had become immunocompromised due to treatment for leukemia. Unfortunately, this was not widely applied to people with AIDS until nearly a decade later. By 1988 many expert clinicians were using Bactrim for PCP prophylaxis. In 1989 the Public Health Service recommended PCP prophylaxis for all those with T4 counts below 200.

It has now been shown conclusively that early use of Bactrim prevents PCP in HIV-infected people. Clinical trials show that HIV-infected people have fewer episodes of PCP and live longer if they use Bactrim. Multiple studies confirm the usefulness of Bactrim both for primary prophylaxis and maintenance (prevention before and after a first episode of PCP).

Various doses of Bactrim are currently in use for PCP prevention. A commonly prescribed regimen is one double-strength tablet of Bactrim taken twice per day.

SELECTED STUDIES SHOWING EFFICACY OF BACTRIM

Study	Year	Purpose and Population	Results
Hughes	1977	Prophylaxis in leukemic children	Showed efficacy
Fischl	1988	Prophylaxis in AIDS-related KS	Showed efficacy
Pierone	1988	Maintenance (with AZT) One double-strength Bactrim twice per day	Bactrim group: 0/11 recurrences, 8% mortality over 8 mos. No drug: 8/11 recurrences, 36% mortality
Neilsen	1989	Maintenance One double-strength Bactrim per day	Only 6.1% recurrence of PCP
Stein	1990	Prophylaxis and maintenance (with AZT) One double-strength Bactrim three times per wk.	1 noncompliant subject out of 64 had an episode of PCP
Ruskin	1991	Prophylaxis and maintenance (with AZT) One double-strength Bactrim three times per wk.	No recurrence of PCP in any of 116 subjects over study period of more than 18 mos.

Bactrim is partly composed of *sulfa* compounds (containing sulfur). Like other sulfa drugs, Bactrim can cause allergies, particularly in HIV-infected people. **Up to half of HIV-infected people will develop Bactrim allergies** that typically cause fever, itchy rash, occasionally leukopenia (a reduction in the number of white blood cells), nausea, and vomiting.

If allergy develops, it typically appears as a widespread itchy red rash with fever eight to fourteen days after beginning the standard dose of Bactrim. If you develop a rash, contact your physician—do so immediately if the fever is high. Your physician will help you decide whether it is necessary to discontinue the medication. The rash and fever are uncomfortable but not dangerous. The symptoms will go away by themselves within a few days after stopping the Bactrim. In the meantime, the rash can be reduced by using Benadryl. Corticosteroids—a class of drugs that are powerful suppressants of allergic reactions—can be used if the reaction is especially severe.

If you find you are allergic to Bactrim, you may be able to tolerate the drug if you start the drug again at very small doses and then build up gradually; this is referred to as **desensitization.** Without desensitization, a substantial fraction of patients have to discontinue Bactrim completely. Attempts to desensitize patients to Bactrim have met with varying success. Desensitization is often done using a liquid suspension of 40 mg trimethoprim and 200 mg sulfa per cc (1 teaspoon), sold commercially as Septra Suspension. One suggested schedule for desensitization is reproduced in the table below. Desensitization carries some risk of causing a second allergic reaction, which in rare cases may be dangerous.

SCHEDULE FOR DESENSITIZATION TO BACTRIM
(Conant in Project Inform Briefing Paper 1, Dec. 1991, San Francisco)

Day #	Dose	Frequency
1–3	20mg TMP 100mg sulfa	0.5 tsp once a day
4–6	40mg TMP 200mg sulfa	1 tsp once a day
7–9	60mg TMP 300mg sulfa	1.5 tsp once a day
10–12	80mg TMP 400mg sulfa	2 tsp once a day
13–15	120mg TMP 500mg sulfa	3 tsp once a day
16–on	160mg TMP 800mg sulfa	1 double-strength tablet once a day

TMP = trimethoprim

Why would anyone recommend using Bactrim if it can cause such allergies? Bactrim has several advantages. It is cheap and convenient for patients, since for PCP prophylaxis it may be taken in pill form. It is easily available, and familiar to physicians from its use in other diseases. We will describe other medications that are delivered only to the lungs through inhalation: in contrast, oral Bactrim is delivered *systemically*— that is, throughout the body via the circulatory system. This provides three advantages:

First, systemic medication is evenly suffused throughout lung tissue, in contrast to inhaled medication. Thus, oral Bactrim reaches parts of the lung that inhaled medication may miss. Some cases of PCP have been reported in the upper (*apical*) lobes of the lungs of people who were taking inhaled medication to prevent PCP. Bactrim prevents such *apical breakthroughs.*

Second, systemic Bactrim may be effective in preventing some other opportunistic infections that occur in HIV disease, such as toxoplasmosis, salmonella, shigella, and sinusitis. Thus, taking Bactrim might kill several birds with one stone.

Third, in rare cases *Pneumocystis* has been reported outside the lung (*extrapulmonary pneumocystosis*). Inhaled medications protect only lung tissue, whereas systemic Bactrim may be able to prevent *Pneumocystis* in the rest of the body as well.

▲ Dapsone

Dapsone is another antibiotic taken in pill form that appears to be very effective in preventing PCP, although clinical studies are not yet complete. Dapsone appears to cause fewer side effects than Bactrim. Those who cannot tolerate Bactrim may be able to take dapsone instead and thereby get the benefits of systemic prophylaxis against PCP.

People taking dapsone may become anemic and so must be monitored by blood tests on a regular basis. Leucovorin (folinic acid) used in combination with the dapsone may help reduce anemia. The usual dose of dapsone is 25 mg four times per day. It can also be given as 50 mg two times per day, or as a single daily dose of 100 mg per day (although in the latter case anemia may be more frequent).

SELECTED STUDIES SHOWING EFFICACY OF DAPSONE

Study	Year	Drug Regime	Results
Metroka et al.	1988	Prophylaxis Dapsone 25 mg four times per day	Only 2 out of 173 got PCP over 9 mos. Suggestive evidence of prophylactic effect against cryptosporidiosis also.
Clotet et al.	1990	Maintenance Dapsone 100 mg twice a wk alone or with pyrimethamine 25 mg twice per wk	0 out of 20 episodes over 6 mos.

Preventing PCP and Other Complications

A number of patients who took both dapsone and the antiviral drug ddI at the same time developed PCP. The failure of the dapsone to prevent PCP in this situation appears to be due to the fact that a citrate-phosphate buffer in the ddI decreases gastric acidity below the level necessary for the absorption of dapsone. In other words, if you take ddI and dapsone at the same time, your stomach will not absorb the dapsone. This problem may possibly be solved by taking the ddI and dapsone at least two hours apart—but some clinicians prefer not to use the drugs together at all.

In some people Dapsone may cause an allergic reaction like that caused by Bactrim. As with Bactrim, desensitization can usually be accomplished by starting with small doses and building up to the standard prophylactic dose gradually. The low doses are achieved by preparing liquid suspensions of dapsone at various dilutions. A suggested desensitization schedule appears below.

SCHEDULE FOR DESENSITIZATION TO DAPSONE (METROKA)

Day #	Dose	Frequency	Total Daily Dose
1–3	0.01 mg	1 per day	0.01 mg
4–6	0.01 mg	2 per day	0.02 mg
7–9	0.10 mg	1 per day	0.10 mg
10–12	0.10 mg	2 per day	0.20 mg
13–15	1.00 mg	1 per day	1.00 mg
16–18	1.00 mg	2 per day	2.00 mg
19–21	2.00 mg	2 per day	4.00 mg
22–24	4.00 mg	2 per day	8.00 mg
25–27	8.00 mg	2 per day	16.00 mg
28–30	16.00 mg	2 per day	32.00 mg
31–33	25.00 mg	2 per day	50.00 mg
34–36	35.00 mg	2 per day	70.00 mg
37–39	45.00 mg	2 per day	90.00 mg
40 and on	50.00 mg	2 per day	100.00 mg

▲ Pentamidine

Another drug used to prevent PCP is pentamidine in an aerosolized form. Pentamidine has been used in hospitals in intravenous form to treat active or acute PCP. Used intravenously as acute-phase treatment the drug is effective, but may cause systemic side effects such as liver problems that make *intravenous* pentamidine unattractive for long-term use to prevent PCP.

Researchers invented another method of administering pentamidine that sidestepped the problem of systemic side effects. A small machine called a *nebulizer* can turn pentamidine solution into a mist that is inhaled directly into the lungs. The advantage of aerosolized pentamidine (aeropent, AP) is that the drug stays in the lungs: systemic side effects such as liver toxicity are for the most part avoided. In fact, aerosolized pentamidine appears to be effective and to have few side effects. Aerosolized pentamidine and AZT are tolerated well together.

A 1990 study of patients who had recovered from an episode of PCP compared the use of Bactrim and the use of aerosolized pentamidine (Ruskin). Bactrim appears to be significantly more effective; patients on aerosolized pentamidine developed recurrent episodes of PCP 3.25 times more often than did patients on Bactrim. Nonetheless, aerosolized pentamidine does provide significant protection against PCP and should be used by those who cannot tolerate Bactrim or dapsone.

Some adverse effects are reported during treatment: a cough and wheezing, mostly among patients who smoke or have history of asthma. This can be reduced by simultaneously using another drug called a bronchodilator (e.g., Alupent, albuterol).

However, recent clinical experience now seems to indicate that aerosolized pentamidine may be less effective than systemic prophylaxis for PCP. People using aerosolized pentamidine sometimes develop PCP in the upper lobes of the lungs (the *apical* lobes), apparently because not enough of the aerosolized drug reaches this area. Get careful instructions in using your nebulizer properly so as to optimize the deposition of drug in the lungs. Also, aerosolized pentamidine will not prevent the rare occurrence of *Pneumocystis* disease outside the lungs *(extrapulmonary pneumocystosis).*

One strategy to minimize apical PCP breakthroughs and extrapulmonary pneumocystosis in those who cannot tolerate Bactrim or dapsone may be to combine aerosolized pentamidine with occasional infusions of intravenous pentamidine. One schedule in use substitutes 300 mg IV pentamidine for aerosolized pentamidine once every three months.

▲ Other Drugs

Fansidar is an antibiotic that has been used to prevent PCP. It may also be effective in preventing toxoplasmosis. It appears to be effective, but in

SELECTED STUDIES SHOWING EFFICACY OF AEROSOL PENTAMIDINE (AEROPENT, AP)

Study	Year	Purpose, Pop'n, Meds.	Results
Bernard and Leoung	1987, 1988	Maintenance AP	Showed efficacy, low toxicity
Girard	1989	Maintenance AZT alone vs. AZT plus AP	61% recurrence without AP vs. only 9% with AP
Montaner et al.	1989	Maintenance AP plus AZT	35% recurrence without AP vs. only 6% with AP
Hirschel	1989	Primary prophylaxis T4 < 200, AIDS, ARC 300 mg AP once a month vs. placebo	*Three* times as many recurrences of PCP in the placebo group as in those taking AP
Leoung	1990	Dosage for prophylaxis 30 mg AP every two wks vs. 150 mg every two wks vs. 300 mg once a month	300 mg once a month is preferable

rare and unpredictable cases it can have very dangerous and even fatal side effects (an allergic response called *Stevens-Johnson syndrome).* Use of Bactrim, dapsone, or aerosolized pentamidine is preferable.

Burroughs-Wellcome is testing a new antiprotozoal drug whose code number is BW566C80 (hydroxynaphthoquinone). So far, data show that the drug is effective in animal studies and safe in humans. Phase I studies of the drug for treating PCP have been completed.

DATA LIMITED ON PREVENTION OF OTHER DISEASES

Primary prophylaxis is not yet routine for opportunistic infections other than PCP. Clinicians and researchers are experimenting with various drugs, but little conclusive evidence is available. You and your physician may decide to try unproven prophylactic strategies, but you should be aware that much less is known about the prevention of other diseases than is known about the prevention of PCP. Maintenance therapy is a different story, however. Expert clinicians routinely prescribe medication to prevent recurrences of many of the infections discussed below. Prevention is discussed for the following infections:

- Toxoplasmosis
- Mycobacterium avium complex (MAC)
- Tuberculosis
- Cryptococcosis and other fungal diseases
- Cytomegalovirus (CMV) disease

- Candidiasis
- Histoplasmosis

▲ Prevention of Toxoplasmosis

(For a complete description of toxoplasmosis, consult pp. 244–48 in Chapter 11: Infections.)

Toxoplasmosis has been a relatively late complication of HIV disease. It is caused by the protozoan parasite *Toxoplasma gondii,* which causes a serious disorder of the brain. HIV-infected people who get toxoplasmosis have generally had T4 cell counts well below 100. One study indicated that the mean T4 cell count within three months of diagnosis with toxoplasmosis was 51. However, toxoplasmosis can occur at higher T4 counts.

You cannot develop toxoplasmosis if you have not been infected with *Toxoplasma gondii.* About one-third to one-half of the people living in the United States are infected by adulthood. A blood test for antibodies to the organism can accurately detect infection. Take this test as part of your initial workup for HIV infection. The result will help your physician diagnose symptoms correctly in the future by either raising suspicion of toxoplasmosis or ruling it out.

If you are antibody-negative for toxoplasma it is useful to take some precautionary measures against infection. Avoid eating rare meats. Use gloves for changing cat litter or gardening or have someone else do it. Wash hands and surfaces that have come in contact with raw meat, and wash all fruits and vegetables.

There are limited data available about primary prophylaxis of toxoplasmosis (prevention before disease). Most of it has been obtained indirectly through looking at people who were in PCP prophylaxis trials. Pyrimethamine (Daraprim) is being tried for prophylaxis for patients with T4 count below 200 and evidence of prior infection with *Toxoplasma gondii* (a positive toxoplasma antibody test). Pyrimethamine is also being used in combination with sulfadiazine, sulfadoxine (see below on Fansidar), clindamycin, azithromycin, Bactrim, and dapsone. Leucovorin (folinic acid) is used in combination with Daraprim to prevent anemia.

Patients who have had an episode of toxoplasmosis should receive maintenance medication to prevent recurrence of the disease. Several drugs are being used for maintenance. They include a combination of pyrimethamine/sulfadiazine, pyrimethamine/sulfadoxine (Fansidar) and leucovorin (folinic acid, sometimes used to control the hematologic side effects of the Fansidar), pyrimethamine/clindamycin, clarithromycin (Biaxin alone and with pyrimethamine), and azithromycin (Zithromax). Trials are under way to compare the efficacy of these drugs. Fansidar occasionally can cause serious allergic side effects. Clarithromycin and azithromycin are particularly promising drugs because they may also be effective in preventing *Mycobacterium avium* complex.

▲ Prevention of *Mycobacterium Avium* Complex (MAC)

(For a complete description of *Mycobacterium avium* complex consult pp. 258–62 in Chapter 11: Infections.)

Mycobacterium avium complex (MAC) is a serious bacterial disease with systemic manifestations (such as fever) that occur late in the course of immune suppression. Patients who develop MAC almost always have T4 counts below 100 (usually below 50) and usually have had a previous opportunistic infection.

Treatment for MAC is still in an early stage. There is no clear agreement about the best way to treat an acute episode of MAC. The treatments that are used now involve multiple drugs, have multiple adverse side effects, and have to be taken on a continuing basis. We need to find an effective prophylaxis against MAC.

A number of different medications are being tried for prevention (primary prophylaxis) and maintenance (secondary prophylaxis) of MAC. Some of the drugs being investigated are ethambutol, rifabutin (Ansamycin), clarithromycin, and azithromycin. There is no clear-cut answer at this point about the best drug or combination of drugs that should be used. Maintenance therapy after an episode of toxoplasmosis is now routine, even though it is not known which of the existing treatments is most effective.

Primary prophylaxis (prevention for those who are at risk for MAC but have not had any acute episode) is not yet routine practice. Some physicians, however, are putting their patients with T4 count below 50 on clarithromycin. The concern with this course of action is that long-term prophylaxis with clarithromycin might make the drug useless for the treatment of acute illness.

▲ Prevention of Tuberculosis

Prevention of tuberculosis among those exposed is standard medical practice but is somewhat complicated. To avoid repeating material, a complete description of preventive and maintenance strategies against tuberculosis appears only on pp. 262–67 in Chapter 11: Infections.

▲ Prevention of Cryptococcosis and Other Fungal Diseases

(For a complete description of cryptococcosis and other fungal diseases consult pp. 272–77 in Chapter 11: Infections.)

Cryptococcus, *Candida albicans* (thrush), and a number of other fungi cause illness in HIV-infected people. Cryptococcus typically causes meningitis, an inflammation of the linings of the brain or spinal cord. It is not clear if cryptococcosis in HIV-infected people is caused by primary infection or reactivation of latent infection. Most patients (96 percent according to one study) who develop cryptococcosis (cryptococcal meningitis) have T4 counts below 100. Some people do develop cryptococcosis at higher T4 counts, however.

Some physicians are starting patients in this category on fluconazole

(Diflucan) or a similar drug, itraconazole (Sporanex). Fluconazole appears to be more effective and to have fewer side effects than the previous standard drug, amphotericin-B (Fungizone). Fluconazole should be used on an ongoing basis after one episode of cryptococcosis. Data on the efficacy of fluconazole for primary prevention of cryptococcosis are limited.

One drug currently in trials is referred to as SCH39304. This medication belongs to the category of antifungal drugs called triazoles. It may also help prevent other fungal infections (histoplasma, candida).

Maintenance with fluconazole can also be used if there are major problems with recurrences of thrush (candida) or possibly *tinea* (jock itch, athlete's foot).

▲ Prevention of Cytomegalovirus (CMV) Disease

(For a complete description of cytomegalovirus disease consult pp. 220–32 in Chapter 11: Infections.)

Cytomegalovirus is a virus that can cause disease in various organs including the gastrointestinal tract and the eyes. It is generally a fairly late complication of HIV disease, typically affecting those with T4 counts below 50. If you have had an episode of cytomegalovirus (CMV) disease, you should have ongoing maintenance therapy using ganciclovir or foscarnet. Studies are now under way for primary prophylaxis of CMV if T4 counts are below 100. A promising prophylactic strategy is the use of high-dose acyclovir (Zovirax, 800 mg five times per day). This regimen appears to cause few side effects. Researchers are also investigating the use of monoclonal (genetically engineered) antibodies against CMV as preventive therapy.

▲ Prevention of Candidiasis

Maintenance drugs being used in clinical practice are fluconazole, itraconazole, and ketoconazole. The drug SCH39304 is under investigation. (For a complete description of candidiasis consult pp. 275–77 in Chapter 11: Infections.)

▲ Prevention of Histoplasmosis

Fluconazole and clotrimazole are under investigation for primary prophylaxis. For maintenance amphotericin B and ketoconazole are used by clinicians, while fluconazole and itraconazole are under investigation. (For a complete description of histoplasmosis consult pp. 249–50 in Chapter 11: Infections.)

Chapter 6
General Health Care

The most significant factors in early treatment of HIV disease are probably the prevention of opportunistic infections and the use of antiviral medication. However, other health care measures can make a significant difference in the course of illness and quality of life. This chapter will describe these steps: e.g., the importance of prompt and aggressive treatment of all symptoms; immunizations (including the crucial topic of immunization against hepatitis B); specialized gynecological care; and dental care. In addition, this chapter will provide information about condom use and needle cleaning; nutrition and food safety; the use of alcohol and other recreational drugs; and how to live safely with domestic animals.

SEEK MEDICAL CARE PROMPTLY AND AGGRESSIVELY

Most people who are HIV infected worry at some point about whether to contact their doctors if a new symptom appears. If you are generally healthy and your T4 count is high, most symptoms do not constitute an immediate medical emergency; nothing terrible is going to happen to you in the next few days. However, it is always a good idea to let your doctor know about any new symptom that lasts more than forty-eight hours. If you find yourself debating whether to call your physician, go ahead and call. It is almost always better to err on the side of being too careful.

Many people put off calling their doctors because they worry about being "hypochondriacs" or bothering their doctors. Many HIV doctors on the other hand seem to report the opposite problem: their patients wait too long to call them with problems. Very few people call their doctors too often; if you are afraid you are doing this, speak about it directly with your physician. If you are becoming too worried about minor symptoms, the solution is not to ignore all symptoms but to get help with your anxiety.

Most people feel a strong impulse not to think about a new symptom. People feel that if something is wrong, even something minor, it could be the start of a larger problem. If you are asymptomatic, you are probably afraid of developing symptoms that could lead to a diagnosis of AIDS. It is tempting for most people to say "If I just wait a few days this may go away and I won't have to worry about it."

Contacting your doctor to report a new problem takes work. Doctors are busy: you may have to make repeated calls and then wait for a return call. Not only is this inconvenient, but during this time your anxiety may increase. (Some doctors have assistants who can give preliminary advice on the phone; this is very helpful).

There are very strong reasons to try to overcome the understandable impulse to avoid calling your doctor if a new problem occurs. Most symptoms will be minor and getting this reassurance from your physician will make you feel better. If you have pushed a worry out of mind it can create anxiety even if you aren't thinking about it consciously. If the symptom requires treatment, it is better to get treatment promptly. Your goal is to stay as healthy as possible; curing infections and other problems as fast as possible will help maintain the proper functioning of your immune system.

If the problem you are experiencing is a symptom of an opportunistic infection, it is crucial that you receive treatment as soon as possible. Opportunistic infections are likely to respond better to treatment when the treatment occurs early in the course of the infection. Early treatment may help you avoid hospitalization; some problems can be treated on an out-patient basis if treatment begins early. More severe illness due to delayed treatment can lead to unnecessary suffering, weight loss, and multiple secondary medical problems. Sometimes early intervention in an opportunistic infection can be lifesaving.

This situation may be particularly difficult if you get your medical care through a clinic. Sometimes the only way to be evaluated between regular visits is to go to the emergency room, a time-consuming and often unpleasant activity. It may be difficult or impossible to get your clinic doctor on the telephone. It is extremely useful to establish contact with a nurse or other health care professional in the clinic in addition to your doctor. This person may be easier to reach and may advise you as to whether it is urgent that you see a doctor.

SYMPTOMS THAT REQUIRE MEDICAL EVALUATION

The symptoms of HIV disease are often the same as the symptoms of common illnesses. HIV-infected people need some way to distinguish run-of-the-mill colds and flus from more serious illness. The following section lists symptoms severe enough that you should call your physician.

Many of these symptoms can occur as a result of depression or anxiety: headache, diarrhea, shortness of breath, confusion, memory loss, nausea, pain, and weakness. If you are feeling very depressed or anxious, your symptoms may be related to these emotional states. However, there is no way to determine if this is the case except by careful medical evaluation of the symptoms. You may be undergoing severe stress and still have physical symptoms that require independent treatment. As doctors say, you must "rule out" physical causes rather than "rule in" psychological causes.

General Health Care

SOME SYMPTOMS THAT MAY REQUIRE MEDICAL EVALUATION

Symptom	Contact your doctor if . . .
Fever	Temperature is above 100°F for 48 hours or longer. Fever indicates underlying illness. Fever is not dangerous in itself unless it is very high. Fever can be lowered with the use of drugs.
Weight loss	Unexplained loss of greater than 10% of your body weight. "Unexplained" means that there is no change of behavior that would logically have caused the weight loss such as dieting, exercising a lot, or not eating because you are depressed or anxious or in love.
Headache	Headache is unusually severe ("worst headache ever"). Headache lasts much longer than past headaches.
Diarrhea	3 or more liquid bowel movements per day. Diarrhea is combined with increased frequency of defecation, stomach cramping, or loss of control of your bowels. Symptoms persist for more than a few days.
Change in stool	Blood or mucus is found in your stool.
Vaginal bleeding	If not during menstruation.
Nausea, vomiting, marked loss of appetite	Nausea or vomiting lasts for more than 1 day. Noticeable but unexplained loss of appetite.
Pain on swallowing	Pain lasts more than a few days. Pain may appear in middle of chest under breastbone (*mediastinal pain*).
Breathing (respiratory) symptoms	Shortness of breath goes on for more than a few days. Look out for unusual shortness of breath on exertion. If normally you can climb flights of stairs and you now notice that you must rest between flights, call your doctor.
Coughing	Dry, non-productive (no mucus) cough goes on for more than a few days.
Severe abdominal pain	Abdominal pain is accompanied by fever, particularly if you have a history of pelvic infection.
Persistent colds or sore throats	Cold or sore throat goes on for 3 weeks or more.
Night sweats	More than 1 episode of night sweats (pajamas and/or sheets drenched). A sweaty neck or scalp is not a night sweat.
Mental changes	Recent onset of confusion or loss of memory.
Rashes	Rash over entire body. Localized rash lasts more than 2 days.
Muscle weakness	Muscle weakness or loss of functioning on one side of your body.
Change in vision	Blurred vision, blind spots, or increased floaters.
Fatigue	Unusual and unexplained fatigue for more than 3 weeks.

(con't. on next page)

Symptom	Contact your doctor if . . .
Vaginal itching or discharge	Symptoms are persistent or unresponsive to self-treatment.
White patches or sores in your mouth	These symptoms are not a sign of any danger to your health but can often be treated easily. Why suffer needlessly?
Swollen lymph nodes	Nodes swell very rapidly, particularly if swelling occurs on only one side of the body.
Purplish or discolored area on the skin	Skin discolorations get darker rather than fading, get hard, or do not blanch when pressed.

COMMON EARLY SYMPTOMS

Some medical problems are quite common in HIV-infected people even before severe immune suppression or an episode of opportunistic disease occurs. Not all HIV-infected people have these symptoms; some remain entirely asymptomatic. Typical problems are swollen lymph nodes, postnasal drip and sinus problems, various skin problems such as warts or seborrhea, problems in the mouth such as thrush, hairy leukoplakia, and aphthous ulcers (canker sores) or, sometimes, constitutional symptoms (fevers, fatigue, night sweats, diarrhea).

The severity of these problems and their tendency to recur usually correlates with your level of T4 cells. The lower your T4 cells are, the more likely it is that the symptom will be more severe, require more extended treatment, possibly require maintenance treatment, and tend to reappear. The higher your T4 cells are, the more likely the problem is to respond to the routine treatment used in non-HIV-infected people. For example, both HIV-infected and non-HIV-infected people can develop herpes. It is only when HIV-infected people become seriously immune impaired that herpes is likely to be particularly extensive and difficult to treat.

If you are HIV infected and develop one of these symptoms, it is likely that you will become anxious about the state of your health. Be assured that most of these problems are treatable and do not mean that you are about to get a life-threatening complication. For example, people with asymptomatic HIV disease who develop swollen lymph nodes (swollen glands) do not progress any faster to AIDS than do people who are HIV infected and do not have swollen glands. Expert physicians believe that swollen lymph nodes should not generally be a cause for alarm unless swelling is rapid and particularly if it occurs on only one side.

IMMUNIZATIONS

In developed countries almost everyone receives vaccinations (injections designed to stimulate a protective immune response). Most vaccinations are given to infants or children. Some familiar childhood vaccines are those used to prevent polio, measles, mumps, rubella, whooping cough, and *Hemophilus influenza* type B (HIB). Other vaccines are usually given later in life to travelers who are going to countries in which a particular infectious disease is common. Examples of this are vaccines against cholera and yellow fever. Some injections that are given to children need to be repeated periodically for adults who are at risk. Examples of these are injections against typhoid, diphtheria, and tetanus.

There are several questions to be answered about immunization for people who are HIV infected. Which vaccines are safe for people who are immune suppressed? Which are unsafe? What vaccines should HIV-infected people get that non-infected people do not routinely get?

(A chart of recommended routine vaccines for HIV-infected adults appears on p. 95. A table of recommendations for travel vaccines appears on pp. 96–97. Recommendations for HIV-infected children are summarized on p. 171 in Chapter 8: Sex, Age, Race, and Ethnicity.)

HIV-infected people are at increased risk of several diseases for which vaccines are intended. **HIV-infected people should be vaccinated against pneumococcal (bacterial) pneumonia at least once and should receive yearly influenza vaccinations (in flu season in November).** Vaccination against bacterial pneumonia and influenza are usually given only to those with increased vulnerability, such as older people or those with chronic illness. These vaccinations are safe and recommended for all people with HIV infection.

There has been concern that since vaccines stimulate the immune system they might therefore provoke T4 cells to divide, making HIV infection worse. However, **no increase of viral activity has been correlated with vaccination of HIV-infected people** in studies of use of vaccines so far and in observation of HIV-infected children who have received the measles, mumps, and rubella vaccines. The side effects of vaccines are largely limited to a sore arm at the site of the injection and sometimes transient fevers.

Immune responses to antigens (substances that provoke immune responses in the body) are not as good in immunocompromised people as in others. However, in limited studies and in clinical practice, **HIV-infected patients generally do respond with protective antibodies to most vaccines.** The ability to respond depends on the degree of immunosuppression. Asymptomatic HIV-infected people are more likely to have a protective response to vaccines than are symptomatic people. It seems possible that vaccines offering long-term protection should be given early in the course of HIV disease. Higher doses and more frequent boosters may be needed.

Hepatitis B vaccination is somewhat less effective in HIV-infected people. However, it is recommended for all HIV-infected people. Antibody response to influenza vaccine in HIV-infected people may be low and is not improved by a booster.

Some vaccines are made from microorganisms that have been disrupted to the point that they cannot reproduce. Since they cannot reproduce, they cannot cause disease. Such vaccines are known as **inactivated vaccines** or **killed vaccines.** Killed-virus vaccines are safe for HIV-infected people.

An **attenuated live vaccine** is made from a microorganism that can reproduce but that has been weakened (or attenuated) so that it cannot cause disease. Attenuated live vaccines are used if inactivated versions cannot provoke a protective antibody response. There is a small risk that attenuated live vaccines may be harmful for immune-suppressed individuals. There have been reports of a few HIV-infected patients who got severe infections following immunization with the smallpox (vaccinia) vaccine. However, most HIV-infected people have not developed atypical adverse reactions to vaccination.

Antibodies (immunoglobulins) can be concentrated from donated blood and injected into those who need protection against certain infectious illnesses. This **passive immunization** provides quick but temporary protection. Once the injected antibodies are gone, there is no native immune response to make more (no activated T cells and no memory B cells for the appropriate antigens; see pp. 33–37 in Part 3: Understanding the Science). The immunoglobulins used may contain many different antibodies (as in the familiar *gamma globulin* shots) or they may contain specific antibodies for specific purposes. For instance, specific passive immunization is given to people who have been exposed to the hepatitis A virus in order to help prevent or limit the development of the disease itself.

Here are some general vaccination tips:

- Do not get vaccinated if you have a moderate to high fever; it is safe to be vaccinated if you have a cold or a low-grade fever.
- Keep track of your record of vaccinations; write down what vaccination you got and on what date. Try to get a record of vaccinations you received as a child. Your mother or other family member or your former pediatrician may have such records.
- Vaccine should be administered by the recommended route (oral, intramuscular, subcutaneous) to increase efficacy and reduce side effects.
- If you wait longer than recommended to complete a series of immunizations and your immune system remains intact, it does not reduce final protective results and you do not need to start

over or get extra doses. However, if you are HIV infected it is good to get protection as soon as possible. Your immune system may be declining so it is best to finish a series of vaccinations in the recommended time. You cannot get doses closer together than recommended or it will reduce antibody response.

• Do not get immunized during the first three months of pregnancy. Avoid conceiving until at least three months after immunization.

As was mentioned earlier, it is recommended that all HIV-infected people be vaccinated against hepatitis B virus, against bacterial pneumonia, and also be vaccinated each year in November against influenza.

The following chart summarizes information about immunizations given to HIV-infected adults.

ROUTINE IMMUNIZATIONS FOR ADULTS

Vaccine	Recommendation	Safety, Efficacy, Route
Measles, mumps, rubella (MMR)	Recommended for all HIV-infected people born after 1956 Vaccination is important: measles can cause severe illness in HIV-infected people	Probably safe: no adverse reactions reported Subcutaneous
Tetanus, diphtheria	Recommended for adults	Booster shot needed every 10 yrs.; pain, swelling may occur Intramuscular
Hepatitis B (Heptavax, Recombavax)	Recommended for adults	Safe 75% response rate in HIV-infected adults Intramuscular
Pneumococcal vaccine (Pneumovax)	Recommended for adults	Safe: pain or swelling at injection site 88% response rate in asymptomatic pts.
Influenza vaccine	Recommended for adults once every year in November	52%–89% response rate in asymptomatic pts. Intramuscular
Hemophilus influenza b polysaccharide vaccine (HbCV)	Recommended for adults	Possibly useful for those not vaccinated in childhood Intramuscular
Hepatitis A immune globulin	Recommended as post-exposure prophylaxis for asymptomatic and symptomatic HIV-infected	Safe Must be used within 2 wks. after exposure
Varicella zoster immune globulin (VZIG)	Recommended as post-exposure prophylaxis for chicken pox	Safe Must be used within 96 hrs. after exposure

Call the Centers for Disease Control (CDC) International Traveler's Hotline at 404-332-4555 for up-to-date health information for travelers, including current areas of infectious disease and current vaccination requirements. Some countries require submission of the International Certificates of Vaccination. Since areas of possible exposure to disease and legal requirements change, they are not listed in the chart below. Call the CDC or have your physician call when you are making travel plans. Almost all of the vaccines are necessary only when traveling to certain geographical areas including the so-called developing countries in Asia, the Middle East, Africa, and Latin America. The following chart summarizes information about travel vaccines.

TRAVEL VACCINES

Vaccine	Recommendation	Safety, Efficacy, Route
Measles, mumps, rubella (MMR)	For travel to developing countries unless already immune	Probably safe: no adverse reactions reported Subcutaneous
Hepatitis A immune globulin	For travel to developing countries unless already immune	Get 3 mos. before or 2 wks. after any live vaccines to avoid interference Effective for 3 to 5 mos. depending on dose
Typhoid (inactivated parenteral vaccine)	For travel to developing countries Do not use live oral typhoid vaccine	Possible redness or soreness at injection site, fever, headaches Two injections at least 4 wks. apart; booster every 3 yrs. if continued exposure
Inactivated polio vaccine (IPV)	Full series for immunization Single booster for travel to developing countries	Subcutaneous
Tetanus, diphtheria	Booster for travel to developing countries	Booster shot needed every 10 yrs. Intramuscular
Meningococcal vaccine	For travel to only certain countries	Booster at 3-yr. intervals Subcutaneous
Plague vaccine	For travel to only certain countries	Redness, soreness, fever Booster interval varies by antibody level Intramuscular
Rabies vaccine	For travel to only certain countries	Booster interval varies Confirm with tests for antibody response Intramuscular

Vaccine	Recommendation	Safety, Efficacy, Route
Japanese encephalitis vaccine	Required only for certain countries, primarily rural area of China, Korea, Indian subcontinent, Southeast Asia	Booster interval varies Confirm with tests for antibody repsonse
Yellow fever	*Not* recommended; preferably avoid travel to endemic areas: jungle areas of South America (especially Bolivia, Brazil, Columbia, Peru) and Africa especially West Africa)	Theoretical risk of encephalitis; no adverse effects reported in practice Confirm with tests for antibody response Subcutaneous
Cholera vaccine	Use only if travel to country at risk (Indian subcontinent; parts of Africa) Current (1991) epidemic in Peru, Ecuador, Columbia	Redness and soreness at injection site, fever 50% efficacy, lasts for only 3-6 mos. Booster at 6-mo. intervals Subcutaneous or intradermal
Bacille Calmette-Guerin (BCG)	AVOID Exception: recommended for asymptomatic HIV-infected children in areas of high risk of tuberculosis	Severe complications seen in immune-suppressed adults
Live oral typhoid vaccine (Ty21a)	AVOID Use inactivated parenteral typhoid vaccine instead	
Smallpox vaccine	AVOID Vaccination is unneccessary, as smallpox has been eradicated worldwide	
Oral polio vaccine (OPV)	AVOID Use inactivated polio vaccine (IPV) instead	

HEPATITIS B VACCINATION

Hepatitis B is a viral disease that can cause serious and even fatal damage to the liver. Vaccination is now available that can prevent infection with hepatitis B. People who are HIV-infected should be screened to see if they are hepatitis B-infected: if infected, they should be monitored (and possibly treated) for chronic infection; if uninfected, they should be vaccinated against future infection. See Chapter 11: Infections for a detailed discussion of hepatitis B.

Hepatitis B screening and vaccination are recommended for:

• Men who have sex with other men
• Health care workers

- Those who share needles for drug use
- People from China, Southeast Asia, tropical Africa, most Pacific islands, parts of the Middle East, and the Amazon basin. Hepatitis B is endemic in these areas, where it is often transmitted at birth.

The vaccine is administered in a series of three injections in the arm. You will get an initial vaccination, one a month later, and one six months later. The timing does not have to be exact. There are few side effects—you may have a sore arm for a day. This vaccine provides an effective level of immunity in 90 percent of cases.

Before you are vaccinated, your blood must be tested to see if you have ever had hepatitis B in the past (remember—you may have had hepatitis B without noticing it). If you have ever had hepatitis B, you have developed natural immunity, cannot be reinfected, and will not need the vaccine. The blood test determines if you've ever been infected by looking for evidence of your immune system's response to the hepatitis B virus (specifically, for antibodies to hepatitis B).

These blood tests also tell you if you are a chronic carrier or have chronic hepatitis. The presence of viral fragments (hepatitis B *antigen*) for more than six months indicates that you are a chronic carrier and are capable of transmitting the virus to others. Further testing can be done to determine your level of infectivity (how likely you are to infect others).

If you are infected with HIV, it is important to get vaccinated against hepatitis B, because acute hepatitis B often produces severe symptoms in those who are HIV-infected. Also, developing chronic hepatitis B is a higher risk if you are HIV infected. HIV-infected persons who develop hepatitis B are at a 19 percent to 37 percent risk of becoming chronic hepatitis B carriers. The vaccine is somewhat less likely to "take"—that is, to provide an effective level of immunity—in those who are HIV infected, but it is effective in the majority of cases. One study indicated that at least 75 percent of asymptomatic patients developed a protective response against hepatitis B.

Hepatitis B vaccine does not transmit HIV, so there is no reason for people to avoid hepatitis B vaccine out of fear of HIV infection or reinfection. There are two kinds of hepatitis B vaccine:

- *Heptavax* is made from human blood and is heat-treated to kill HIV
- *Recombivax* is synthesized using recombinant DNA technology. Since it is not made from human blood there is no danger of contamination with HIV.

OBSTETRIC AND GYNECOLOGICAL ISSUES

For a longer discussion of the health concerns of HIV-infected women, refer to pp. 159–65 in Chapter 8: Sex, Age, Race, and Ethnicity. Following is a summary of the obstetric and gynecological recommendations found there:

Women who are HIV-infected may be more prone to cervical disorders than uninfected women. Expert clinicians have recently recommended that an initial exam include *colposcopy* (magnified visual inspection of the cervix) and cervical cytology (Pap smear), followed by a Pap smear every six months.

Although it was initially thought that pregnancy might increase an HIV-infected woman's risk of developing symptoms, recent studies contradict this. The pregnancy of an infected woman has a 25 percent to 30 percent chance of resulting in a child born with HIV infection. If you are pregnant and HIV-infected, you may want to seek counseling about whether to continue your pregnancy. If you carry the fetus to term, get obstetrical care from a physician knowledgeable about HIV infection. Newborns may sometimes be infected through drinking breast milk: in areas where it is possible to obtain and prepare hygienic breast-milk substitutes, do not breastfeed. Since newborns carry their mother's antibodies, all infants born to HIV-infected mothers will initially test positive for HIV antibodies: however, only some are actually infected. Pregnancy may necessitate the modification of standard treatment regimes because some drugs used in treating HIV-related illnesses may cross the placental barrier and adversely affect the fetus. Studies are under way.

DENTAL CARE

See the discussion of mouth problems in Chapter 10: Organ System Complications, for a description of typical dental problems in those who have HIV disease.

Because people with HIV disease have an increased incidence of problems with gums, it is important to take particularly good care of your teeth and gums. This means following routine dental hygiene (tooth brushing and flossing) and seeing your dentist regularly, at least once a year.

Unfortunately, this is not as easy as it sounds. Many people are limited in their ability to get adequate care because dental care is very expensive and is not covered under many insurance policies. If dental insurance is available to you through your job and you can afford it, it usually turns out to be a good bargain. If you do not have insurance and cannot pay for dental care out-of-pocket, check on what clinic resources are available to you at a medical center near you that has a dental school affiliated with it.

Registering at a dental clinic can involve time and red tape. It is better not to wait until an emergency to become a registered patient at a dental clinic.

If you are in bad pain from a dental problem, cannot afford a private dentist, and are not a clinic patient, you can always go to an emergency room for dental care, although this is likely to be time-consuming and not very pleasant. Call the hospital before you go and make sure that it has a dental department.

An additional problem with dental care is that many people have faced discrimination. Some dentists overtly refuse to treat HIV-infected patients. If this happens to you, consider calling your local AIDS organization for information about legal recourse. Dentists or technicians may also subtly discriminate, for instance in attitude. It is important to counter discrimination but it is also important to get your health care (including dental care) in as comfortable a setting as possible. Few people feel comfortable confronting their dentists about a troubling attitude. The realistic option may be to switch to a dentist who is better informed about HIV disease.

Many people worry about whether to tell their dentists that they are HIV infected. There is no need for you to do so in order to protect your dentist. Your dentist should be following routine infection-control measures such as wearing gloves and mask and sterilizing instruments. This protects both dentist and patient. If your dentist is not following these procedures you should find a new dentist.

On the other hand, there are some reasons to tell your dentist about your HIV infection. Many people feel uncomfortable keeping a part of their medical condition hidden from a provider. If you have not told your dentist, you have no way of predicting her or his reaction if you develop symptoms. Also, HIV-related problems are often manifested first in the mouth. A dentist who is aware of your HIV infection and knowledgeable about oral symptoms in HIV disease can be helpful to you.

In some big cities there are dental practices that welcome HIV-infected people and specialize in their care. Call your local AIDS organization or ask friends to get information about such dental practices.

NUTRITION AND FOOD SAFETY

Issues regarding nutrition vary widely in HIV-infected people depending on their state of health. The same "well balanced" diet is recommended to asymptomatic HIV-infected people as to anyone else. People with more advanced HIV disease may need a special diet, often to control weight loss (and the various factors that lead to it).

Good nutrition should maintain *lean body mass* (muscle as opposed to fat) and should provide adequate vitamins and minerals. Malnutrition complicates the course of HIV disease. Therefore, early intervention to prevent malnutrition is important.

Some drugs used in the treatment of HIV disease may interact with certain nutrients. Whenever you start a new medication, ask your physician about any diet modifications that might be useful.

Learn about nutrition. There are a number of books that you can consult; one standard available in many bookstores is *Jane Brody's Nutrition Book* (Bantam Books, 414 E. Golf Road, DesPlaines, IL 60016; phone 212-765-6500).

In addition, there are a number of pamphlets available to the public that provide up-to-date information specially tailored to people with HIV disease. You can get these pamphlets by calling the National AIDS Information Clearinghouse (phone 800-458-5231). The Cutting Edge, P.O. Box 392, Fremont, California, 94537 (phone 415-797-9768), can provide referrals to HIV-knowledgeable nutritionists and a database of available articles and pamphlets on nutrition and food safety in HIV disease.

A balanced diet consists of varied foods with adequate calories, protein, vitamins, minerals, and fluids. It is possible to get good nutrition from either a vegetarian diet or one that contains meat. If you are HIV infected, it is a good idea to learn the basics of good nutrition and try to modify your diet to conform.

Some people who have HIV disease believe that a special diet or dietary supplements may help maintain health. Use your judgment carefully when changing your diet. Any diet that limits the variety of foods eaten may make it harder to get complete nutrition. In addition, limited diets may contain some substances in harmful amounts.

Some of the special diets that have been tried seem to be harmful rather than helpful. A macrobiotic diet must be monitored very carefully to assure sufficient calories and protein. A very-high-fiber diet may lead to diarrhea. A yeast-free diet has shown no evidence of effectiveness and is very restrictive.

If you feel that a special diet may help you, you must approach this with the same rigor as any other experimental program. That is, you have to be sure you understand the pros and cons of the diet you are trying.

Unfortunately, most physicians are not knowledgeable about nutrition. Consulting with a registered nutritionist may be a better idea. However, many nutritionists do not know much about HIV disease. The ideal consultant is a nutritionist who has specialized in counseling patients with HIV disease. You can ask your doctor or nearby AIDS organization for referrals. If you are hospitalized, you may be able to get a nutritional consultation at no extra fee.

Taking a daily vitamin pill is a good idea to make sure you are getting 100 percent of the Recommended Dietary Allowances (RDA) of **vitamins**

and minerals as set by the Food and Nutrition Board of the National Academy of Sciences. It is safe to take up to two or three times more than the RDA of vitamins and minerals. Amounts higher than these may cause problems, particularly with vitamins A, D, E, and K. There is no information for or against taking moderate extra amounts of vitamin B_{12}; however very large doses of fat-soluble vitamins (such as the B vitamins) may cause inflammation of the liver. There is no evidence that use of very large amounts of vitamin or mineral supplements ("megadoses") is helpful in HIV disease. It is safe to take up to 200 grams per day of vitamin C (ascorbic acid). Higher doses of vitamin C may lead to gastrointestinal symptoms such as diarrhea.

Trace minerals in high dosage can also be toxic. For example, zinc used ten times more than the RDA can lead to diarrhea, vomiting, reduced serum copper levels, and anemia. High levels of selenium can also cause cardiac problems.

Food safety is an important issue. HIV-infected people are particularly susceptible to infections from microorganisms in food. Infectious organisms include salmonella, campylobacter, shigella, *Clostridium perfringens, Staphylococcus aureus,* and *Clostridium botulinum* (which causes botulism), as well as others. These infections occur more frequently and tend to be more severe and more long-lasting in people who are HIV-infected. For this reason, food safety precautions that help prevent infection are important for those with HIV disease.

Following are some essential food safety precautions:

- Do not eat raw meat, chicken, shellfish, or eggs. Examples are steak tartare, uncooked oysters or clams, and homemade mayonnaise or other dishes made with uncooked eggs. These foods are more likely to contain infectious organisms. There has been debate about the safety of raw fish such as sushi. Avoid undercooked meat, chicken, poultry, fish and shellfish, and eggs. The temperature of any meat, poultry, or fish should reach 165 to 212 degrees F.
- Be careful in food preparation not to contaminate cooked foods with raw meat, fish, or poultry. For example, do not cut cooked meat on a cutting board that you have used for raw meat. (Plastic cutting boards are easier to clean. After using a cutting board for preparing raw meat, clean it with diluted bleach.) If you are using a marinade in which meat has been placed raw, you can use the marinade as part of the finished product, but only if the marinade is also cooked.
- Thaw frozen meat in the refrigerator. Do not stuff chicken in advance.
- Fruits and vegetables are much less of a problem than meat, poultry, or fish. However, fruits and vegetables can contain

bacteria. Wash all fruits and vegetables thoroughly. Buy fruits and vegetables with unbroken skins.

- Wash hands frequently when cooking and always after handling raw meat, chicken, or fish. Keep all utensils in contact with food clean.
- Keep hot foods hot (above 140 degrees F). Keep cold foods cold (below 40 degrees F). Reheat leftovers.
- Use packaged luncheon meats within three to five days after opening.
- All milk and milk products should be pasteurized. Make sure frozen foods you buy are frozen solid. Make sure refrigerated foods are cold.
- Do not keep leftovers too long. If you are in doubt, discard it.
- Be careful with food that may have been outside for a long time or carelessly prepared. This includes foods brought on picnics or purchased from street vendors.

SAFER SEX AND CONDOM USE GUIDELINES

Gay men have made significant strides toward safer sexual behavior. Other sexually active people also need to learn about and adopt risk-reduction behavior.

It is never too late to begin protecting yourself against HIV. Even if you have already been infected, it is always to your benefit to follow sexual risk-reduction guidelines since repeat exposure to HIV (possibly to a more virulent strain of the virus) or exposure to other sexually transmitted infections may help to trigger illness. Follow the risk-reduction guidelines below in any future sexual encounter.

Safer sex in one sentence: use a condom for every episode of intercourse, from start to finish, whether vaginal or rectal.

More detailed risk-reduction guidelines divide common sexual behaviors into three categories of risk for transmitting HIV: high risk, lower risk, and no risk. Behaviors in the high-risk category generally involve contact of blood or semen with a mucous membrane. Mucous membranes include the linings of the rectum, vagina, mouth, and urethra (the tube through which urine is passed). Contact of blood or semen with a mucous membrane has a *high risk* of transmitting HIV if one partner is infected—avoid sexual activities involving such contact.

If there is no contact between one partner's bodily fluids and the other partner's mucous membranes, there is *no risk* of infection—transmission of HIV cannot occur. No-risk sexual activities are therefore completely safe even if one or both partners are infected.

The situation is less clear-cut in the case of the lower-risk category. Behaviors in this category involve some risk of mucous membrane contact with bodily fluids other than blood and semen. These fluids occasionally contain HIV, but at a low concentration that makes infection much less likely. Saliva is almost certainly safe, and it is unlikely that the virus enters the body through the mucous membranes of the mouth. It is impossible to prove that lower-risk behaviors will never transmit the virus, but these behaviors are much less dangerous than those in the high-risk category. In cases where one or both sexual partners may be carrying the virus, the partners should carefully discuss exactly which lower-risk activities are acceptable to both of them.

In the following pages, common sexual activities are described with a brief explanation of why they are considered high risk, lower risk, or no risk.

▲ High-Risk Activities

High-risk activities have a high probability of transmitting HIV infection. If you are infected, avoid high-risk sexual activities.

Vaginal or rectal intercourse without a condom: If ejaculation (coming) occurs while the penis is inside the vagina or rectum, the mucous lining of the vagina or rectum is exposed to semen, which may contain a high level of HIV. Use adequate lubricant to reduce abrasion or other damage to the vagina or rectum; infection can happen even if no abrasion occurs. Using a condom to contain the semen lowers the risk of infection considerably, but condoms may break or leak. If ejaculation occurs and semen escapes, there is a risk of infection. For this reason, intercourse with a condom is safer if the penis is withdrawn before ejaculation.

Being the receptive partner during unprotected rectal or vaginal intercourse has been highly associated with contracting HIV infection. Being the insertive partner during unprotected vaginal or rectal intercourse can also lead to HIV infection, probably via exposure to secretions or menstrual blood in the vagina, or to blood in the rectum. During intercourse, the insertive partner's urethral lining may be exposed to infected fluid that enters through the opening in the tip of the penis.

If you are HIV infected you can infect your sexual partner during unprotected intercourse, vaginal or rectal, whether you are the insertive or receptive partner. Use condoms and, for men, withdrawal before ejaculation.

Fellatio is stimulation of the penis with the mouth. There are a few documented cases of infection where HIV was transmitted by a man ejaculating (coming) into his partner's mouth, but this has been quite rare. **Fellatio is high risk if the lining of the partner's mouth is exposed to semen.** However, saliva contains components that inactivate HIV. The risk is considerably lowered if the man wears a condom or if the penis is withdrawn before ejaculation. See the section on fellatio that follows under "Lower-Risk Activities."

Cunnilingus is stimulation of a woman's genitals with the lips and tongue. **Cunnilingus during menstruation** is high risk for the partner performing cunnilingus because there may be a high concentration of virus in menstrual blood. See the section on cunnilingus that follows under "Lower-Risk Activities."

Oral-anal contact (rimming) is stimulation of the anus with the lips and tongue. It is high-risk because blood that may be present in the rectum may contact the lining of the mouth. The risk is for the partner performing the oral-anal contact. This may not be a likely route of transmission of HIV but is very likely to transmit intestinal parasites which can produce serious medical problems and exacerbate an existing HIV infection.

▲ Lower-Risk Activities

These activities have only a small chance of transmitting HIV infection. Discuss lower-risk sexual activities with your sexual partners.

Condoms are an effective barrier to virus transmission. Using a condom during vaginal or rectal intercourse lowers the risk of infection considerably. However, condoms may break or leak. If ejaculation occurs and semen escapes, there is a risk of infection. Be sure to use condoms correctly (see the section on condom information, pp. 106–07). **Intercourse with a condom is much safer if the penis is withdrawn before ejaculation.**

Fellatio without ejaculation into partner's mouth: Even if the risk of infection through oral-genital sex is low, semen may contain a relatively high concentration of virus, so it is wisest to avoid contact of semen with the lining of the mouth. Two studies have attempted to assess the relative danger of oral sex for HIV transmission. The subjects in these (small) studies did not become infected or ill from performing receptive fellatio (sucking, or giving a blow job).

If fellatio is not continued to ejaculation, the mucous membranes of the mouth are not exposed to semen. This lowers the risk of fellatio considerably. However, it is not known whether pre-ejaculatory fluid ("pre-cum") contains virus. (Pre-ejaculatory fluid is a viscous, clear fluid that is secreted from the penis some time prior to the ejaculation of semen itself.) The risk is further reduced if the head of the penis is never placed in the mouth or if a condom is worn. Kissing or licking the shaft of the penis is perfectly safe.

During **cunnilingus performed when menstruation is not occurring,** the mucous membranes of the mouth are not exposed to blood. This lowers the risk of infection during cunnilingus considerably. However, vaginal and cervical secretions sometimes contain a low concentration of virus. The small risk associated with cunnilingus is lowered still further if an effective barrier such as a square of latex or plastic wrap (called an "oral dam") is used to separate the genitals from the partner's lips and tongue.

Oral dams (also known as "dental dams" from their use in dental surgery) are hard to find; they are sold in dental supply stores. You can more easily make one at home by cutting off the tip of a condom and then cutting the condom lengthwise. It will unroll into a square of latex. Use unlubricated condoms for this purpose.

The risk associated with oral-anal contact (rimming) is made much lower if an effective barrier is used to keep the lips and tongue from contacting the partner's anus.

Deep kissing (French kissing, tongue kissing): Studies have indicated that the virus is sometimes present in saliva but only at very low levels. There is no evidence that exchange of saliva transmits the virus, even in prolonged deep kissing. No cases of AIDS transmitted by kissing alone have been reported.

▲ No-Risk Activities

Mutual masturbation, rubbing bodies, and kissing skin are examples of sexual activities that carry absolutely no risk of transmission of HIV. If no bodily fluids contact any mucous membranes, infection with HIV is impossible.

▲ Condom Information

Condoms can prevent the transmission of HIV and also provide protection against diseases such as gonorrhea, chlamydial infections, syphilis, and herpes. Other methods of birth control, such as using a diaphragm with spermicide, do not provide adequate protection against the transmission of HIV infection and other sexually transmitted diseases. Condoms can be bought at drugstores (no prescription is needed), or ordered through the mail. Condoms may also be bought from vending machines in public toilets and other places.

Be sure to use condoms correctly:

- Condoms are either latex or animal-membrane sheaths that fit over the erect penis and act as a barrier to prevent semen or pre-cum from escaping while the penis is inside the vagina or rectum. Latex condoms are preferable. Do not use condoms that are ribbed or textured to increase stimulation since these condoms may cause damage to genital tissues that, while unnoticeable, may make infection more likely.
- Store condoms in a cool, dry place, out of direct sunlight. Condoms kept in wallets may become damaged after a period of time. Condoms are considered good for two years after their date of manufacture, which is sometimes printed on the package.
- The condom should be put on the penis after it is erect, not before. Put on the condom before the penis comes in contact with the genitals or the anus. If the penis is uncircumcised, retract the foreskin before putting on the condom.

- Condoms come packaged either rolled up or loose. If the condom is rolled up, determine which side is the inside of the condom, place that side against the tip of the penis, and roll the rest of the condom down to the base. The condom should fit snugly so that it does not slip off during intercourse. If the condom is packaged unrolled, draw it over the penis like a glove.
- When putting on a condom, pinch about one-half inch of the condom's tip to leave a small air-free space—this will help keep semen from bursting the condom upon ejaculation.
- If intercourse is continued to ejaculation, the penis should be withdrawn promptly afterward. Since condoms may break or leak, ejaculation inside the body presents a risk of infection.
- In any case, the condom-covered penis should be withdrawn from the vagina or rectum before the penis becomes soft. During withdrawal, hold the rim of the condom firmly against the base of the penis so that the condom cannot slip off and no semen can escape.
- Do not reuse condoms.

Lubrication is important to avoid tearing the condom or abrading body tissue. **Always use a water-based lubricant** such as *K-Y™ Jelly* or *Surgilube™*. **Never use oil-based lubricants such as hand-lotion,** *Vaseline™, Crisco™,* baby oil, vegetable oil, mineral oil, suntan lotion, *Albolene™, Elbow Grease™, Lube™,* or *Shaft™,* since these may damage the latex of the condom. Put a drop of lubricant inside the tip of the condom before it is put on the penis. Too much lubricant inside the condom may lead it to slip off during intercourse. Use a generous amount of lubricant on the outside of the condom.

A spermicide called Nonoxynol-9 is found in some contraceptive jellies and creams as well as in some lubricants. **Preparations that contain at least 5 percent Nonoxynol-9 provide extra protection** when used with condoms since this concentration has been shown to kill both free HIV and virus living within white blood cells. A water- and glycerin-based lubricant called *ForPlay™* will not weaken or damage the latex of condoms and contains 5% Nonoxynol-9. Some brands of condoms now come coated inside and out with a 5 percent Nonoxynol-9 lubricant. One such brand is *LifeStyles Extra-Strength™ Condoms with Nonoxynol-9.* A number of contraceptive creams, jellies, and foams contain Nonoxynol-9, but not all contain enough. Also, most products intended as spermicides dry out quickly and so do not make good lubricants.

▲ Additional Guidelines

Sex toys (dildoes, vibrators, etc.) should not be shared. Clean sex toys thoroughly with soap and water. Wash the genitals with soap and water after sex. Douching or enemas immediately before or after sex do not help protect you against infection and may even increase the risk of infection by damaging natural protective barriers of the vagina or rectum. Do not put chemicals not intended for internal use into your vagina or rectum.

Urine may contain the virus. Do not allow urine to enter the mouth or come in contact with open cuts on the body.

If you have sores or abrasions on your genitals, anus, or mouth, avoid activity that brings these into contact with your sexual partners. Also, if you have another sexually transmitted disease, have only no-risk sex until you are healthy. The presence of any one of a variety of sexually transmitted diseases may increase the risk of transmission of HIV infection.

If a partner's semen accidentally gets inside your vagina or rectum, you may use spermicide (possibly containing Nonoxynol-9) to reduce the risk of infection. If semen gets in your mouth, spit it out and gargle with fresh mouthwash, toothpaste (or even soap and water, if nothing else is available).

▲ Adapting to Risk Reduction

If you are HIV-infected, the primary way to protect sexual partners from infection is to use condoms and withdrawal carefully every time you have intercourse. Limiting the number of your sexual partners is not precaution against infecting others with HIV or becoming reinfected yourself. Only safe sex prevents transmission.

Even if you have only one sexual partner, you can infect that person if you have unprotected intercourse. Repeated unprotected intercourse with one infected partner exposes you to a high risk of being reinfected yourself or developing other sexually transmitted diseases.

The issue of **talking about safer sex with a partner** is a difficult one for people who are HIV infected. (See Chapter 7: Your State of Mind for further discussion of this). When will you tell your prospective partner that you are HIV-infected? For most individuals, this raises both an ethical and an emotional problem.

Some people feel that it is their partner's right to know about their HIV status prior to any sexual activity, no matter how safe. Others feel that if they are practicing safer sex, they have no particular need to disclose their HIV status. Still others feel that the need to disclose depends on the degree of risk in the activity they are practicing. It is important for you to think out in advance what you believe is right and wrong. Impulsivity followed by guilt is an uncomfortable choice.

You need to think also about how your disclosure will affect your relationship with the prospective sexual partner. It is true that you may be rejected by a partner if you disclose that you are HIV-positive, either because of fear of infection or fear of a relationship with an HIV-infected person. On the other hand, your partner may feel angry or misled if you do not disclose your status prior to the first contact. In addition, you are likely to become anxious about this issue if the relationship progresses and you have not told your partner of your status.

Strike a balance in your sexual behavior. Some HIV-infected people are so afraid of infecting others or of others' reaction to hearing they are HIV-infected that they give up sex, or alternate abstinence with occasional impulsive episodes of high-risk sex. An extreme of behavior (anxious and fragile abstinence) may lead to a very high risk of infection. You need not give up your sex life, nor should you expose partners or yourself to high-risk sexual activity. Many people have been practicing risk reduction for several years now. They report that although it was sometimes difficult at the beginning, they are now able to enjoy sex that is both safe and satisfying.

Plan for risk reduction. Learn how to come to an agreement with your partner about the sexual activity you will have together. Think through the issues in advance. This will help you avoid impulsive decisions and give a clear and consistent message to your partner. Have condoms available if you plan to have intercourse. Women hesitant to purchase and carry condoms should be aware that women now buy half of all condoms sold. The use of alcohol or other recreational drugs often impairs judgment; do not make decisions about sexual activity while you are intoxicated.

Try to talk about risk reduction with your partners before sexual excitement interferes. Many have found that prospective partners interpret raising the subject of risk reduction well before sex as a sign of intelligence and prudence. Others prefer to wait until they are actually involved in explicit sexual activity; follow this course of action only if you can stick to your decisions about risk reduction and if you know that your partner will respect your wishes.

Ask yourself the following questions:

• Have I been practicing risk reduction *consistently?*
• If not, what issues or circumstances interfere?
• How can I resolve these issues or avoid these circumstances?

If you are having difficulty avoiding high-risk sex, get help and support from an AIDS organization in your community. Many such organizations run "safe-sex workshops" designed to help with this problem.

Men who have sex with both women and men face difficult issues regarding risk reduction. Ideally, discuss your sexual history with all your partners, both male and female, so that they may make informed decisions about risk reduction. Practice risk reduction with both women and men to avoid infecting yourself or others.

Frank discussion of risk reduction may be difficult for men who have not told their female partners about their sexual relations with other men. If your sexual contact with men has never involved the exchange of bodily fluids, you pose no special risk to your female partners. However, if you are infected you must practice risk reduction with your female as well as your male partners: at a minimum, use condoms. If you feel you cannot tell your female partners, seek counseling from an AIDS organization in your community.

NEEDLE-SHARING AND NEEDLE-CLEANING

An estimated 1.2 million Americans use IV drugs regularly. The proportion of IV drug users in treatment programs who have been found to be HIV infected varies from 0 percent in Cheyenne, Wyoming, to 61 percent in New York City. Existing treatment programs can accommodate only one in every twelve IV drug users. In New York City, the average waiting period to get into a methadone maintenance program is one to three months. The waiting period to get into a drug-free program where addicts are kept "clean" of all drugs is up to six months.

Studies show that education about AIDS and clean needles leads IV drug users not only to adopt HIV-safer injection techniques but to come into treatment for their drug problem. A leading medical and public health authority on IV drug abuse offers the following recommendations:

- Large-scale expansion of drug-abuse treatment programs
- Face-to-face health promotion activities conducted by former IV drug users
- More teaching of needle-cleaning methods and/or distribution of sterile needles
- Support of self-help groups of IV drug users who work to legitimize safe sex and the refusal to share needles

The National Academy of Sciences has also recommended experimenting with legalization of sale and possession of sterile disposable needles and syringes as a public health measure to reduce HIV transmission through needle sharing.

If you are already infected, drugs themselves increase the chance that your infection will make you ill. Just shooting up—even if you aren't sharing needles—can damage your immune system and encourage the virus to multiply. HIV-infected intravenous (IV) drug users who continue to shoot drugs have a worse course of illness than do those who stop using needles. If you are now using IV drugs, make use of every resource available to help you quit.

If you continue to use IV drugs, it is crucial that you **do not share IV drug equipment** ("works," "gimmicks," "sets"), including syringes, rubber bulbs, needles ("points"), "cookers," or cotton. If you buy new works, clean them *before* using them. **If you must share works, clean them before you or the next person uses them.** Blood may be in your works even if you can't see it. Clean your works either with rubbing alcohol

110

(available in drugstores), a household bleach solution (3 tablespoons of bleach in a cup of water), or boiling water. To clean your works:

- Pour the alcohol, bleach solution, or boiling water into a clean glass.
- Pull liquid up into the syringe, shake well, then squirt the liquid out again. Repeat this several times.
- Take your works apart, separating the plunger and needle from the syringe.
- Let them soak in the alcohol, bleach solution, or boiling water for ten to fifteen minutes.
- Rinse the parts of your works well under running tap water.
- Put your works back together. Pull clean water up into the syringe, then squirt it out again. Repeat a few times.

If you can't wait, use the bleach solution, skip the soaking step, and be sure to rinse thoroughly with water.

Remember: You face a high risk for HIV infection if you have shared needles, whether to inject or "skin-pop" heroin, cocaine, speed, or any other drug. And, no matter how you got infected, you can still pass it on through sex.

TRAVEL

Generally speaking, there are few purely medical reasons that restrict the travel of HIV-infected people both within the United States and internationally. However, travel may take extra planning, depending on the state of your health, the location to which you are traveling, and the length of time you will be away.

Most people who are HIV-infected are asymptomatic. They have normal energy and stamina and have to make only minor provisions for their special health needs when traveling. Developed countries pose no greater risk of infectious disease than is found in the United States. Special planning needs to be done in advance for travel to developing countries where certain infectious diseases may be more common. Obviously, a very long trip requires making arrangements for routine health care and medication.

Certain countries have regulations that allow them to restrict the entry of HIV-infected travelers. Ironically, the United States—with more AIDS cases reported than any other country—is the only major developed country to have such laws on the books. Check on the rules that apply to the country to which you are traveling. You can do so by calling the Washington, D.C., embassy or local consulate of the country to which you intend to travel.

If you are asymptomatic (or have only minor symptoms) and your trip is of less than three months' duration, you are very unlikely to need medical care while away from home. In most developed countries, you can obtain adequate emergency care. Most geographical locations are easy to return from if you develop more serious medical problems.

Plan for emergency and routine health care. You are unlikely to need these arrangements, but it can be reassuring to know they are in place. Work out in advance a plan for return home if it should be necessary. For continuity of care and for psychological and financial reasons you may prefer to return home to get any major medical care (including hospitalization) even if such care is available in another location. Make sure that you bring enough money to purchase a flight or other rapid transportation home if this should be needed.

If you will be away from home for more than three months or if you currently have major medical problems, ask your doctor for the name of an HIV-expert physician in the area to which you are traveling. If your doctor cannot help you with this, call a local AIDS organization in the area to which you are going. If this is not possible, find out what the nearest major medical center is. If you think you might require major medical care, it is obviously best to travel only to areas where such care for HIV-infected people is available.

HIV-infected people face special risks of infectious disease when traveling to some countries. The presence or increased incidence of infectious disease in these countries may be due to tropical climate or to inadequate health care and poor sanitation secondary to poverty. Generally the risk is greater in Latin America, Africa, parts of the Middle East, the Indian subcontinent, parts of Asia, and Southeast Asia. However, travel to western Europe, Australia, Japan, and Canada present no additional risk to United States travelers. Epidemics of infectious diseases come and go in different areas. In order to find out about risk of infectious disease in a particular geographical area you need up-to-date information. Your best bet: check with the CDC International Travelers Hotline at 404-332-4555.

The most common diseases in travelers are caused by microorganisms in food and water contaminated with infected feces. Diseases caused by microorganisms that enter via the gastrointestinal tract are known as *enteric* infections. It is estimated that at least forty percent of travelers to developing countries suffer from enteric infections. In many of these developing countries the indigenous population suffers chronically from these infections and lacks adequate resources for prevention and treatment such as an uncontaminated water supply, sanitation facilities, refrigeration, medications, etc.

The most common symptom of these diseases is diarrhea, often referred to as "traveler's diarrhea." The symptoms of traveler's diarrhea are increased volume of unformed bowel movements, urgency, cramps, fever, malaise, and nausea. Traveler's diarrhea often has an abrupt onset and usually lasts for three to seven days, although it can be longer.

People with HIV disease are particularly vulnerable to many enteric infections and have an increased risk of developing severe forms of the illness. The most common enteric infections are *E. coli* diarrhea, salmonellosis, campylobacteriosis, cryptosporidiosis, hepatitis A, and shigellosis. People with HIV disease have increased risk of developing serious symptoms with all these diseases, particularly campylobacteriosis, shigellosis, and salmonellosis. There are a number of other diseases caused by contaminated food and water including poliomyelitis, cholera, and typhoid fever.

There are several strategies to control enteric infections. They include sanitary measures to avoid exposure to the infectious organisms, immunization, and prevention of illness through the use of antibiotics, antimicrobials, or immune globulins. Medications exist to prevent the development of some infections, but not others.

Prevention is the best way to deal with the possibility of developing an infection while traveling. **Caution about food and water is the main method of prevention.** In poor, developing countries where sanitation and refrigeration are likely to be inadequate, follow the suggestions below:

- Do not drink tap water or use ice. Drink bottled water and use it for brushing your teeth. Soda, beer, wine, and hot tea or coffee made from boiled water are safe to drink. It is better to drink from a can or bottle than from a container that might have been washed with contaminated water. Wipe the outside of the bottle or can.
- If bottled water is not available, you can treat water. The best method is to boil it vigorously, then allow to cool. Do not use ice to cool boiled water. Chemical disinfection is also possible with either iodine or chlorine, preferably iodine. Tincture of iodine or iodine tablets are available from sporting-goods stores and pharmacies. If the water remains cloudy after treatment, strain it through a clean cloth and use double the number of disinfectant tablets. Mechanical filters have not proven to be reliable.
- If you eat raw fruit or vegetables, eat only those that you have peeled yourself. Eat only thoroughly cooked eggs, meat, and fish. Do not eat unpasteurized milk or dairy products. Do not eat prepared food from street vendors. Restaurant food that is cooked and still hot is generally safe.

If you are HIV-infected and traveling to a developing country where enteric infection is likely, discuss medication with your doctor. **The risk of enteric infections may be reduced by taking preventive medications** such as norfloxacin, ciprofloxacin, Bactrim. The advantage of prophylaxis with these drugs is that they can prevent from 65 percent to 90 percent of traveler's diarrhea. The disadvantage is that some bacteria may be resistant to some drugs, and many drugs do not work against campylobacter and protozoa (parasites). In addition, it is possible that in some instances these drugs might actually worsen infection by disrupting normal intestinal bacteria. HIV-infected people are at increased risk for adverse side effects from these drugs.

If you are traveling to a developing country and you decide not to begin a course of preventive medication, you should nonetheless get and fill a prescription to take with you in case you develop traveler's diarrhea. You should get careful directions from your doctor on what to do if you develop diarrhea. An expert on travel disease recommends ciprofloxacin or norfloxacin rather than Bactrim because of the high rate of allergic reaction in people taking Bactrim and the increasingly high rate of organism resistance. If you are already taking Bactrim for PCP prophylaxis, you should use a different drug for dealing with enteric diseases. These drugs are taken for three to five days.

If you develop **traveler's diarrhea,** it is important to avoid further infection. Be even more careful about food and water precautions. It is also important to avoid dehydration by drinking plenty of fluids. Fruit juices and caffeine-free soda are ideal. Eat salted crackers to help you retain fluids.

You should seek medical help if you have a fever over 102 degrees F, bloody diarrhea, dehydration, shaking, or any symptoms of long duration.

Various drugs such as Bactrim and doxycycline can be used to treat traveler's diarrhea and shorten the time symptoms are present. Lomotil or Imodium can be used to control symptoms—but do not use them if you have a high fever or blood in your stools.

Hepatitis A is another disease which is transmitted by the fecal-oral route and is common in certain developing countries. HIV-infected people are no more susceptible to hepatitis A than are other people. Nevertheless, HIV-infected travelers can benefit from an injection with hepatitis A immune globulin (*passive immunization*). Passive immunization against hepatitis A is effective, has few side effects, and can prevent an uncomfortable illness that lasts several weeks.

Other health measures for travelers:

- If you take a long trip on an airline you may develop respiratory problems due either to recirculation of air in the cabin or to the very dry atmosphere on board. Ear infections or sinus problems may get worse due to changes in airplane cabin pressure that take place at take-off and landing. It may help to use a decongestant or nasal spray.
- While on long airplane trips, get up and walk around if possible. This will help reduce blood clots, particularly in those taking EPO (a medication against anemia).
- The flu season may be different in another geographical area. Check to see when you should get your influenza vaccination, if it is available.
- HIV-infected persons do not seem to develop particular problems

114

with malaria, but any traveler who is going to an area where malaria is a danger should take medication to prevent the disease and take precautions against mosquitoes that spread the disease. Several drugs are used (for example, mefloquine, doxycycline, chloroquine). Your doctor or you should check on what type of medication is best to use. This depends on your destination since resistance to antimalarial drugs differs geographically. You can get this information by calling the Centers for Disease Control International Travelers Hotline: 404-332-4555.

• Use of condoms for intercourse is crucial in all countries. Bring an adequate supply of condoms and lubricant, no matter where your destination. Condoms may be in short supply or of inferior quality.

See the chart on **travel immunizations** on pp. 96–97.

AVOID SUNBURN

People who are HIV infected, especially those who are taking certain medications—such as sulfa drugs, nonsteroidal antiinflammatory drugs, or doxycycline—can have heightened sensitivity to the sun. This shows itself as bad sunburn or itchy, scaly patches. It may spread to areas of the skin that have not been exposed to the sun. It is caused by shortwave ultraviolet radiation (UVA).

If you are HIV infected, use sunscreen and protective clothing to avoid bad sunburns. This is desirable also because ultraviolet radiation increases the activity of HIV, at least in the test tube. If you are photosensitive and exposure to sunlight is inevitable, consult your physician about suspending the use of medications that contribute to photosensitivity. A medium- or high-potency topical steroid (such as hydrocortisone cream) will reduce symptoms of bad sunburn and encourage quicker healing.

ALCOHOL

Many people who are HIV infected use alcohol. Does this damage the immune system? Is it correlated with faster progression to AIDS? No studies answer these questions definitively. Consumption of large amounts of alcohol damages the body (including psychological damage). This has been proven in countless studies of non-HIV-infected people. Therefore, if you are HIV infected and fighting to maintain the best health possible, you may impair your health further by drinking too much.

People with chronic active hepatitis should not drink alcohol at all. People taking ddI should drink alcohol only in limited quantities because alcohol increases the risk of pancreatitis.

Alcohol dependence and abuse is extremely common in the United States; estimates are that 13 percent of the population are alcohol abusers or dependent. What is excessive use of alcohol? This is a difficult question to answer. It cannot be simply quantified by amount. For some people even a relatively small amount of alcohol can cause adverse effects both physically and psychologically.

Here are some questions to ask yourself to help you figure out if you are using alcohol in a way that is harmful to you:

- Have you ever had a blackout? (A blackout is a period of time when you were intoxicated and cannot remember what happened.)
- Have you ever been arrested for drunken driving or any other crime while under the influence of alcohol?
- Have you done anything you seriously regret when you were drinking?
- Have you ever been involved in violence while drunk?
- Have you had unsafe sex while drunk?
- Do you frequently fail to take prescribed medication when you have been drinking?
- Are you frequently hungover?
- Have you missed multiple days of work or school due to aftereffects of alcohol?
- Have you ever lost a job due to alcohol use?
- Have you ever lost a friend or lover due to alcohol use?
- Do you spend so much time drinking or recovering from being drunk that you have given up previously important social and recreational activities?
- Do you have any alcohol-related medical problems?
- Has use of alcohol caused you financial problems?
- Have you made unsuccessful efforts to cut back or eliminate alcohol use?
- Do you drink every time you feel anxious or depressed?
- Have other people complained about your drinking or told you that you drink too much?

If you answer yes to one or more of the above questions, seek further help in assessing a possible problem with alcohol. There is one important resource for alcohol problems that is available almost everywhere throughout the United States and in many other countries. That is Alcoholics Anonymous (AA). Even if you are not sure if you have a problem with alcohol, you can go to an AA meeting and learn more about the problem from people who are expert in alcohol problems—recovering alcoholics.

AA is a self-help group. It is free and anonymous. Although some people feel uncomfortable with certain aspects of the AA program, the fact remains that AA has been the single most successful program in helping people deal with alcohol problems. Almost every town has an AA chapter. If you live in a big city you will have a choice of multiple AA groups. For example, many cities have several gay AA groups. In addition, in New York, San Francisco, and Los Angeles you can go to an AA meeting specifically intended for HIV-infected people. Call your local AIDS organization for information about these meetings. Some contact numbers for Alcoholics Anonymous Intergroup include: 212-683-3900 in New York; 415-661-1828 in San Francisco; and 213-387-8316 in Los Angeles.

In addition to AA, there are a number of professional resources available to help individuals evaluate or treat alcohol problems. You can get information about these from calling either a local AIDS organization that maintains a resource directory, a local AA information number, or the psychiatry department of a local hospital, or possibly from your doctor.

OTHER RECREATIONAL DRUGS

Many other recreational drugs are used by people who are HIV infected: cocaine, heroin, so-called designer drugs such as Ecstasy (MDMA) or Special K (ketamine), marijuana, tranquilizers (such as Valium and Librium), sedatives such as Quaaludes or drugs intended for sleep, and amphetamines (speed), to name only a few. It is beyond the scope of this book to talk in any detail about the problems of drug use. Following are a few recommendations if you are concerned that you may have a problem with a recreational drug.

• Ask yourself the questions listed in the alcohol section (pp. 115–17) substituting the drug with which you are concerned.

In addition, ask the following questions.

• Am I sharing needles for drug use? Like intercourse without condoms, this puts you at risk of re-infection with new, perhaps more dangerous, strains of HIV as well as other blood-borne diseases.
• Am I injecting drugs? Even when needles are not shared this is probably a poor idea because of the possibility of infection and because injection of drugs may activate the immune system, possibly promoting the progression of HIV disease.
• Am I facing the possibility of legal trouble because of the use of illegal substances?

It is a tragedy of American society that despite the loud talk of the dangers of drug abuse, there is a disturbing lack of services to help people stop using drugs. Nonetheless, you should try to get help if you feel you have a drug problem. Some insurance policies pay for in-patient and/or out-patient treatment of drug abuse. There are some free drug programs sponsored by government and by private philanthropies. These may have waiting lists. Many people who use drugs are able to get help from going to AA meetings, even when their problem is a drug other than alcohol. Some communities have Narcotics Anonymous (NA) groups modeled on AA. For specific information, see what referral resources are available near you. Possibilities are an AIDS organization, a drug hotline, a state or locally run information service, the psychiatry department of a local hospital, or your doctor.

SMOKING TOBACCO

There is no definitive information available about the effect of smoking tobacco on HIV disease. Studies done so far on the effect of smoking on T4 cell levels have produced contradictory results. However, tobacco has a multitude of bad effects on health. Many of the opportunistic infections in HIV disease affect the lungs. Your lungs will be in better shape and better able to resist damage caused by disease if you do not smoke. If you are HIV infected and trying to take the best possible care of your body, you may want to consider stopping smoking.

PETS

Some animals harbor organisms that are transmissible and may cause harm to people with HIV disease. For example, cat feces may contain *Toxoplasma gondii*. Other animals that may spread harmful organisms are birds, turtles, and tropical fish.

This does not necessarily mean you have to give up your pet. Your veterinarian can determine whether your cat carries the toxoplasma parasite. Cats that have never been outdoors are less likely to be infected with toxoplasma. If you want to keep a toxoplasma-infected cat, have someone else clean out the litter box or wear gloves and a mask when you clean it. Wear gloves when cleaning a fish tank or handling fish, birds, or turtles.

Chapter 7
Your State of Mind

The first part of this chapter examines ideas and feelings HIV-infected people may have about the disease and discusses factors that may influence these ideas. Thinking about the sources of distressing emotions may help you feel better.

The second part describes types of professional help that you may use to cope with psychological problems. It covers both talk therapy and psychoactive medications.

PSYCHOLOGICAL ISSUES

In the course of HIV disease you may experience a variety of psychological dilemmas. Your experience of HIV disease is unique for three reasons. First, no two people have the same course of illness. The kind of disease, type and duration of symptoms, and response to medication vary from individual to individual.

Second, many social and economic factors affect your experience of HIV. Can you support yourself even though you are ill? Can you afford decent medical care? Do you have comfortable housing? Do you have friends? Is your family involved and helpful? Do you have caretakers if you need them? Are you facing prejudice or hostility because of your disease, sex, age, race, appearance, drug use, or sexual orientation?

Third, your mental life crucially determines your response to HIV. "Mental life" means all your attitudes, feelings, thoughts, and reactions. Your mental life evolves through an interaction between what you were born with (your body, your disposition, your circumstances) and your life experiences.

There can be no universal psychological response to HIV disease. However, HIV-infected people do share some typical experiences, conflicts, problems, and states of mind. These dilemmas may have no common solution, but increased awareness of the problems may make you feel better and more in control.

Potentially troubling areas include:

- Your image of AIDS
- Feelings about being sick
- Relations with other people
- Misplaced guilt and other unhelpful feelings

119

YOUR IMAGE OF AIDS

What do you picture (or fear) when you think about "having AIDS"? Your image of AIDS cannot be limited to some neutral medical definition. Rather, it is an entire complex of thoughts and feelings, only parts of which are conscious. Your image of what it is to "have AIDS" is constructed from direct experiences with friends and acquaintances who have had AIDS and from images from the media (newspapers, TV, movies, books). In addition, it will be influenced by seemingly unconnected ideas that are associated with AIDS by some linking thought.

The psychological term for this type of image is "fantasy." In everyday speech we usually use the word fantasy to mean a daydream, often one with sexual content. In psychological language a fantasy is a set of images, ideas, and thoughts that may be conscious or unconscious and that in some way express a wish. Unconscious fantasies strongly influence the way in which we interpret everyday events. When you become aware of unconscious fantasies about AIDS, you reduce their power to upset you.

Fantasies about having AIDS have many sources and start as soon as you become aware of the disease. Such fantasies can only become more intense when you realize that you are at risk for infection, or when you test HIV positive. Because some of the ideas and feelings attached to AIDS are not conscious, they do not have to be "logical" in our usual sense of the word. You may have several contradictory ideas about your infection at the same time. Some of these will be formed by your current knowledge about HIV disease. Other ideas derive from old experiences and childhood ways of understanding misfortune.

For example, you or someone close to you has probably been quite ill at some point. The details of this experience influence your picture of illness in general (including AIDS). To pick a different kind of example, most people have had the experience of feeling unwanted or like an outsider. The thought or fear of being ill with HIV disease (and therefore different from many people around you) may bring back some aspect of these feelings. If you are gay you may have spent years of your life feeling different from other people. In the past you may have felt bad about being gay, even if your current attitude toward homosexuality is positive. Your fantasy of having AIDS may inherit distressing emotions of being different or not belonging from your past feelings about your homosexuality.

It is medically useful to be HIV tested and to get early medical treatment if you are positive. Early intervention and all that it entails—keeping up with regular doctor's visits, getting lab tests, learning about HIV disease, taking medication, paying medical bills—makes you more aware of your illness. **Treatment means confronting unpleasant fantasies of AIDS.** As thoughts of AIDS gain emphasis you may unconsciously blur the distinction between your actual situation and your worst fears associated with AIDS.

Some people may be consciously preoccupied with thoughts of developing AIDS. Others may not be aware that these ideas are on their mind but will nonetheless be affected by distressing feelings connected to their idea of AIDS. Organizing appropriate medical care for HIV disease usually requires not only practical work but the emotional work of dealing with heightened fantasies about AIDS. As a result, you may notice a period of increased depression, anxiety, or anger when you begin to take medical action to deal with HIV disease.

Fantasies may distort your ability to look at HIV disease realistically. Think consciously about some of your fantasies that are attached to AIDS. When you worry about HIV disease, you have some picture(s) in mind of an unpleasant eventuality. Some parts of this picture may be realistic and some unrealistic. Some parts may be conscious and others unconscious. Some of your worst fears may actually be determined more by your past experiences than your current situation. However, understanding your fantasies may relieve distress.

For example, an HIV-positive man was panicky at the idea of hospitalization when he thought about "getting AIDS." He had been hospitalized before, at the age of 3 following a bad car crash. In the hospital he experienced pain. He also was separated from his parents and consequently felt rejected, unprotected, and abandoned. Because he was an infant he had limited ways to understand his distress. As an adult (and with the help of a psychotherapist) he thought about the impact of this childhood experience and was able to separate it from his actual situation. He realized that hospitalization as an adult need not be as frightening as when he was a helpless infant. As an adult he would be able to understand what was happening to him. He would realize that hospitalization is not a punishment and need not mean abandonment and rejection. Although he remained realistically anxious, his panic subsided.

Past trauma in your life may affect your experience of having HIV disease very specifically, as in the example above, or in more general ways. HIV disease is commonly associated with sexuality, loss, death, separation, abandonment, and rejection. In your mind the idea of HIV disease may attract a huge range of thoughts, feelings, and emotional conflicts. Whatever has been difficult for you in the past psychologically may rear its head again in the course of HIV disease. Consider your past experience. Try to remain aware of how it may unnecessarily amplify the distress you feel at your actual situation.

YOUR REACTION TO BEING SICK

Your psychological reaction to being sick may in and of itself cause you distress. Despite improvements in treatment, HIV disease remains a very serious medical problem. You do have an increased chance of sickness and early death. This grim fact necessarily colors the psychological state of many people with HIV disease. An upsetting preoccupation with being sick is probably inevitable during medical crises. Use whatever support you have available to get through these periods.

However, people with HIV disease do not necessarily spend all their time thinking about death and dying. You do not have to accept or live with continual or extreme fear. Painful preoccupation with your illness is potentially treatable: get professional mental health assistance. (See the discussion of psychotherapy and medication later in this chapter.) In addition, many anxious people are helped by talking with other HIV-infected people. Some people also find comfort in work or other accomplishments, relationships with other people, art, or spiritual beliefs.

▲ Age-Inappropriate Feelings

Many people with HIV disease are angry about a feeling of loss of control over their own lives. You must accommodate the disease in many aspects of your daily routine. You have to take medication at certain times. You may feel compelled to stay at a disliked job to maintain your health insurance. You may need to avoid certain foods. For many people this feels like a reduction in the amount of control they have over their own lives. In addition, the illness makes it harder to think of yourself as independent. You must wait to see your doctor. You may need more emotional support from those around you. You may worry about having someone to take care of you if you become very ill. **Feeling less able to control your life and feeling more dependent on others may make you feel like a child again.**

In old age, every human must confront changes in appearance, limits on physical activities, medical problems, and the deaths of friends and loved ones. **The grief, caution, and infirmity of old age may be forced prematurely on many HIV-infected people.** The problems of age are hard for the old as well as the young, but the old have more time to prepare and to adjust. A long life may also bring with it a sense of accomplishment and wisdom that helps make growing old more tolerable.

HIV-infected people may feel that the future holds nothing to look forward to. If you are HIV infected, your future is necessarily uncertain. Anxiety about your future causes two problems: it spoils the pleasures of the present and weakens the motivation to work now for distant goals. Some people get distracted by morbid thoughts: whenever they have fun they worry that this may be the last time. A summer day at the beach may become melancholy as a result. Being HIV infected may also make it more difficult to plan for the future. Consider the dilemma of people who are getting some kind of advanced educational degree. This often requires much work and yields little money. The payoff is what you will be able to achieve when the educational project is finished. Should you stick to this plan or do something else that is more rewarding in the short term? Sticking to the plan may create a feeling of deprivation in the face of a possibly shortened life span. Giving up your plans may create a feeling of loss, failure, and despair.

▲ The Changing Body

Knowledge of your **HIV infection may change the way you feel about your body, even if you have had no symptoms whatsoever.** Our greatest pleasures and anxieties are derived from our experience of our bodies.

Images of the body's fragility, betrayal, and contamination may amplify anxiety. Some people with HIV disease experience their infection as a kind of "time bomb." You may be unnerved by the sense of a virus living inside you, "lurking" and waiting to cause trouble. This can add an unpleasant element of suspense that might not be present with illnesses that follow a more predictable course. Although many diseases function in the same way, HIV has been given a special status in the public mind as a dangerous intruder, as "the enemy within." Minor symptoms which in uninfected people may be easily dismissed frequently become a source of profound anxiety. You are entitled to ask for frequent consultations with your doctor to get information and possibly reassurance about any symptom.

Many people with HIV are likely to be predisposed to feeling that their body has betrayed them. Gay men may have been encouraged to regard their sexuality as a defect or problem. People who share needles for intravenous drug use may have experienced the grip of addiction. Hemophiliacs infected through the use of clotting factor have survived a lifetime of medical problems. In our culture, women are encouraged to feel anxiety about their bodies. Given this type of history it is all the more likely that an HIV-infected person would react badly to changes that threaten the body's integrity.

HIV disease has a very slow and uncertain course. **Should you think of yourself as sick?** During most of the course of the disease you feel healthy and look healthy. Despite this you must devote serious attention to your health. The distinction between sick and healthy becomes confused. Are you sick or well? Neither is precisely true. It may be depressing to think of yourself as "sick," but it may also feel bad to think of yourself as healthy while having to worry and make sacrifices to deal with medical issues. This dilemma is shared by all those with chronic illness.

What should you tell other people about your health status? **Should others think of you as sick?** If other people do not acknowledge your illness you may feel very lonely. On the other hand, if others regard you as sick when you feel perfectly healthy you may feel stigmatized, discriminated against, or forced prematurely into a "sick" role.

The paradox of medication arises if you begin to take antivirals early on in the course of the disease. Side effects are rare in people with higher T4 counts, but some healthy people may briefly feel worse than they did before beginning medication. Even with no side effects, simply swallowing the pills on a regular schedule may upset you by reminding you that you are ill. If you are so distressed that you neglect medication or other treatment that you need, seek professional help.

RELATIONS WITH OTHER PEOPLE

As we have described, HIV disease may profoundly affect the way you think about yourself. Some aspects of the illness may make it harder to maintain your self-esteem. This in turn affects your relations with other people. It is an accurate assessment of reality on the part of HIV-infected people that some people will reject them, discriminate against them, or scorn them on the basis of their infection. However, even without rejection, **infected people may feel less worthy of attention, respect, or love from others.** You may magnify existing feelings of insecurity, self-doubt, or self-hatred. Some infected people have reported feeling like "damaged goods" due to HIV.

You are likely to spend significant energy deciding whether and how to talk to other people about your HIV infection. **Some infected people feel burdened by a terrible secret** and become preoccupied with hiding knowledge of their illness from others. Some derive a sense of freedom and power from being openly HIV-positive. Most people take the middle road, telling those closest to them while preserving a degree of privacy.

You have a lot on your mind and may be in a terrible mood at times. People may avoid you because of your moodiness. This may then make you feel rejected and lead to a vicious cycle in which a feeling of rejection increases your grouchiness and your irritability causes people to avoid you all the more.

▲ Sexual and Romantic Partners

HIV disease definitely interferes with the formation and conduct of sexual and romantic relationships.

There are a number of difficult decisions facing you regarding when and how you should tell **new sexual partners** about your infection. There is no one right course; you have to find answers that are comfortable to you. Thinking about these issues in advance will help you figure this out, as will talking with other HIV-infected people. You have to figure out whether to tell every sexual partner even if you are using condoms for intercourse, and at what point to bring up the subject in the course of meeting someone. For some people this means grappling with the moral issues that are connected to disclosure and with the fear of rejection. Telling every sexual partner may feel intimidating, too public, unsexual, or may make you feel vulnerable. Not telling may make you feel guilty, secretive, and afraid of the moment of disclosure.

The uninfected can be irritatingly smug and self-absorbed. An HIV-infected man tells the story of meeting a prospective sexual partner one evening. After a pleasant hour of conversation, the man thought it responsible to mention the fact that he had AIDS. The prospective partner responded by exclaiming, "Why do these things always have to happen to *me!*" Not everyone responds so badly, but the story demonstrates an attitude that is not rare.

You may feel increased pressure to find a "spouse." This may be partially motivated by feelings of loneliness exacerbated by the disease and by the desire to find a partner who will be with you and care for you if you become ill. These pressures may lead you to work hard at having a relationship that will open new possibilities for closeness. On the other hand, it may increase your ambivalence as you ask yourself, "Would I stay with this person if I were not HIV infected?" Such questions are not answerable in this form but are expressions of grief at changed circumstances and a feeling of narrowing choices.

If you have an uninfected sexual partner, then **the two of you must decide what sexual practices you will do together.** Uninfected partners will have varying reactions to your illness: some may request stringent limits on your sexual activities, some may have illogical preferences (such as having protected intercourse but not kissing), and some may even seek sex with you *because* of your illness. On your side, you may be disproportionately afraid of infecting your partners, or shy or angry about making sexual requests. To understand sexual (or indeed any) behavior, look for psychological interpretations, not logical explanations. (For detailed guidelines on the reduction of the risk of HIV transmission during sex, refer to pp. 103–10 in Chapter 6: General Health Care. Particularly note the discussion on how to adapt to risk reduction, pp. 108–10.)

HIV infection throws conflicts about emotional commitment and care-taking into high relief. Fights over who takes care of whom move from metaphor into ugly actuality. If your partner is HIV negative, you may worry about whether she or he will care for you if you become seriously ill. You may worry that you will be a burden to your partner. If your partner is also HIV positive you may be in the position of coping with simultaneous illness. An infected partner understands your situation. However, it is upsetting to have to worry about the health and survival of someone you love. Some partners may fall into bickering over who feels worse on a given day. HIV is likely to intensify both the existing strengths and the conflicts of most relationships.

▲ Friends

Friends can be a tremendous source of emotional and practical support. Many gay men and lesbians have constructed intricate webs of friendships that provide love, companionship, and resources for caretaking in addition to the biological family. Heterosexuals may also have friends who can step in if the biological family is unsupportive. The AIDS epidemic has seen many moving examples of heroic friendship, particularly in lesbians and straight women who (though as a group less hard hit than men in this country) have come forward in great numbers to care for the infected.

Is it prudent or desirable to tell friends that you are HIV positive? There are practical and emotional risks to discussing your infection publicly, yet how can you feel close to your friends if they are ignorant of something so central to your life? It is burdensome to have to tell a lot of people, talk about the issues over and over, and often cope with odd or unsympathetic responses. A response on the part of the other person of fearfulness, despair, or pity may make you feel temporarily worse. Your friends are entitled to be upset when you tell them this piece of news, but then to some extent you have to deal with their feelings as well as yours. On the other hand, friends who struggle to maintain equanimity in the face of learning of your HIV infection may make you feel as if they don't care.

Telling your friends may be upsetting, difficult, or irritating. Once you have told a number of people, it is probably unrealistic to think that knowledge of your infection can be kept totally private. This is going to be particularly worrisome if, by virtue of your geographical, social, or vocational position, you are likely to face discrimination if the information becomes widely known.

However, it is impossible to get support from people who don't know of the problem. It is difficult to feel intimate with people who are ignorant of something so central to your life. Maintaining secrecy can be complicated and emotionally taxing.

Issues of commitment and caretaking arise in intimate nonsexual friendships as well as between romantic or sexual partners. In this time of the epidemic, many people have multiple friends with HIV disease. This complicates both practical and emotional demands, as many people find themselves feeling overwhelmed.

Most people with HIV disease have more than one friend who is HIV infected. This is generally helpful because you will feel more understood and less alone. However, it can be distressing to deal with friends who are developing serious medical problems, and you may feel burdened by the need to provide practical and emotional support for sick friends when you yourself are dealing with HIV disease.

▲ The Workplace

If you are diagnosed with HIV disease, you may feel increased uncertainty about your work life. Some of the questions that arise are: Can I work? Will I be able to support myself and maintain my health insurance? Should I continue with my current job? If I should lose or leave my job, will my HIV status make it difficult for me to find a new job? What kind of career goals are realistic? Should I change my plans regarding work? Is my work life being damaged by my HIV status? If I am sick, should I go on disability?

You may have little choice about your work life. Many working people with HIV disease are forced by economic necessity to continue at jobs they may not like or feel are too stressful. They may also have to worry about being laid off and losing both income and crucial medical benefits. Many others who wish to work and need the money and benefits are unable to find jobs. Some people work in jobs with an uncertain future, such as freelance or temporary work, self-employment, or artistic endeavors.

Women with HIV disease are often in the most difficult situation regarding work and money. Women typically earn less money than men and usually carry the burden of housework and child raising. Women who are infected with HIV may find themselves—like many other women—essentially doing two jobs. At the same time, they are faced with their own health problems and sometimes with caring for a child with HIV disease. "Choice" about work would be a luxury.

However, even if you are in a position to make some choices about your work life you may find decisions difficult. Work is central for most of us. It takes up a large part of our time and often defines how we think of ourselves. If you are HIV infected you may find yourself making many choices about how hard to work, whether to change jobs, or whether to stop working and live on disability. For information on the types of benefits that may be available to you, consult Chapter 21: Money to Live On.

Some people worry about whether their current job is too stressful. You may be a relatively young person who is working many hours a week to establish a career. If you are HIV infected you may be concerned about whether this is putting too great a stress on you and consequently potentially damaging your health.

Lack of sleep, physical exhaustion, and lack of time to take care of your medical needs can have a negative impact on your health. However, there is no evidence that hard or challenging work is harmful. It seems likely that if your job is demanding but enjoyable and satisfying, the stress will not harm you.

If you are working at a job you do not like, there are psychological as well as practical reasons why **it may be difficult to change your job or go on disability.** Finding a new job may seem stressful in itself; it takes time and energy and you may worry about disclosure of your HIV status. It can be hard to contemplate change at a time when so much of your life is in flux. Time and planning are usually the best answers to these problems. Don't make decisions about job or career changes impulsively or during times of great stress.

You may also be concerned about whether you will be able to maintain past standards on your job. You may be concerned that preoccupation with your medical problems, fatigue, or even some change in your mental functioning could cause a decline in your performance. Fear of failure may lead you to leave the field before necessary.

If you have significant medical problems that make it difficult for you to work, going on **disability** may be the best option. However, some people feel that going on disability is "giving in" or equivalent to becoming an invalid. Some people express the fear that if they stop work they will become more severely ill: "You called yourself disabled, okay, now *be* disabled." This is a magical idea that may partly reflect guilt about not working.

In addition, it can be difficult to go on disability because many of us define ourselves in terms of our work. What will you do with your time? How will you answer the question "what do you do?" Will you be bored? Will you feel that you are unimportant?

What do you give up for future gain? You may be working at something partly because of the payoff (emotional, intellectual, artistic, social, financial) that you hope to get in the future. This becomes problematic if you have an illness that may limit your future. How much should you "live for the moment"? What does this mean about investing in a career or giving priority to other activities or relationships?

Many people who are HIV infected find themselves asking what they want to do with their lives if they have only a few years to live. This question itself can be distressing or liberating; few of us know what would be ideal let alone what would be achievable. Thinking about this is likely to raise questions about what gives your life significance. Although these issues may be painful, facing them can add to the richness of your life.

How are you treated at work? People with HIV disease arrive at many different answers to the question of disclosing their HIV status on the job. Many people choose not to tell anyone on the job or to tell only a few trusted supervisory personnel or good work friends. This discretion guards your privacy and prevents discrimination. However, it can be difficult if you are facing significant medical problems and require time off for sick days or doctors' visits. The feeling of having a secret or fear of your infection being revealed may be uncomfortable.

Sometimes, if you are having significant medical problems, it becomes impossible to keep the information private. The most serious problem following disclosure is actual harassment or discrimination. This can be fought legally—Chapter 22: Some Legal Matters contains a sketch of legal protections against HIV-related discrimination.

Even if you do not face discrimination or hostility regarding your HIV infection, it can be difficult to have your HIV status known at work. It is a loss of privacy. You may feel that people see you in a different way, treat you as if you are breakable, write you off, or do not take your work and abilities as seriously as they once did.

However, there may be advantages to having your health situation known on the job, at least by some people. It can be a relief not to feel you are constantly keeping a secret. Many people feel good about the support they receive from colleagues at work. If your status is known, you are in a position to ask for the accommodation you may need to any health problems you have.

Before you tell people at work about your HIV infection, think through the advantages and disadvantages. Get legal advice if you are concerned about possible discrimination, if you need to make arrangements for disability payments, or if you need your employer to make some accommodation to a disability you may have developed. If you have a trustworthy colleague at work, discuss this issue and get help planning the best possible strategy for disclosure. It is your decision (not your employer's) whether to disclose your HIV status.

▲ Family

Family relationships are always complicated. Your bad news is likely to upset all those who love you. However, many people who were afraid of a bad reaction have been surprised by their family's loyalty and support. It bears repeating that, as with sexual and romantic partners, HIV is likely to intensify both the existing strengths and conflicts of most family relationships. If your family is usually loving and supportive, they likely will remain so after learning of your infection. If you do not get along with your family, HIV may not improve matters. If your family charac-teristically gives you more grief than support, you may decide you are better off keeping your infection secret.

You have a number of choices about **when to tell your family:** you may tell them as soon as you test HIV positive; later, after you get somewhat used to the idea; or at some medical transition point (such as when you begin taking antivirals or PCP prophylaxis, at a particular T4 count, or if you develop an opportunistic infection). You may also decide never to tell certain family members.

If you tell your family before you have serious symptoms, your family will adjust to your news with less stress. Keeping your infection secret puts distance between you and your family and denies you your family's practical and emotional support.

Some people decide not to tell their families, either due to alienation or to avoid distressing members of the family. This may be appropriate with elderly parents, very young children, or other family members who may be more vulnerable. Some HIV-infected people find it harder to tell the family about HIV infection because that would require open discus-sion of sex or drug use.

If your family is aware of your risk for HIV infection, they may ask you directly whether you are infected. You may or may not be ready to talk to them—prepare a response in advance. Be prepared also for late but well-intentioned efforts to protect you from infection, such as heart-to-heart talks about condom use.

When you talk to your family, remember that reactions, beliefs, and

129

emotions may be very deeply held, and consequently hard to amend through education or persuasion. If you have a reasonably positive relationship with your family, explain to them how their attitudes and comments affect you. Some people can change with time and education. Tell your family as clearly and calmly as possible what you want and need. In return, try to understand what they want and need. Most of us have had some trouble talking with our families about difficult topics: be realistic about your family's ability to change.

Many people who are HIV infected want solicitude and involvement from their families, but also feel pained by their worry. Many HIV-infected people report that their mother or father now say "how *are* you?" in a tone of voice that seems new and different. Worry and curiosity are entirely understandable from your family's point of view. However, your family's worry may make you feel anxious rather than comforted. Alternatively, your family may be so anxious that they avoid the topic of HIV altogether, with the result that you feel isolated or abandoned. Emotional discussions may feel too upsetting. Calm "neutral" discussions may feel too cold.

HIV-infected people often find themselves in the position of teaching the uninfected basic facts about the disease, such as the lack of transmission through casual contact. This is necessary but may feel tedious and irritating. Your family may be quite ignorant about HIV disease. They may be afraid that you may infect them or other people. They may be naive about what kind of medical care you should get. **Get help from some other person or group in providing your family with information about HIV disease.**

Your family also needs to talk about their anxiety, grief, and sense of isolation. Explaining feelings (or even medical facts) to your family may be the last thing you feel like doing while you are striving to maintain your own emotional stability. **Involve other people in talking with your family.** A longtime friend who can talk to your family may play a useful role. In some areas, support groups may be available for families— unfortunately, few support groups have been organized for families of people at earlier stages of illness. You may be able to encourage your family to get some kind of professional counseling.

If you involve others, your family will be able to get information and emotional support without overburdening you.

The battle between feeling dependent and feeling abandoned can be a serious issue. An individual's assertion of independence from parents or family is a major developmental step. HIV disease may provoke the return or resurgence of conflicts over independence from your family. You may need financial and practical help from your family. You may then feel that you are burdening them. Any increased dependence on others may feel like a poignant loss of an aspect of adulthood won with great struggle. Of course, you also want to feel that someone will take care of you: you may wish that you could exchange some of the burdens of adulthood for the security of childlike dependence. Either of these reactions is natural. Depending on circumstances, you may be able to find a creative balance between independence and security.

A slightly different situation arises if you find yourself depending on people who live very differently or have different values. For instance, if you are gay, you may need help from someone who disapproves of your sexuality. In such cases you must calculate your options as dispassionately as possible.

Your HIV infection is traumatic for you but also grievous for your family. One of the oldest and strongest human reactions to trouble is to seek a scapegoat. **Assigning blame** for calamity allows the fortunate to believe there is justice in the vicissitudes of an indifferent and meaningless universe. It would be surprising if your family's attitude toward AIDS had no tinge of fear or blame.

This lurking sense of blame may fasten on to old sources of conflict. If you are gay, telling your family about your HIV status may involve discussing your sexual orientation for the first time, the famous "double whammy." If you have already come out to your family, this news may revive old arguments about your sexuality. If you have been infected heterosexually you may also find yourself defending your sexual and romantic choices. Issues of profound disapproval may also arise if you were infected by sharing needles for drug use. Some family members may blame you for your infection in some way, while others may somehow blame themselves. Later we will discuss how to handle your most harmful accuser: yourself.

Problems with your family are more likely to take the form of **unconscious knee-jerk behavior rather than deliberate cruelty.**

One man's family responded to the news of his infection with kindness and acceptance. He later saw them wince when a young niece wanted to share her ice cream cone with him. The family was instinctively afraid that he might transmit HIV through sharing food, although they knew this was impossible. This family did not mean any harm, yet they managed to hurt deeply the person they loved.

Another man told his fundamentalist family about his HIV disease. Although they did not reject him or blame him directly, they offered prayers for him and enjoined him to come back to their church. They did so not to hurt him but because they were scared. Nonetheless, this was the same church whose threats of eternal damnation for homosexuals had made his adolescence a living hell. His parents request that he return to their church reawakened this torture at a time when he wanted to be close to them and needed their help.

Stop your family from hurting you by making them aware of the problem. You or a professional may be able to alert your family to the meaning and impact of their hurtful actions.

Your family affects you for good or for ill. No matter how negative your family's attitude toward your having HIV disease, you will probably still want their love, attention, and support. Even if your parents respond to your news with direct blame, criticism, or rejection, do not expect it to be easy to write them out of your psychological life.

MISPLACED GUILT AND OTHER UNHELPFUL FEELINGS

Emotional responses occur for definite reasons. Patterns of emotional response are determined by disposition and personal history. Circumstances change, however, and responses learned in the past may no longer be appropriate or useful. The responses and impulses themselves are difficult to alter, but you may be able to change some behavior based on these responses.

▲ Guilt and Shame: "The Wrath of God"

You do not deserve to be HIV infected, just as those who experience earthquakes or tidal waves do not deserve these disasters. You were infected in the course of trying to conduct your life as best you could in the face of a world filled with accidents waiting to happen. Despite this, you may be troubled by feelings of guilt or shame. These feelings may take many forms. At some level you may blame yourself for being HIV infected. You may feel as if your illness confirms a view of yourself as irresponsible, worthless, self-destructive, or dangerous to others.

HIV-infected people sometimes ascribe their infection to a supposed character flaw such as irresponsibility, lack of self-control, disobedience to authority, or even immorality. You may recognize such statements as:

- I must have done something wrong to end up HIV infected.
- I'm paying for my wild period when I was younger.
- I got HIV infected because I was just out of control.
- I should not have sinned.

Some people associate their infection with a sense of worthlessness in the eyes of others. This is most often seen in rueful comments such as:

- I knew I'd turn out to be infected because I was such a slut.
- See what happens when you stay single?
- This is what I get for being promiscuous.

Some people associate HIV infection with a pattern of self-destructive behavior. The sense of self-inflicted doom provokes shame and a feeling that you have no right to complain of misfortune:

132

- My parents always told me I'd come to a bad end.
- I should have known better. I had been told about safe sex. It's all my fault.
- I did drugs, so I deserve to be infected.
- If I had cancer I could tell people, but I'm ashamed of HIV. I did it to myself.

You may feel "dangerous," or develop worries or fantasies about infecting others accidentally or deliberately. Do you recognize these feelings?

- I'd better stay away from the kids.
- I'd love to stick Jesse Helms with a hypodermic full of my blood.

You would not be human if you did not feel angry at your bad luck. You should be aware that your anger may be overt (see the section on p. 135 on anger) or unconscious. In unconscious form your anger may only be noticeable as a reaction of guilt or caution, such as in the exaggerated desire to protect young relatives in the example above.

HIV disease seems to be a powerful magnet for feelings of shame. HIV-infected people sometimes feel that their bodies are dirty. People who are infected sometimes see their semen or blood as contaminated and talk about those who are not HIV-infected as being "clean." Sometimes, despite knowledge to the contrary, HIV-infected people become unrealistically concerned about infecting other people through casual contact, as if their very presence were a contaminant.

Unfortunately, such thoughts are common among people who are HIV infected. Some people consciously believe that they should feel guilty about or ashamed of their HIV infection. Most people reject this reasoning consciously, but continue to feel a pervasive sense of "badness" or self-blame. Why is guilt so common among people with HIV disease?

One of the main reasons you may feel guilty about HIV disease is that **you are repeatedly told you are guilty**—that the disease is your fault and that you have reason to feel ashamed of yourself. This view is common in public discourse about AIDS.

Theories of HIV disease that attempt to scapegoat those affected have been common since the beginning of the epidemic. HIV disease is seen as a consequence for various forms of unacceptable behavior, such as drug use, homosexuality, or sexuality in general. The crudest version of this actually argues that AIDS is a moral punishment, a "visitation" from God.

Subtler versions implicate irresponsibility rather than immorality. "Promiscuity" is frequently blamed for AIDS. The word promiscuity is often used not only in popular discussion but also (disappointingly) in medical and scientific literature. The word lacks a scientific or sociological definition. Rather, it is a term borrowed from the language of moralizing. It denotes no specific information, but simply serves to punish those to whom it is applied through implication of wrongdoing and sin. HIV is transmitted via unprotected vaginal and anal intercourse: the number of partners is not directly relevant.

Moral accusations made by the media, religious figures, or by politicians are harmful, but it is the accusations of those we care about that hurt the most. Many people with HIV disease are directly rejected by their families and told by them that their disease is their fault. Even families who respond supportively to news of HIV disease may have a history that makes this support problematic for the infected person.

However, the blame of other people (even your family) does not adequately explain **why you blame yourself.** What are some of the fantasies that lead to guilt in the individual and make one susceptible to self-blaming propaganda? Why are they so powerful and so hard to resist?

One way of approaching the problem is to think about how children experience illness. Clearly there is an age when children are too young to understand the physiological nature of painful symptoms. All they know is that they are being hurt. For them there is essentially no distinction between being purposely hurt by someone and feeling pain. Consequently, children experience the suffering of illness as an act of aggression directed against them. They often **imagine illness to be a punishment for some action of their own.**

Adults have other models of understanding pain, yet the old ideas linger in the unconscious mind. We may not consciously *think* of pain as a punishment, but may nevertheless *feel* it as a punishment. When we are under periods of great stress—such as being sick—we tend to return to earlier, more familiar patterns of experiencing the world around us. Thus, it becomes easy to construct an (unconscious) scenario in which HIV disease is punishment for wrongdoing.

Some illnesses are more likely than others to be felt in terms of this unconscious fantasy of punishment. Because sexual impulses and activities are a ripe area for guilt in most of us, illness associated with sexuality is even more likely to be interpreted as punishment for transgressions. This is especially true for "unacceptable" sexuality. Almost all of us grew up being taught that homosexuality is unacceptable. (The same kind of thinking applies to drug use, which is an illicit activity in our society). However, virtually any source of guilty feelings about sex can stimulate the fantasy of HIV disease as a punishment for sexual activity or even thoughts.

When you are faced with something unknown and try to make sense of it, you will probably explain it according to models of the world you already possess. **If the unknown is threatening, this increases the urgency of the need to explain.** If it can be explained, perhaps it can be controlled, fought, or seen not to be a threat to you as an individual or to those you most care about. You are likely to develop a viewpoint, a theory, that (perhaps unconsciously) fits your model of the way the world is organized.

These theories are often built around some kind of moral system and particularly the kind of absolutist moral system common among children. Explanation is made in terms of fault and punishment, right and wrong. **Assignment of blame becomes a primary goal.**

The sheer "unfairness" and relative randomness of HIV disease—or any other serious disease—is hard to tolerate. It makes people feel unimportant and too much a powerless object of fate. It is a reminder of the limited control we all have over our lives. Moralistic theories of the causation of AIDS can (temporarily) serve to make you feel more in control. This is true even if it requires categorizing the self or past behavior as "bad." At times it feels better to say, "This happened because I was bad," rather than to say, "This just happened."

▲ Anger: Your Own Wrath

One of our more difficult psychological tasks is controlling aggressive impulses or actions. A child may think sickness is punishment for angry thoughts at the parents. Again, although most of us do not consciously employ this model as adults, it is likely to affect us emotionally, especially when our mental reserves are being tested by the stress of illness. This probably plays a part in the terrifying image some HIV-infected people have of their genitalia as a "loaded gun" and of their sexual fluids as poison, capable of killing with a single orgasm.

You may find yourself feeling angry more often than in the past. This is not surprising. The anxiety, limitations, inconveniences, and uncertainties associated with HIV disease are tremendously frustrating. Governmental neglect and lack of access to medical treatment should enrage us all. The sheer "unfairness" of fate contributes to anger.

You cannot and should not eliminate feelings of anger from your life. But consider whether the anger you feel (or the way you express it) is damaging you. Are you so angry that you alienate all your friends, commit physical violence, or increase your use of alcohol or other drugs? If anger has become a problem, there are many things to try. Consider a support group, counseling, or at least sitting down and talking with a friend about your anger. Some people feel better when they can channel their anger appropriately and productively, for example by doing political work with an organization such as ACT UP to fight the injustices associated with AIDS. (See the appendices for contact information for political organizations.)

▲ Defenses and Denial

A defense is an unconscious mental process that helps control anxiety and resolve emotional conflict. It allows you to deal with an emotion or idea without directly confronting the content and/or impact of that idea or feeling. Defenses have both a helpful (*adaptive*) side and a harmful side.

Mental life always involves the use of defenses. Without them we would be paralyzed with anxiety and emotional conflict. We could not reconcile our impulses with the demands of reality. Useful defenses help you cope. Harmful defenses redirect anxiety into self-destructive behavior.

The defensive process called *denial* **can be useful or harmful.** Denial resolves conflict and anxiety by blotting out awareness of some upsetting aspect of reality. Denial is necessary. Without denial we would feel overwhelmed by all the troublesome aspects of reality. On the other hand, denial can be dangerous if it distorts the accurate perception of the external world that we need to function safely.

A simple example of denial is when you are able to "forget" about your medical problems while you are busy taking an exam for school. In this example, denial is helpful to you. This "forgetting" allows you to concentrate on your academic work for a period of time without being distracted by other concerns. Another example of denial is when you have a severe cough for a few weeks but keep "forgetting" to call your doctor. In this example, denial is probably harmful to you because it would be better for your health to report the symptom to your doctor and receive treatment if necessary.

Ask yourself these questions to decide whether the denial you are employing is helpful or harmful:

- Are you unable to think about your situation long enough to make appropriate plans?
- Do you alternate never thinking about HIV disease with periods of acute anxiety?
- Do you feel you want to avoid everyone else with HIV disease?
- Are you staying calm by avoiding appropriate medical care?
- Do you delay reporting symptoms to your physician?
- Do you neglect medication or doctor's appointments?
- Are you unable to think about HIV disease enough to keep up-to-date with developments in treatment?

If you are answering "yes" to many of these questions on a sustained basis, it is likely that denial is interfering with your ability to cope with HIV disease. In this case, sitting down and thinking about the issues—by yourself, with a friend, in a support group, or with a therapist—may help you reach some more satisfactory approach.

Try to strike a balance between denial and preoccupation. Thinking more about these issues may upset you temporarily. It may be worthwhile tolerating a period of distress if it will improve your chances of health sufficiently. For example, most people who test HIV positive report that the benefits of appropriate medical care are worth the psychological difficulty.

On the other hand, if you are going to go about your normal daily life, function at work, have relationships, and have some fun, you cannot be thinking every minute about having a serious disease. Sometimes the term denial is used as if it were necessarily a bad response. In fact, denial is both inevitable and sometimes useful in facing HIV disease. If you are HIV-infected and getting early intervention, you have to walk a narrow line between thinking about HIV disease and its most serious consequences and keeping enough distance from the thoughts so that you can go on with your life.

If you find it difficult to maintain this balance, it is not because you are inadequate or doing something wrong. It is a tremendously difficult task. No one can do it perfectly all the time. Too many forces exist that may disrupt your equilibrium.

You may go through some periods of anxiety or depression or a period of being less thorough about your medical care. For example, you may forget to take medication. **When you are feeling depressed or anxious, remind yourself that your state of mind is likely not to be permanent.** It's cold comfort, but it can help you keep things in perspective.

Changes in your medical status or personal behavior may trigger psychological distress. Some of these changes are starting safer sex or safer injection practices, HIV antibody testing, T4 counts, starting medication, developing an HIV-related symptom, having an invasive diagnostic procedure done, being hospitalized, becoming disabled (even in minor ways), being diagnosed with AIDS, telling someone significant about your infection, or having to make a change in your plans to take HIV disease into account. You may react strongly to the illness or death of others.

Adapt your responses to the circumstances. In times of change, try to increase the support you get from others. Reduce other stresses when possible. Avoid making major life decisions—though circumstances may sometimes force this on you. What feels useful at one point may be stressful at another moment. For example, being involved with other people with HIV disease, doing AIDS political work, subscribing to newsletters, and belonging to HIV support groups are all valuable sources of information and at times will make you feel more comfortable and secure. However, at other times these same activities may make you feel more anxious because they cause you to focus on HIV disease and its possible consequences. Do what you need to do.

▲ The Problem of "Positive Thinking"

"Positive thinking" is another outgrowth of the need to try to gain control by inserting HIV disease in a moral system. It is widely and uncritically believed that hopeful, optimistic thoughts have a beneficial physical effect on the body, perhaps even strengthening the immune system. This idea is comforting because it restores the self to a position of control and power by asserting that your thoughts can directly influence the course of the illness in some beneficial way. Positive thinking *can* sometimes be seen to alleviate emotional distress, but no physical effect on the immune system has yet been demonstrated. Connections between mental attitude and the immune system will probably prove to be quite complex.

Try positive thinking if it alleviates distress, does not interfere with more proven treatment, and does not in itself cause harm. However, positive thinking can cause harm if massive denial is required to maintain unrealistic optimism. It has sometimes kept individuals from getting needed medical care. A more subtle danger is that positive thinking can turn into a "blame the victim" attitude that can backfire on the self. That is, we may hold the unconscious idea that "people who have a good attitude do better. He's getting sicker. There must be something wrong with his attitude. I'm not like that." But then this can become, "I'm getting sicker. There's something wrong with the way I'm thinking. It's my fault."

PROFESSIONAL MENTAL HEALTH SERVICES

During the course of HIV disease, you may have periods when you feel upset, worried, anxious, or depressed. There are a number of different approaches to understanding and lessening emotional distress and they are not mutually exclusive. You may be able to get help from a variety of sources. Professional mental health services fall into two broad categories: psychotherapy and the use of psychoactive medications.

There are numerous misconceptions about psychotherapy and psychoactive drugs. In our culture many people associate psychotherapy and the use of therapeutic psychoactive drugs with shame, loss of passion or feeling, numbness, passivity, and sedation. There are many reasons for this misconception, but the truth is that good use of therapy and medication generally increases feeling, awareness, and activity. Psychotherapy does not rob you of your identity or passion any more than setting a broken leg does—quite the contrary.

A specific suspicion sometimes voiced is that psychotherapy and the use of therapeutic psychoactive drugs may make you "docile" and interfere with your ability to fight for your political rights. **Therapy and medication are completely compatible with political awareness and political action.** Distress is not just the consequence of psychological conflict: external events profoundly affect your emotional life. These include sickness, changes in your body, and the possibility of dying. They may also include the problems of getting medical care, the unpleasant experience of being a patient, and the social problems of lack of money, discrimination, homophobia, racism, and sexism.

It can be emotionally helpful to clarify reality by better understanding the medical and political issues. It may also make you feel better (as well as useful) to try to change the current reality with political work or social service work. Consider working with your local AIDS organization or ACT UP, or some of the other groups in the AIDS treatment movement (see pp. 409–16 in the appendices for contact information). Becoming involved with these activities will also put you in a position where you are more likely to be up-to-date on treatment developments and will have the comfort of getting to know people who share your situation and concerns.

PSYCHOTHERAPY

It can be emotionally helpful to better understand your psychological state and to identify the influence of your own particular history and conflicts. Support groups and psychotherapy are useful for this purpose. Both also provide you with a chance to talk about upsetting feelings, to feel the comfort of being understood, and to alleviate anxiety and depression at times of particular stress.

Psychotherapy is actually a disparate group of techniques designed to improve emotional well-being, and usually involve some kind of verbal dialogue between patient and therapist. Because of the **broad range of practices described as psychotherapy** it is difficult to discuss the use and efficacy of therapy in a coherent fashion. Furthermore, because the human mind and emotions are so complex, it is extremely difficult to develop objective measures for judging the utility of therapy. Therapy even within the same "school of thought" varies tremendously from practitioner to practitioner.

Some kinds of therapy currently in use are psychoanalysis, psychoanalytically oriented psychotherapy, family and couple therapy, group therapy, cognitive therapy, and behavior therapy. These therapies are based on divergent views of the mind, behavior, and the pathways of change. We will concentrate on describing psychoanalytically oriented psychotherapy and will only briefly describe the other types of therapy mentioned above.

Frequency and duration: Psychotherapy most often takes the form of regular one-on-one meetings with a therapist that occur one to four times per week. Individual therapy sessions typically last from forty-five to sixty minutes. Group therapy and support group sessions may last longer, up to about two hours. Treatment may continue from months to years depending on the nature and goals of the therapy.

A tremendous problem with psychotherapy is the **cost.** Because it is often an ongoing activity, the fees can mount up. Some insurance policies pay for some therapy, but usually this covers a limited amount of the cost. Some therapy at low cost or covered by Medicaid is available through clinics (usually associated with hospitals, medical centers, and social service agencies).

▲ Guidelines for Choosing a Therapist

It is extremely difficult to give advice on how to find a therapist. The referral you get will depend on the point of view and experience of the person who gives you the referral. Obviously, you should seek a referral to psychotherapy from a person you trust. Good sources of referrals include your medical doctor, the psychiatry department of a well-respected hospital or medical school, or perhaps a local AIDS organization. Guidelines for choosing a therapist appear below.

You are entitled to ask therapists about their training, **credentials, experience, and therapeutic approach.** You should not expect personal information or a long, detailed discussion of therapeutic philosophy. This is generally seen as bad for the therapy.

Anyone can call himself or herself a psychotherapist; there are no legal requirements to use this title. Many therapists practicing in the United States are either psychiatrists, social workers, or psychologists. All three do psychotherapy; only psychiatrists prescribe medication. Training within each of these groups varies widely; some clinicians in each category are highly trained while others have little specific training in the practice of psychotherapy. State licensing is required for each of these professions. This means that if you see a licensed psychiatrist, social worker, or psychologist, you have the reassurance of knowing that they have met some standard of education and ethical practice. However, the requirements are variable and merely being licensed is no proof of competence.

Generally speaking—but not always—more training is better than less, and training at a recognized and respected training institution is desirable. If you are attending a clinic where you are being seen by someone in training, this person should be supervised.

Avoid therapists who make extravagant claims for fast cures.

It is helpful if your therapist is somewhat knowledgeable about HIV disease and has some experience in treating patients who are HIV infected. You may be able to find such a therapist if you live in a large metropolitan area with a high incidence of HIV disease. If your therapist does not have experience in this area you may have to do some extra explaining in your therapy. Therapy can still be very helpful.

Homophobia is a problem that has dogged some areas of psychotherapy, particularly in the United States. If you are lesbian or gay, you need a psychotherapist who is not homophobic. This can be difficult to establish. As a minimum, reject any therapist who believes that homosexuality is a disease or maladjustment or who seems overtly insensitive to lesbian or gay issues.

If you have had problems with **substance abuse,** it is often helpful to find a therapist who specializes in this kind of problem. Generally, therapy in combination with some kind of "twelve step" program (on the model of Alcoholics Anonymous, or AA) is the treatment of choice.

You are entitled to **total confidentiality** from your therapist. This means that a therapist can never communicate any information about you to anyone without your explicit permission. This includes doctors, insurance companies, and family members. The only exception is if you are in danger of physically hurting yourself or someone else, in which case your therapist is required by law to communicate this information in order to prevent this.

There should never be any sexual activity between therapist and patient. Frank discussion of sex is part of many therapies, but sexual activity in therapy is always inappropriate. If this occurs in your therapy, you should discontinue therapy and report your therapist's behavior to the relevant professional organization.

Following is some information regarding various types of psychotherapy.

▲ Psychoanalysis and Psychoanalytically Oriented Psychotherapy

Psychoanalysis and psychoanalytically oriented psychotherapy (sometimes referred to as *psychodynamic* psychotherapy) are oriented toward change through increased understanding of the self. Basic concepts are the *unconscious* (feelings and ideas out of consciousness that affect one's ideas, emotions, and behavior) and the relationship between internal *conflicts* and the development of emotional distress and symptoms. The therapy consists of regular dialogue between you and your therapist during which you and the therapist seek a serious and complex understanding of your life.

There are several misconceptions about psychoanalytically oriented therapy. Psychoanalytically oriented psychotherapy focuses on your mental life and personal experiences. There is an inaccurate stereotype that this kind of therapy is interested only in the past and childhood experiences. This is not true. The goal of psychoanalytically oriented psychotherapy is to understand how your present view and experience of the world has been constructed. If this is clarified, then you are in a position to examine how well your view and interpretation of reality serves you at the present time. Change occurs through the development of this insight in the emotional context of a close involvement with another person, the therapist.

Another inaccurate stereotype is that psychoanalytically oriented psychotherapists never talk, but instead sit in stony and mysterious silence. This is not true. Psychoanalytically oriented therapists talk when they have something to say to further the goals of the therapy. They will not generally share details of their personal life, give advice, or chat. You can get advice and conversation from friends for free; psychotherapy follows particular rules in order to make it an effective vehicle for insight and change.

Psychoanalytic theory in its most important elements is not homophobic. However, in the United States, homophobic attitudes and theories are common. If you are gay, even subtle homophobic attitudes on the part of a therapist may adversely affect your treatment. You are entitled to ask an analyst some questions about his or her attitudes toward homosexuality.

Psychoanalytically oriented psychotherapists follow a certain method that has different rules from those of polite everyday social interaction. The implicit agreement that you make with your therapist is that you will **try to talk about *all* your thoughts and feelings,** however trivial, irrelevant, aggressive, embarrassing, or shameful they may seem to you. In return, your therapist will not hold you accountable for your thoughts. That is, the therapist will distinguish thoughts from actions and will not judge fantasies as if they were reality. The therapist expects that you may have hostile or sexual thoughts about him or her.

In psychoanalytically oriented therapy, **therapists provide emotional support by listening.** They do not give you advice, tell you how to live, make decisions for you, or interfere with your life. Nonetheless, this type of therapy can be extremely supportive. It is comforting and encouraging for many people to know that their therapist is attentive to the details of their illness and life. Many people with HIV disease find that it is difficult to get someone to listen to their more upsetting feelings and thoughts. In therapy, it is a relief to know that there is someone who is prepared to listen to an account of how you feel and what your life is like no matter how difficult your situation is and how painful your feelings are.

Frequency of therapy varies. However, generally speaking, people see psychoanalytically oriented therapists one to four times per week. Sessions usually last fifty minutes. Therapy may last a few months to deal with a crisis or can go on for some years to provide ongoing support and self-awareness. Social workers, psychologists, psychiatrists, and others function as psychotherapists. Psychoanalytic training is a valuable component of a therapist's education, although it is uncommon in some parts of this country.

▲ Family (or Couple) Therapy

Family therapy is psychological treatment aimed at helping a family or couple reach a better level of functioning. ("Family" can refer to your family of origin or to whatever group of people with whom you share your life.) A couple or members of a "family" meet regularly with a therapist. Many good family therapists combine psychoanalytic principles and an understanding of the individual in the context of family relationships.

If you experience difficulties in a relationship in the face of illness, then you and your partner may benefit from talking together to a therapist. For example, some couples find that seeing a therapist for a period of time is a good way to work out sexual problems that arise in a relationship or to discuss the troublesome issues of caretaking and support that may arise when illness is present. If you are closely involved with your family of origin, talking with a family therapist may help reduce tension for you and your family.

▲ Support Groups

Groups of people meeting together to discuss common issues have been particularly helpful to those with HIV disease. These groups can be run by a professional therapist, a peer counselor, or without a leader. One advantage of these groups is that in many locations they are available free of charge. They allow you a chance to talk about your situation with others who know firsthand about some of your problems. As with psychotherapy, you can gain a sense of being known and understood and a reliable place to go in times of crisis. Consult your local AIDS organizations for referral to such groups.

▲ Cognitive Therapy

Cognitive therapy is based on the theories of Aaron Beck. He believed that stereotyped thoughts lead to distortions in the way people see themselves and the world. This leads to "self-defeating" behavior. The therapy operates by identifying "negative cognitions." The patient is asked to understand when these occur and what assumptions they are based on. Cognitive therapy focuses on examining these assumptions and seeking a more accurate representation of the world and the self. Treatment is usually fifteen to twenty sessions over three months. Patients are usually given "homework" to do between sessions.

This type of therapy has been used with some success in treating depression. Cognitive therapy views depression as based on a "cognitive triad": a negative view of the self, a negative interpretation of past experience, and a negative view of the future.

▲ Behavioral Therapy

Behavioral therapy is based on the position that behavior can be changed without any effort to understand its underlying causes.

Behavioral therapy has been used with some success to treat certain kinds of anxieties (such as fear of flying). It works best when used with specific problems such as quitting smoking and overcoming phobias or compulsions. One kind of behavior therapy operates by "desensitizing" the patient. Desensitization involves exposing the patient to anxiety-provoking stimuli so that the patient may gradually learn to overcome them.

You should be aware that a form of behavioral therapy called *aversion therapy* has at times been misused to attempt to forcibly change a homosexual orientation to a heterosexual orientation.

On the positive side, techniques based in behavioral therapy have inspired useful methods for relaxation and stress reduction such as biofeedback.

MEDICATION

Medication can sometimes provide enormous relief from specific symptoms of emotional distress. This is particularly true with certain kinds of depression and anxiety. Medications that affect you psychologically are called *psychotropic* drugs or *psychoactive* drugs.

Some people have unrealistic fears regarding psychoactive drugs. Common fears include the notion that taking medication means that you are "crazy," that medication will sedate you into being a zombie, change your identity as a person, or disarm appropriate anger at social injustice. These fears are unrealistic. Psychoactive drugs are appropriate for people with wide ranges of problems, not just people who are "crazy." People who are generally well-functioning psychologically can have transient periods of extreme anxiety or depression, particularly when confronting the stress of HIV disease. There is no reason why you should suffer such distress when safe, effective medication can reduce the burden you have been forced to carry.

While some drugs used to treat severely disturbed people are sedating, the drugs normally prescribed for milder problems are not. Drugs used to treat depression restore you to normal mood rather than blunting or blurring all feelings. Antianxiety medications restore normal calmness without robbing you of emotion or passion.

Like other drugs, psychoactive medications have some side effects. These side effects are typically noticeable only at the beginning of a course of medication and disappear after a few weeks. When prescribed correctly, psychoactive drugs do not dull your intelligence or your ability to perceive reality. Anxiety and depression inhibit your ability to see the world clearly and act effectively. By reducing anxiety and depression, drugs help some people clarify their thinking and become more active.

One healthy asymptomatic HIV-infected man was suffering from panic attacks (extreme anxiety, sobbing, palpitations, the sensation that he could not get enough air to breathe, and the conviction that he was about to die). These attacks would occur several times each week and last for a few hours. He was prescribed antianxiety medication, which relieved the panic attacks. He described the experience as follows:

I used to feel as if I were in a closed room filled with water. In order to breathe I had to stand on tiptoe and stretch my neck to stick my nose out to get air. I felt overwhelmed by the struggle. The drug didn't change anything really. It just lowered the water level to the point that I could stand normally and breathe easily. It didn't take my problems away—it just made them easier to stand.

You can learn about medical and social issues, be active politically, understand yourself better psychologically, *and* take medication to alleviate symptoms. These activities are all compatible. The combination that will be helpful to you depends on your social situation, health, access to care, and particular emotional needs. The mix of strategies you use to improve your state of mind is likely to evolve over time in response to changing circumstances.

Everyone is anxious or depressed sometimes. If you have HIV disease, you may have good reason to be anxious or depressed. No drug can make this go away entirely. **However, when anxiety or depression becomes very intense and interferes with your daily life for a protracted period of time, the use of psychoactive medication may help reduce suffering.** Medication is not a substitute for human contact or talking with lovers, families, friends, in support groups or psychotherapy.

To decide whether you should seek professional help with anxiety or depression, consider the extent and duration of your anxiety or depression, its interference with functioning, its potential for danger, and the degree of suffering it causes. If the anxiety or depression is not so bad as to interfere with functioning but it goes on for months and makes you miserable, seek help. If it is very severe, is a major interference with functioning, or causes you to do something self-destructive, get help promptly.

Effective medication depends on correct diagnosis. Diagnosis of psychological symptoms requires specialized training. There are a multitude of perspectives on the cause and development of symptoms and consequently a variety of diagnostic classifications in use. All diagnoses are artificial constructs developed to increase technical understanding of emotional problems: their origin, cause, course, development, prognosis, and treatment. In the United States today, medication for psychological symptoms is commonly prescribed using diagnostic categories defined by the American Psychiatric Association (APA). These categories are published in the APA *Diagnostic and Statistical Manual, Version III, Revised* and are therefore known as *DSM-III-R* criteria. *DSM-III-R* criteria do not capture the richness of mental and emotional life, but they are useful in determining whether currently available medications might reduce your symptoms and, if so, which medications should be tried. We will discuss medication for anxiety and depression primarily in terms of *DSM-III-R* diagnostic criteria.

Prescription of psychoactive drugs requires experience. The issue of dosage is critical, and the choice of effective drugs can be subtle. **It is important to see a psychiatrist who is well trained and up-to-date on the use of psychoactive drugs.** You may want to consult a psychiatrist who specializes in the use of such medications, called a *psychopharmacologist.*

145

Psychopharmacologists are more likely to choose the most suitable drug for you and are more likely to prescribe appropriate doses. They are trained to have an organized strategy to try different drugs if the first is not successful.

Sometimes physicians who are not psychiatrists may prescribe antidepressants or antianxiety medication. Physicians (and even some psychiatrists) inexperienced with medication sometimes prescribe antidepressant or antianxiety drugs at doses that are too low. This may mean that the drug never has a chance to work or takes a long time to build up to a therapeutic dose. Nonspecialists may also give up if the first medication does not work.

Consultation for medication generally involves several closely spaced visits (usually weekly) with a psychiatrist while you start medication, and then occasional more widely spaced visits to monitor your progress on the drug. Your contact with the psychiatrist need not necessarily be as frequent or regular as visits for psychotherapy.

If you are seeing a psychotherapist who is a psychiatrist, she or he may do both the psychotherapy and the drug therapy. If your therapist is a psychiatric social worker or psychologist, you may also see a psychiatrist for consultation about medication and periodic checkups. Your therapist and psychiatrist should consult with each other.

A psychiatrist or psychopharmacologist who has experience in treating patients with HIV disease will give you the best advice. This is less important if you are physically asymptomatic and more important if you have major medical symptoms.

Most drugs, both therapeutic and recreational, can cause depression, anxiety, or problems with thinking on rare occasions: this includes alcohol or alcohol withdrawal, amphetamines, cocaine, and most of the drugs used to treat HIV disease. In addition, a number of diseases can adversely affect mood and thinking. Depression or anxiety caused by a medical problem is treated by treating the underlying problem, if possible. At times, it is also appropriate to use psychoactive drugs to relieve symptoms in addition to treating the underlying illness. Keep track of the time of your anxiety in relationship to development of infections or other symptoms or use of new medication.

If you see a psychiatrist for a medication consultation, you should be able to give him or her a clear picture of your current and past illnesses and medications. It is useful to have the psychiatrist talk to your physician, especially if the psychiatrist does not have extensive experience in treating people with HIV disease.

▲ Depression

To feel depressed is a common experience. People describe it as feeling unhappy, down, blue, sad, or hopeless. Following are guidelines about when to consider seeing a psychiatrist to get medication for depression.

Again, this is likely to work best in combination with some kind of talk therapy or group support.

One of the common symptoms of depression is a feeling of hopelessness. If you are seriously depressed, you may feel that it is impossible to get any help and that you will never feel better. You may feel that you have always been in this mental state. This hopelessness can lead to failure to get help. If friends comment on your depression or suggest that you get professional help, take them seriously.

If your symptoms fit the *DSM-III-R* criteria of "major depressive disorder," talk to a psychiatrist about the possibility of medication. Depressive disorders are also referred to as *affective disorders.*

Basic criteria for **major depression** are (literally) one symptom from column A and four symptoms from column B, lasting for at least two weeks.

CRITERIA FOR MAJOR DEPRESSION

One from Column A	Four from Column B
• Feeling depressed most of the day and almost every day. (Down, sad, blue, hopeless.) It can evolve gradually over a few weeks or suddenly after great stress, *or* • Loss of interest and pleasure in things that are usually interesting and pleasurable; this can be partial or complete. Some people may not be able to feel better no matter what the circumstances; others may periodically respond to positive things by feeling better.	• Loss of appetite and/or weight loss without dieting or medical cause, or increase in appetite and/or undesired weight gain. • Insomnia (Waking up early and not being able to fall back asleep; difficulty falling asleep). Sleeping too much. This happens to everyone from time to time. It can be a symptom of depression if it is persistent. • Being slowed down physically or mentally. You and other people notice that it takes you longer than usual to accomplish activities. • Being agitated (restless, can't sit still, pacing, wringing hands, rubbing head). • Fatigue, loss of enegy. • Feeling excessively guilty or worthless. • Difficulty in concentrating. Feeling that your thinking is slowed down. Increased difficulty in making small decisions. • Persistent thoughts about suicide.

You may find that you are skipping days of work or not going to work. If you are a student, you may stop studying. You may avoid friends or your usual social activities, hobbies, or recreations. You may neglect yourself physically (in terms of grooming and hygiene). You may forget things. You may cry a lot or feel like crying without knowing why. You may get into arguments easily. If someone in your immediate family has had an episode of severe depression, you face an increased risk of developing this kind of depression.

All of these symptoms can be caused by various medical problems. If there is an underlying physical cause, the first step is to diagnose and treat the illness. However, whether or not an underlying medical problem can be identified, psychoactive medication may still be useful.

Dysthymic disorder is a term used in psychiatry to describe an ongoing depression that may not be as severe as a major depressive disorder, but is chronic, often lasting for years—and, for some people, as long as they can remember.

The symptoms may be similar to that of major depressive disorder, but milder—that is, fewer and less severe symptoms. The diagnosis is usually made when the symptoms have lasted for at least two years.

According to *DSM-III-R,* dysthymia requires that you feel depressed most of the time on most days, and that, while depressed, at least two of the following symptoms be present:

• Poor appetite or overeating
• Difficulty sleeping or sleeping too much
• Low energy or fatigue
• Low self-esteem
• Poor concentration or difficulty making decisions
• Feeling hopeless

Medication for major depressive disorder is extremely effective. In the general population, this kind of depression when untreated typically lasts for many months. Use of medication can dramatically shorten this suffering. In general, two thirds of patients with a major depressive disorder will respond positively to the use of medication within two weeks to two months. Most of the rest will get better when they try other antidepressants. Major depression is one of the most treatable of medical conditions. In recent years, cyclic antidepressants have been successfully used to treat dysthymic disorders.

Antidepressants belong to several different categories. Although much is known about the effects of these drugs in the body, the mechanism of antidepressant action is not clearly known. It is thought that they work by their effects on the function of certain neurotransmitters (chemical messengers) in the brain.

A group of drugs referred to as *cyclic antidepressants* are the most commonly used for treating major depressive episodes. They are extremely effective.

These cyclic antidepressant medications vary primarily by side effects. Some are more sedative than others—that is, they make you feel sleepy or fall asleep. This can be useful if you are suffering from insomnia or troubling if it interferes with your daily activities.

These drugs have what are referred to as *anticholinergic* side effects, some drugs more than others. These side effects include dry mouth, constipation, blurred near vision, and difficulty in urinating. Dry mouth is the most frequent symptom. It can be alleviated by sucking on hard candies (preferably sugar-free ones for the sake of your teeth).

Sometimes cyclic antidepressants cause a drop in blood pressure associated with change in posture that can lead to fainting or dizziness. This is referred to as *orthostatic hypotension.* Standing up slowly after being in a prone position can help prevent this.

People with a few specific cardiac problems should avoid the use of cyclic antidepressants. These conditions are *bifascilar block, left bundle branch block,* or a *prolonged QT interval.* Your psychopharmacologist will help you avoid any medication that might be dangerous.

The following cyclic antidepressants have the fewest anticholinergic side effects:

- Desipramine (Norpramin)
- Nortriptyline (Pamelor, Aventyl)
- Protriptyline (Vivactil)

Desipramine is probably the least sedating of the cyclic antidepressants. It is often the first choice among the cyclic antidepressant drugs for several reasons. It has a good history of efficacy and safety and relatively few side effects. It can be monitored in the blood with blood tests to determine if a therapeutic level is being reached. In addition, it is a relatively inexpensive drug because it is available generically.

The following drugs do not usually make you sleepy or give you dry mouth or constipation. However, they can increase the possibility of developing seizures. For this reason they should not be used in people with a prior seizure disorder, certain metabolic dysfunctions or a cerebral mass lesion, or who are withdrawing from benzodiazepines (such as Valium). They are rarely the first choice of antidepressant drugs.

- Amoxapine (Asendin)
- Maprotiline (Ludiomil)

Amitriptyline (Elavil) is one of the most sedating of these drugs and causes the most severe anticholinergic side effects (such as dry mouth) and orthostatic hypotension (lowered blood pressure leading to dizziness).

Other similar drugs that usually cause fewer of these problems are:

- Imipramine (Tofranil)
- Trimipramine (Surmontil)
- Doxepin (Sinequan)

Trazadone (Desyrel) is the most sedating of the cyclic drugs and is useful for treating severe insomnia. It is sometimes used in combination with other antidepressant medication to treat insomnia.

Monoamine oxidase inhibitors (MAOIs) are usually used in patients who have not responded to other antidepressant drugs. They are not usually the first choice but can be very effective. They seem to work well in certain patients who are considered to have atypical depressions. They are particularly useful for people who have depression combined with panic disorder, although other antidepressants work for this purpose also. The following MAOIs have comparable effectiveness and similar side effects. If one does not work, another may.

- Tranylcypromine (Parnate)
- Phenelzine (Nardil)
- Isocarboxazid (Marplan)

MAOIs have significant side effects. They provoke dangerously high blood pressure when combined with a substance known as *tyramine,* which is contained in some food, beverages, and drugs. If you take MAOIs you must entirely avoid cheese, liver, cheese pizza, Chianti wine, beer, herring, bologna and some other sausages, and a number of other foods as well as many cough and cold medications. Any meat you eat must be fresh. Coffee and chocolate should be consumed only in small amounts. If you are taking holistic remedies for HIV disease and do not know their ingredients, avoid MAOIs or stop taking the holistic remedy. If you take MAOIs you must get a dietary restriction list from your doctor. If you eat a "forbidden" food with no problem, you may still develop a severe reaction if you eat that food again.

Other antidepressants: Fluoxetine (Prozac) is a newer drug that is now widely used because it seems very effective and has fewer side effects. It is used for treating both major depressive episodes and dysthymic disorder. It does not cause sedation, weight gain, dry mouth, or constipation. It can cause nervousness and insomnia, restlessness, and increased gastrointestinal activity.

Bupropion (Wellbutrin) generally has mild side effects and is not sedating. It may cause mild anxiety, sleep difficulties, insomnia, or nausea. It sometimes exacerbates the risk of seizure disorder if central nervous system lesions or certain metabolic abnormalities are present.

General comments: Antidepressant medications are usually taken for at least six to nine months. The drug dose is usually started low and built up. Major improvement should occur in two to six weeks after taking a therapeutic dose of the drug; do not expect it to work immediately. If one antidepressant does not work, another (especially from a different category) may be effective. Inadequate dosage or inadequate length of time on the drug is the most common cause of treatment failure. There is no evidence that use of antidepressant medication suppresses the immune system.

A number of antidepressant medications cause sexual side effects such as delayed orgasm, difficulty in achieving orgasm, and decreased interest in sex. These problems often disappear after a period of time on the medication. Be sure to inform your psychiatrist of any such problem.

Psychostimulants: Amphetamine (Dexedrine and generic) and methylphenidate (Ritalin) seem useful in medically ill patients, especially those who are withdrawn and apathetic, and in depressed people in general who do not respond to other medication. They are generally not used in depressed people who are medically asymptomatic. They are energizing and work more rapidly than cyclic depressants or MAOIs. Dexedrine appears to be more effective than Ritalin.

Side effects are jitters, insomnia, and loss of appetite. When used for recreational purposes, these drugs have a high potential for abuse and addiction, which is why they are not widely prescribed. This problem may be outweighed by their utility in seriously ill patients (those with major symptomatic medical problems). An overdose may lead to paranoid episodes with loss of ability to judge reality.

▲ Mania and Bipolar Disorder

Mania, like depression, is a disorder of mood, an affective disorder. It presents itself as a state of extreme excitement, euphoria, or intense irritability. Some patients who have serious depressions at other times have manic episodes. This is referred to as a *manic-depressive illness* or *bipolar affective disorder.* Mania is not nearly as frequent as depression. Bipolar affective disorder, like other affective disorders, seems to be inheritable.

Symptoms are:

• Elevated, expansive, or irritable mood
• Being highly talkative, racing thoughts, a decreased need for sleep, increased activity, agitation, distractability, poor judgment about spending money, unrealistic planning, grandiosity, and hypersexuality

When these symptoms are severe, interfere on an extended basis with work or daily life or require hospitalization, the disorder is classified as mania. If the symptoms are less severe, it is classified as *hypomania.*

Mania and hypomania can be caused by a number of medical problems and side effects of medication. Some drugs that cause mania or hypomania are amphetamines, cocaine, and steroids. There have also been rare reports of syndromes resulting from AZT that resemble mania. Any infection or cancer that affects the brain and causes organic mental disorder can manifest itself as mania or hypomania. Treating the illness or discontinuing the medication that causes the symptoms is the first order of business. Medication is commonly used for helping people through acute mania.

As with depression, your ability to assess the need for treatment may be impaired. Try to listen to your friends.

Drugs that are used to treat mania: For people who have a pattern of manic and depressive episodes, bipolar disorder, a drug called lithium is often very helpful. It can be used in combination with antidepressants to help someone in the depressed state of bipolar illness. Other medications that are used to treat bipolar disorder are carbamazepine (Tegretol), valproate (Depakote), and clonazepam (Klonopin).

For treating acute mania (and sometimes chronic mania), drugs of the neuroleptic category can be used, especially during the initial period of treatment. These include haloperidol (Haldol) or Mellaril, Prolixin, Trilafon, Stelazine.

▲ Anxiety

Almost everyone has had the experience of being anxious. It is sometimes referred to as nervousness, being upset, being freaked out, or "losing it." It is characterized by worry, restlessness, a sense of emotional discomfort, and is often accompanied by a variety of physical signs.

Transitory anxiety is part of everyday life, especially in response to stress. The question is whether anxiety is severe enough or frequent enough to merit treatment with medication.

The psychiatric definition of various anxiety disorders (according to *DSM-III-R*) states that the anxiety is not a response to an immediate situation or that the anxiety is unrealistic or excessive. However, this aspect of the definition of anxiety is confusing and in the end probably not very useful. For example, how much anxiety is unrealistic or excessive when you are told you have AIDS? Having HIV disease puts you in a chronically anxiety-provoking situation, with many occasions for more acute anxiety.

Most people respond to bad news with a period of anxiety. This is not a sign of abnormality or instability. Give yourself time to feel better. It usually helps not to be alone during a period of anxiety. Spend time with friends, especially people with whom you can talk openly. If possible, distract yourself. If possible, try to avoid major decisions or changes while you are acutely anxious. Take care of yourself: try to rest, eat, and exercise. However, a sleepless night or a period of feeling unable to eat will not do you any lasting medical harm.

Following are situations when you may want to consider medication:

A *panic attack* is an episode of extremely severe and disabling anxiety, often accompanied by physical symptoms. Occasional panic attacks are very common; probably 20 percent of people will at some point in their lives have one or more panic attacks. They are often referred to as *anxiety attacks.*

If you have multiple panic attacks, this is referred to in *DSM-III-R* terms as ***panic disorder.*** Some of the criteria for panic disorder according to *DSM-III-R* are:

• A discrete period of extreme fear, sense of impending disaster

This is associated with a few of the following physical symptoms:

• Shortness of breath or a feeling of smothering or choking
• Dizziness, fainting
• Rapid or pounding heart beat
• Trembling or shaking
• Excessive sweating
• Nausea or stomachache
• Numbness or tingling in hands or legs
• Hot flashes or chills
• A feeling that you are unreal or your physical surroundings are unreal
• Fear of losing control
• An inexplicable conviction that you are about to drop dead or go crazy

These symptoms escalate rapidly over a short period of time—usually just a few minutes. The peak of the anxiety may last up to a half-hour and leftover feelings of nervousness may last for up to a few hours. Some people wake up from sleep with a full blown panic attack (particularly a feeling of being unable to breathe) and may not have them at other times.

These panic attacks respond well to medication. (See below for specifics). The experience of a panic attack is very unpleasant. If you have multiple panic attacks, you might become generally fearful of recurrence. This is referred to as "anticipatory panic" and may lead you to avoid situations in which they might occur. This is a destructive cycle and is an important reason to seek help early on.

Anxiety can appear in many other forms. What other types of common anxiety might be helped with the use of medication? Anxiety that is less severe and episodic than panic attacks can often be helped with medication.

Although less intense than panic attacks, this anxiety is also often accompanied by physical signs including trembling, muscle tension, fatigue, shortness of breath, dizziness, sleep problems, and difficulty in concentrating. For our purposes, we will not separate further the various technical diagnostic categories for anxiety other than panic disorder.

If you are HIV infected, you may find that you may develop extreme anxiety at times of increased stress. Examples of this kind of stress are finding out that you are HIV infected, waiting for T4 cell test results or other test results, being given a diagnosis of some illness, going to the hospital, or dealing with a friend's death from AIDS.

We are not suggesting that the only or best response to this kind of stress is to take medication. Often, acute anxiety reactions go away on their own with a little time. Turning to a good support system in times of stress is the most effective way of dealing with short-term anxiety. However, occasional use of medication for severe anxiety can alleviate suffering and have very few side effects. Medications used to treat this kind of anxiety include benzodiazepines and buspirone (Buspar).

The first choice for treating panic disorders are drugs that are often referred to as antidepressants. This may seem surprising. They were developed for use in treating depression but turned out to be effective in preventing panic attacks. They are suitable for people who have had multiple episodes of panic because they function as prophylaxis rather than treatment for an acute episode. It may take several weeks for antidepressants to stop anxiety attacks.

Antidepressant drugs are not addictive. Side effects are generally few after you are accustomed to the drug. Both cyclic antidepressants and monoamine oxidase inhibitors (MAOIs) can be used; generally cyclic antidepressants are first choice because they are easier to use. The drug most extensively studied is imipramine (Tofranil), but most of the drugs in this category are probably equally effective. Other commonly used antidepressant drugs for anxiety are desipramine (Norpramine) or nortryptiline (Pamelor, Aventyl).

The most commonly used antianxiety drugs are benzodiazepines. There are many different types of this drug available in the United States including diazepam (Valium), lorazepam (Ativan), chlordiazeapoxide (Librium), alprazolam (Xanax), oxazepam (Serax), temazepam (Restoril), flurazepam (Dalmane), triazolam (Halcion) among others.

In general these drugs are fairly safe—that is, it is hard to take a dangerous overdose either purposely or accidentally. However, they can be dangerous when taken in combination with alcohol. They may not be a good choice if you are having breathing difficulties or if you have been diagnosed with AIDS dementia complex (see Chapter 10: Organ System Complications), because they may exacerbate these problems.

The advantage of benzodiazepines is that they rapidly lessen the symptoms of anxiety. They do not have to be taken on an ongoing basis and are a good choice for a very anxious short-term reaction to anxiety-provoking events.

Using benzodiazepines for a few days may help you get over a difficult period of anxiety. They are also appropriate for sporadic use when you know in advance that you will be in an anxiety-provoking situation. For example, taking a benzodiazepine would be appropriate if you become anxious after being told of the diagnosis of an opportunistic infection, or if you were very anxious about an upcoming doctor's visit.

If you are having occasional disturbing anxiety in response to particular stresses, you might ask your physician for a prescription for a limited amount of benzodiazepines to use from time to time when you develop extreme anxiety or anticipate that you will be in a situation that will cause extreme anxiety. You have to be careful not to use these drugs too often, because they can be habit forming. (See below.)

If you can afford a consultation with a psychiatrist, this is the best way to get the most appropriate antianxiety medication for your particular needs. Your regular medical doctor may prescribe these medications, but if you are using them for a prolonged period, you should definitely get a consultation with a psychiatrist because you may not be taking the right drug.

The side effects of benzodiazepines are relatively few and consist mostly of sleepiness and difficulty in concentrating and occasionally loss of balance. However, there is a major disadvantage to the use of benzodiazepines. These drugs may be habit forming. It appears generally to take several months of daily use in order to develop dependency, but dependency can sometimes occur more quickly. Withdrawal after long-term use can lead to multiple symptoms including increased anxiety, insomnia, tremor, and even, in severe cases, seizures. Because of this potential for addiction and because the benefits of these drugs diminish with continuing use, these drugs should be used only for short-term or periodic use. If you have used these drugs on a regular daily basis for at least several weeks, you should taper off carefully and with the advice of a physician. If withdrawn properly, stopping the use of benzodiazepines should not be a problem.

These drugs vary somewhat in the side effects they produce, the difficulties of withdrawal they present, the length of time they take to work, how long they continue working, and the tendency to accumulate in the body. A psychiatrist must take into account all of these factors in figuring out which is the best benzodiazepine with which to treat you.

For example, one of the benzodiazepines that is widely used now is clonazepam (Klonopin). The advantage of clonazepam (Klonopin) is that the sedating effects are low, the drug does not leave you feeling hung-over and it needs to be taken only twice a day. On the other hand, if your anxiety is particularly marked by difficulty sleeping, you may do better with a more sedating medication taken before bed.

Buspirone (Buspar) is another drug, not a benzodiazepine, that is used to treat generalized anxiety disorders. Unlike benzodiazepines, Buspar is not addictive. It is not sedating and has minimal effects on ability to think clearly and react rapidly. Unfortunately, Buspar is not effective for many people and must be taken three times a day to be effective. Buspar is not particularly helpful for insomnia.

Some drugs should almost always be avoided. Secobarbitol (Seconal), phenobarbitol (Nembutol), and glutethimide (Doriden) have been used to treat anxiety in the past but now should rarely be used to treat anxiety. These drugs are much more addictive than the benzodiazepines and lethal overdose is easier than with benzodiazepines. Some of them are used to treat other medical conditions.

▲ Sleep Problems

Anxiety, depression, and medical illness are common causes of sleep problems. Another frequent cause of sleep disturbance may be a movement disorder such as "restless leg syndrome." You may not be aware of such movement disorders. Consequently, the way to lessen insomnia is to reduce anxiety and depression or to treat the movement disorder. Physical illness and many medications (including AZT) interfere with sleep. It is always hard to sort out the role of anxiety from the side effects of medication.

Following are some practical things you can try if you are having trouble falling asleep or staying asleep:

- Avoid alcohol and other recreational drugs; they can interfere with sleep.
- Reduce caffeine as much as possible. Caffeine is in coffee, tea, and cola drinks.
- Go to bed and get up at approximately the same time each day. An erratic sleeping schedule can make it difficult to sleep.
- Exercise during the day—this frequently improves sleep.
- Avoid daytime naps.
- Make your bedroom as comfortable as possible: cool temperature, comfortable bed.
- Use ear plugs if noise disturbs you.
- Use your bed for sleep and sex only. Do not read or watch television in bed.
- If you cannot fall asleep after half an hour, get out of bed and do something else for a while. If you lie in bed and worry about your insomnia, your bed becomes a place to worry rather than a place to sleep.

Medication plays a limited role in the treatment of sleep disorders. A major drawback of sleep medications is that the benefits usually diminish over time. In addition, after you stop sleep medication you may have increased insomnia or anxiety for a few days. Sleep medication should be used only on a short-term basis; you should not take sleeping pills on a regular daily basis for more than three weeks.

The first choice for sleep medication is a benzodiazepine that works quickly and has an appropriate duration of action so that it does not leave you feeling hungover or sleepy. Such medications include temazepam (Restoril), lorazepam (Ativan), flurazepam (Dalmane), and triazolam (Halcion).

Triazolam (Halcion) is the most widely used sleeping pill in this country because it does not cause a sleepy feeling on the following day.

However, it appears that Halcion may cause more memory problems than other benzodiazepines. There have also been reports of violent behavior and psychosis with the use of Halcion. There is not sufficient evidence to indicate whether Halcion was the cause of these behaviors.

While all sleep medications have some potential for addiction, when used properly and under a psychiatrist's supervision, addiction is uncommon. However if the decision is made to stop these drugs and they have been used on a regular daily basis for several weeks, they should be tapered off rather than abruptly stopped in order to avoid withdrawal symptoms.

▲ Pain

The drugs most commonly used to relieve mild pain are aspirin (acetylsalicylic acid, ASA), acetaminophen (Tylenol), and ibuprofen (Advil or Motrin). Unlike narcotics, these pain relievers do not work on the central nervous system. These drugs are available without prescription and have few side effects. They can cause problems when used in very large quantities. Ringing in the ears while taking aspirin is a sign of overdose.

The most effective medications for serious pain are narcotics, drugs that come from opium or resemble it. The most commonly used narcotics are codeine, morphine, and demerol. These pain medications are addictive. However, they do work to reduce pain. Narcotics frequently cause sleepiness, lethargy, and constipation. Pain medication must be correlated with your weight; bigger people need more pain medication.

Many studies have indicated that physicians underestimate the amount of pain medication needed to control pain and overestimate the danger of addiction. Consequently, many patients are routinely and unnecessarily undermedicated for pain. You should take the question of addiction seriously but without overemphasizing it or ignoring other factors. Prolonged or severe physical pain is demoralizing and debilitating. **You may have to be assertive in order to get pain medication; do not let your doctor or pharmacist make you feel like a "junkie" if you ask for pain medication.** Studies in which patients essentially control the amount of pain medication they use suggest that this method is effective and does not lead to abuse. Some people feel worse, with a sense of loss of control, from these drugs than they do from the pain. It is your choice whether to use pain medication.

It is a good idea to take pain medication prior to the development of severe pain, if this is predictable. It is more effective and requires lower doses.

If you are hospitalized, ask in advance about the pain medication ordered for you. Nurses need your physician's written permission in the chart to give you certain pain medications. Find out whether the pain medication will be given to you on a regular basis or whether you have to ask for it. If the latter is the case, find out how frequently you can get it.

157

Be sure you ask your physician at the beginning of a hospitalization if there is a pain-medication order for you in the chart. Otherwise, it will be difficult to get pain medication if your doctor is not available.

If you are suffering a great deal of pain and suspect that you are not being adequately medicated, ask for a consultation with a liaison/consultation psychiatrist. These are psychiatrists who specialize in helping people with medical illnesses. They are usually well informed about pain medication.

For **chronic moderate pain,** some people have found relief with the use of the cyclic antidepressant amitryptiline. This is can be useful for neuropathy. Usually a considerably lower dose is used than when the drug is taken to treat depression.

▲ Other Techniques for Countering Anxiety, Sleep Problems, and Pain

A number of other methods have been very useful to some people in reducing anxiety, sleep problems, and pain. These methods include hypnosis, acupuncture, meditations, massage, and various relaxation techniques. These methods are often referred to as "alternative" or "non-Western" treatment because many of their roots lie in ancient and respected traditions of other cultures.

It is beyond the scope of this book to describe or evaluate these treatments in any depth. You may be able to get referrals from your local AIDS service organization.

The advantages of these techniques are that they have few or no side effects and often increase a sense of well-being and control. They do not conflict with the use of any of the medications described above. Many people find it a relief to do something to help themselves that is outside the inconveniences and frustration of the medical care system.

Many of these techniques require time to learn and put into effective use. For example, hypnosis has been used by some people to control nausea that may occur as a side effect of medication. In order to do so, you usually need to spend some weeks in learning and practicing the technique before you can put it into use. This requires some planning ahead. If you are going to use either hypnosis or acupuncture, make sure that your treatment is done by a licensed practitioner.

Chapter 8
Sex, Age, Race, and Ethnicity

In the United States the majority of people diagnosed with AIDS so far have been white (Caucasian ethnicity). In addition, over 90 percent of people with AIDS in this country have been adult males. Even if one were to ignore the effects of racism and sexism, these statistics imply that most physicians' experience of HIV disease has been among white male adults. Activists have pointed out that research and health care must include women, children, and people of color. Both fairness and pragmatism motivate this inclusion, since these groups represent a steadily increasing proportion of new cases of AIDS. (For example, people of color represented 51 percent of new cases of AIDS reported in New York City in 1991.)

Most of the information presented elsewhere in this book is relevant to all HIV-infected people, independent of sex, age, and race or ethnicity. This chapter presents some medical information specifically relevant to women, children, and people of color.

WOMEN WITH HIV

In 1991 women accounted for 10 percent of cases of AIDS in the United States. AIDS is the fifth leading cause of death among women aged 15 to 44 in this country. It is the leading cause of death among women of color in New York and New Jersey and the leading cause of death for all women aged 30 to 34 in New York City. Yet, AIDS is still often seen as exclusively a men's disease. If you are a woman who has had unprotected vaginal or rectal intercourse or who has shared needles, you have some risk for HIV infection. If medical care is available, you may want to get the HIV antibody test so that you can benefit from medical treatment if infected.

▲ Undercounting of Women With AIDS

The Centers for Disease Control (CDC) developed the formal diagnostic definition of AIDS by observing symptoms that occurred in the first cases—which in the United States happened to occur in men. Because of this historical accident, some conditions that should probably be AIDS-defining for women have not been counted as AIDS. For example, cervical cancer and persistent severe vaginal candidiasis in HIV-infected women indicate profound immune suppression and yet as of early 1992 do not officially confer a diagnosis of AIDS. Some women have died of HIV-related problems without meeting the formal governmental definition of AIDS: these women have not been counted as cases of AIDS.

More and more women are diagnosed with AIDS every year, even under the current definition. Yet, women remain underdiagnosed and undercounted in AIDS figures. Women undeniably sick with HIV-related illness but who lack a formal diagnosis of AIDS may be denied financial benefits or the chance to participate in studies of experimental drugs. These problems may be solved if the Centers for Disease Control alter the criteria for diagnosis with AIDS to depend on underlying immune deficiency as measured by T4 cell count rather than on specific diseases or symptoms.

▲ Information Lacking on Nongynecologic Clinical Differences

There is little information available about special medical issues for HIV-infected women. This is due partly to the inherent demographics of the disease and partly to racism and sexism. Ten percent of people with AIDS are women—90 percent are men. In this country, most women with HIV are impoverished women of color who historically have received inadequate health care. In addition, women are underrepresented in almost all areas of medical research.

The differences between women and men in survival, course, and response to treatment are unclear. Some studies have shown that women have a shorter survival time after an AIDS diagnosis than do men; other studies have disagreed. If women have shorter survival time than men it is probably because of social rather than biological differences. Generally, women are sicker at the time of diagnosis than men with AIDS because, as a group, women with AIDS are poorer than men. Poorer people are not well connected to the health care system and so get medical care later in the disease. At this point, women with HIV are sicker for many reasons related to poverty: infectious disease, malnutrition, poor health care, and multiple medical problems due to nonsterile intravenous drug use.

Large studies intended to document the ordinary progress of HIV disease have been done entirely among men and may not reflect how the disease operates in women. It is possible that a woman's sex may affect her course of illness and response to treatment. Estrogen and progesterone production are different in men and women and these hormones affect the functioning of the immune system. In addition, the relation of HIV to gynecological issues such as sexually transmitted diseases and cancers is not well understood.

No systematic studies have been done to see whether the incidence of any **nongynecological opportunistic infections** is higher in one sex than the other. Clinical experience suggests that women have an increased incidence of esophageal candidiasis. Kaposi's sarcoma is rare outside men who have sex with men, and particularly rare among women. As with men, most women with AIDS are first diagnosed because of an episode of PCP. No difference in the course (as opposed to incidence) of opportunistic infections has yet been reported, but data are limited.

Few women are studied as subjects in drug trials generally. This is also true of studies of drugs used to treat HIV disease. Drugs may have different effects on women. Without specific data on women, results from drug trials on male subjects may not apply. For example, anemia is more common among healthy women than among healthy men. Thus, women may have more hematological problems with AZT and other drugs, but existing studies provide no solid information.

Pregnancy and paternalism: Sometimes researchers design trials that explicitly exclude women. Some researchers argue that a female subject may become pregnant, and that the experimental drug may endanger the fetus. This argument infringes on women's autonomy. Women have a right to choose to undergo the possible risks and benefits of an experimental drug trial.

Women are seen as less reliable subjects. Poor, minority, or drug-using experimental subjects are perceived as unreliable or uncooperative. Since the majority of HIV-infected women at this point are poor or have a history of drug use, this perception contributes to the exclusion of women from trials.

In addition, **trial design lacks features necessary to attract women.** Few studies have provided services such as child care that would allow impoverished women to participate as subjects. Neglect of such considerations effectively denies this population access to trials.

▲ Specific Gynecological Issues

Despite the current lack of information about HIV disease in women, there are ways to improve your situation if you are an HIV-infected woman. You need thorough and regular gynecological care. Try to find a gynecologist who is experienced in treating HIV-infected women or who at least is willing to learn. Several problems specific to HIV-infected women are outlined below.

Candida albicans is a type of fungus called a yeast. It is always present in the body in small amounts, but is usually kept under control by the immune system. Candida can sometimes grow and cause problems, even in people with healthy immune systems. This is particularly common in the vulva and vagina. Symptoms of ordinary vaginal candidiasis are itching and irritation of the vulva and vagina, and a small amount of cottage cheese-like white discharge. **Ordinarily, vaginal candidiasis improves either spontaneously or with medication.**

Candida causes a variety of problems among people with immune impairment. In HIV disease candida can appear in the mouth, the esophagus, the vagina, or elsewhere. Several studies have shown a high rate of vaginal candidiasis among women who are HIV infected. **HIV-related vaginal candidiasis can be much more persistent and severe than** vaginal candidiasis among healthy women. It has been reported that symptoms of vaginal candidiasis among HIV-infected women have been painful enough to interfere with walking.

The first time you develop symptoms of vaginal candidiasis, see a physician to get an accurate diagnosis. Because vaginal candidiasis often occurs among HIV-negative women and because HIV is (at present) less common among women, physicians treating severe or persistent vaginal candidiasis may not realize that HIV is a possible cause. This may mean that a woman's HIV infection may go unrecognized and untreated.

Treatment of vaginal candidiasis is usually done first with topical antifungal creams (clotrimazole, ketoconazole) used on tissues of the vulva and vagina. Because these medications are now available over the counter (under the brand names Gyne-Lotrimin and Monistat), you can buy medication and treat yourself if symptoms recur.

If your vaginal candidiasis is severe or persistent, systemic oral antifungal medications may be helpful. Ketoconazole (Nizoral) is available for this purpose in pill form. Two newer medications, itraconazole (Sporanox) and fluconazole (Diflucan), are also available in pill form and may be superior.

Cervix means "neck" in Latin. The anatomical cervix is the narrow end (or neck) of the uterus that opens into the vagina. For a variety of reasons the cervix is prone to certain disorders. **In all women, whether HIV infected or not, a percentage of cervical disorders leads to cancer of the cervix.**

Major questions remain regarding three major issues relating HIV, cervical disease, and cervical cancer.

- Do HIV-infected women have a higher rate of cervical infections and other problems?
- Does HIV infection increase the risk that cervical disorders become cancerous?
- Are the diagnostic tests called *Pap smears* reliable in this population for detecting cervical disorders? What other diagnostic tests should be used?

Studies have shown an association between HIV infection and cervical disease. **HIV-infected women, especially those who are symptomatic, show an increased rate of cervical disorders on Pap tests.** However, there were problems in the methodology of these studies that make the results questionable.

Women who acquire HIV through unprotected sexual intercourse may also have acquired other sexually transmitted infections. These infections or possibly HIV infection itself may increase the risk of cervical disorders.

Cervical dysplasia is abnormal cell growth in the tissues of the cervix. It is detected on microscopic examination of cells obtained via PAP smears and biopsy. Cervical dysplasia is not actually a cancerous condition, but it may become cancerous. A recent study in New York City showed that HIV-infected women had about a ten times greater prevalence of cervical dysplasia.

One cervical disorder is condyloma acuminata, or genital warts, caused by the **human papilloma virus, HPV.** This infection is a serious concern because certain types are associated with increased risk of cervical cancer. Certain strains of HPV are more likely than others to lead to cervical cancer. Unfortunately, there's no easy way to know which strain you have.

At least one study (Feingold) has indicated a high rate of HPV infection among women who are HIV infected. There are two possible reasons for this: either unprotected intercourse increases the risk of both infections independently; or infection with one virus makes infection with the other more likely by disrupting normal mucosal barriers to infection or reducing the vigilance of the immune system.

Use of condoms for intercourse will reduce risk of both HPV and HIV infections. HPV may occasionally be transmitted despite condom use, because warts are not limited to the areas protected by the condom.

Although the rate of cervical disorders is higher, it is not yet clear whether HIV-infected women are at increased risk for cancer. No studies have been done. **HIV may accelerate the progression of cervical cancer.**

The best way to detect cervical disease is with regular gynecological care including twice-yearly Pap smears. To obtain a Pap smear, the gynecologist inserts a tool called a *speculum* into the vagina to hold the vagina open, permitting access to the cervix. Cells are then gently scraped off the cervix to provide material for the smear. Only mild discomfort is involved. Pap smears can usually detect cervical abnormalities early on.

Because Pap smears may be less reliable in women who are HIV infected, expert physicians argue that women who are HIV infected should also have an examination called a *colposcopy,* which is a visual examination of the cervix through a magnifying instrument, sometimes done in combination with a biopsy of a small piece of the cervix. The recommended frequency of colposcopy varies. In general, colposcopy probably needs to be performed only every six months. If a Pap smear is at all abnormal or difficult to interpret, a colposcopy should definitely be performed. If abnormalities are present, your gynecologist may want you to get Pap smears and colposcopies more frequently.

Treatment of cervical disorders: Since viral typing for HPV is not yet widely available, it is important to treat all genital warts to minimize the risk of development of cervical disease. If detected early, cervical disease can be treated with cryosurgery, laser surgery, or other local treatment. Cervical cancer should be treated aggressively: surgery may be considered.

Pelvic inflammatory disease (PID) is a generalized infection of organs in a woman's pelvic area. The infection starts in the vagina and cervix and spreads upward to the endometrium (lining of the uterus), fallopian tubes, and contiguous structures. Generally the organisms that cause PID are *Neisseria gonorrhoeae* and *Chlamydia trachomatis.* These organisms are transmitted sexually. PID can be a very serious disease, causing infertility, chronic pelvic pain, and ectopic pregnancy (pregnancy outside the uterus). Symptoms are abdominal pain and fever. Treatment often requires hospitalization and sometimes surgery to remove abscesses caused by infection.

Women infected with HIV may have also contracted gonorrhea or chlamydia during unprotected intercourse. It is reasonable to expect high rates of PID among HIV-infected women and some small studies have indicated that this is true.

No real information is available about the effect of HIV on PID. It appears that PID may be more severe in women who are HIV positive, requiring more surgery.

Women who are HIV infected should make every effort to avoid PID. Condoms for intercourse can prevent new infections that might lead to PID. Early intervention for chlamydia and gonorrhea can stop these infections from progressing to PID. If you are an HIV-infected woman, it is crucial to see your gynecologist regularly and to report promptly all symptoms of possible infection. These symptoms include itching, burning, pain, painful intercourse, and vaginal discharge. It may be particularly hard to get rid of an infection if you are HIV infected. Take the entire course of medication your doctor prescribes and return for follow-up visits.

There have been anecdotal reports of persistent, difficult-to-treat **genital ulcers** in HIV-infected women. These ulcers were not caused by syphilis, chancroid, or herpes simplex. These ulcers have responded to treatment with AZT. They may be caused by HIV or an unidentified virus.

▲ Pregnancy

Risk to the fetus: The pregnancy of an HIV-infected woman has a 25 to 30 percent chance of resulting in an HIV-infected newborn. Consequently the decision to carry through a pregnancy if you are HIV-infected must be given careful thought.

Risk to the woman: The effect of pregnancy on the health of an HIV-infected woman is not clear. Pregnancy does affect immune status and T4:T8 ratio is decreased during pregnancy as well as by HIV. However, there is no clear evidence that pregnancy makes HIV disease worse. Studies have not been adequate. Careful T4 cell monitoring during pregnancy is important: T4 cells counts may be more rapidly variable.

Treatment recommendations during pregnancy: It is generally recommended that AZT and PCP prophylaxis not be started during the first fourteen weeks of pregnancy when it might affect formation of the fetus. After that, both are recommended to pregnant women who have T4 cell counts of below 200. There is disagreement about AZT for pregnant women who have T4 cell counts between 200 and 500. Dosage of AZT is not different during pregnancy. Bactrim does not seem to adversely affect the fetus. With aerosolized pentamidine, the risk to the fetus is low because there are low levels of the drug in blood.

Opportunistic infections may worsen rapidly among pregnant women. It is important to try to sort out medical problems (such as fatigue, loss of appetite) that can be caused both by pregnancy and by HIV. Pregnant women who are HIV infected should be assessed for syphilis, gonorrhea, chlamydia, hepatitis B, cytomegalovirus, herpes, and toxoplasmosis. This information may be useful for both the mother and baby as some of these diseases can be transmitted in utero or during delivery or can cause damage to the fetus. Symptoms should be reported promptly.

Since not all babies born to HIV-infected mothers will be HIV infected it is important to avoid potential infection to the baby during delivery. Your doctor should avoid as much as possible any contact between the mother's vaginal secretions and fetal blood. For example, scalp-blood sampling of the fetus or scalp electrodes for monitoring fetal heartbeat could inject infected fluid into the fetus and so should be avoided.

All infants born to HIV-infected mothers will test seropositive for HIV antibodies for a period of time. It is therefore **difficult to tell if an infant is HIV-infected at the time of birth.** More sophisticated testing by a pediatric AIDS specialist may help make the determination.

Infants have occasionally been infected with HIV via **breast feeding.** In developed countries such as the United States, HIV-infected women should avoid breast feeding. In many developing countries the risk of bottle feeding without adequate sterilization may outweigh the risk of HIV transmission by breast feeding. (Infants may sometimes be able to acquire HIV via the mouth because their immune systems are not fully developed. This contrasts with adults, in whom HIV infection via the mouth is quite rare.)

PEDIATRIC ISSUES

(The authors are indebted to Samuel Grubman, M.D., for his many contributions to the information presented in this section.)

Children under the age of 13 account for about 2 percent of cases of AIDS reported in the United States. Studies of newborns suggest that about 1.5 infants among 1,000 are born to HIV-infected mothers. This country currently has 10,000 to 20,000 HIV-infected children.

About 84 percent of AIDS cases in children are due to mother-to-fetus (*perinatal*) transmission and 15 percent are due to direct injection of blood or blood products. The proportion of cases due to infection from blood and blood products has been shrinking since screening of the blood supply began in March 1985. In 1990, 87 percent of new cases of pediatric AIDS were due to perinatal transmission and 9 percent to blood products.

Over 80 percent of pediatric cases occur in children under 5. AIDS is one of the ten leading causes of death in children. The prevalence varies both geographically and by race and ethnicity. One study done in the Bronx, New York, indicated that one in forty-three births was to an HIV-infected woman. More than 70 percent of children with AIDS are African-American or Latino. Nationwide, 24 percent of all children are African-American or Latino.

▲ Diagnosis and Course of Illness

Not every child born to an HIV-infected mother will become HIV-infected. The pregnancy of an HIV-infected woman has a 25 to 30 percent chance of resulting in an HIV-infected child.

All newborns of HIV-infected mothers will test positive for antibodies to HIV because they passively carry maternal HIV antibodies. An infant can be diagnosed by ELISA testing confirmed by Western blot at the age of 15 months or older. New tests are being developed for the purpose of earlier diagnosis. HIV culture or polymerase chain reaction testing (PCR, DNA amplification) are both promising possibilities. Detection of a specific class of HIV antibodies that does not cross the placenta (immunoglobulin A, IgA) may also allow earlier identification of HIV-infected infants, although this method is effective only in infants over 3 months of age. An infant below the age of 15 months is also considered HIV infected if the infant is HIV-antibody positive, has an impaired immune system, and certain symptoms. Diagnosis should be performed by a pediatric AIDS specialist.

Elevated immunoglobulin levels are often the first lab abnormalities seen in HIV-infected children. T4 cell abnormalities usually develop before symptoms. The absolute number of T4 cells in young children is normally much higher than in adults, although the ratio of T4 cells to total lymphocytes is the same as in adults. T4 cell levels and immuno-globulin levels need to be judged according to age-appropriate norms. Multiple other laboratory abnormalities occur during the course of disease.

▲ Manifestations

Children with HIV disease present a wide spectrum of symptoms and degrees of illness. Virtually every organ system can be affected. The diagnostic criteria for AIDS in children are different from those for adults.

There are two typical patterns of illness in HIV-infected children. It is not known why a particular child follows one pattern or the other.

About one-third of HIV-infected children develop severe, life-threatening illness in the first year of life. PCP is the most common opportunistic infection. Encephalopathy (deterioration of the brain) is also seen. These infants have a high risk of death in the first year.

About two-thirds of HIV-infected children have a slower course of illness. They do not develop symptoms until after 1 year of age and their illness tends to be less severe. They tend to suffer from a series of characteristic illnesses (described below). They have a much increased length of survival compared to children who become ill in the first year of life. Although these children may be diagnosed with AIDS, this does not mean that they will die within a very short period of time. It is difficult to provide any better estimates of survival time.

As with adult HIV disease, the group of children with slower-developing disease are likely to have medical problems arise before the development of a specific opportunistic infection. These symptoms include enlargement of the liver and spleen and chronic swollen glands (generalized lymphadenopathy). Other early common signs are oral thrush (candidiasis), allergic skin reactions, inflammation of the salivary gland (*parotitis*), recurrent fevers, and chronic or recurrent diarrhea.

Recurrent severe bacterial infections are a serious problem for HIV-infected children. Various bacteria typically cause infections in small children, whether HIV infected or not: *Hemophilus influenzae, Streptococcus pneumoniae, Staphylococcus aureus,* and *Salmonella.* These bacteria can cause localized infections such as *otitis media* (ear infection), sinusitis, or *impetigo,* a skin rash. When immune-suppressed children are exposed to bacteria for the first time they have neither the previously established antibodies that protect immune-suppressed adults nor the healthy immune system that protects immune-competent children. An HIV-infected child must be treated promptly and thoroughly to prevent the development of severe *disseminated* (generalized throughout the body) life-threatening illness. Thus, severe manifestations of common childhood illnesses may be AIDS-defining conditions in an HIV-infected child. Also, because such children do not have a normal antibody response, they may have recurrent episodes of these diseases.

Children with HIV disease can develop life-threatening cases of illnesses from normal diseases of childhood, such as measles and chicken pox (*varicella*). Prolonged chicken pox in HIV-infected children may lead to serious problems in the lungs, liver, pancreas, or brain. Some HIV-infected children have died from measles.

Lymphoid interstitial pneumonitis (LIP), a lung disease, is another illness more common in children, occurring in 30 to 40 percent of HIV-infected children. It is an AIDS-defining illness in children. Characteristic changes in X rays are used to diagnose LIP, but other infections must also be ruled out. A child with LIP may have mild symptoms or become severely ill with chronic lung disease. LIP in children causes *hypoxemia,* insufficient oxygen in the blood that may lead to a chronic disorder of the airways (*bronchi*).

Kidney problems occur in 10 percent of HIV-infected children. Cardiac abnormalities may also be present, but less frequently.

Many of the opportunistic infections that occur in children are the same as those that occur in adults. *Pneumocystis carinii* pneumonia (PCP) affects about 65 percent of children with HIV disease, occurs at much higher T4 counts than in adults, and may often be the first HIV-related illness. Other common opportunistic infections are esophageal candidiasis, disseminated cytomegalovirus infection (CMV), disseminated *Mycobacterium avium* complex (MAC), cryptosporidiosis, and disseminated herpes simplex.

Some opportunistic infections (toxoplasmosis, cryptococcal disease, and disseminated fungal infections) are rare in HIV-infected children. Cancers are rare, occurring in only 1 to 2 percent of HIV-infected children. Kaposi's sarcoma (KS) is virtually never seen in children.

HIV and many of its associated disorders interfere with an infected child's physical and mental development. Development is measured by multiple factors: height, weight, motor skills, cognitive ability. Some babies with HIV disease suffer from *failure to thrive,* a condition in which they do not gain weight or do not grow according to established normal growth curves for age and sex. These neurodevelopmental disorders are a central problem in children with AIDS.

Neurological problems vary. Delays in development occur in 50 to 90 percent of children with HIV disease. Most children have some amount of developmental delay that affects both motor skills and learning ability. The pattern of these problems is widely variable; children may show delay of development, loss of previously gained abilities, or (with antiviral treatment) neurodevelopmental improvement. Some children with AIDS develop degenerative brain disease (*encephalopathy*), which often presents as weakness of legs and trunk and the loss of previously gained developmental milestones. Encephalopathy may or may not be progressive. Seizures and loss of movement or sensation are other common neurological symptoms.

▲ Access to Care

Although the prognosis for HIV-infected children is currently poor, treatment can extend life and improve the quality of life. Tragically, children with HIV in the United States generally have inadequate access to appropriate health care because they are usually among the poorest people in our society.

The recommendations for care described below require both access to medical care itself and a social situation that allows for appropriate practical, educational, and emotional help for sick children and their families. At the present time most HIV-infected children do not get this kind of care and support.

It is highly desirable for a child to be treated by a team of health care practitioners. Social services, educational advice, and psychological services are a crucial part of the care of HIV-infected children. The family as well as the infected child requires care. Most HIV-infected children have HIV-infected mothers. This tremendously complicates practical and psychological issues. Many HIV-infected children come from families where substance abuse is or was a problem. The majority of families with HIV-infected children face problems of poverty and racism.

The same suggestions that apply to finding a physician for an adult generally apply also to pediatricians. Seek a pediatrician expert in HIV disease. The best resource is to find out if there is a hospital in your area that is a center for research and treatment on HIV disease in children. Most pediatricians do not accept Medicaid patients with no other form of insurance; most clinics will accept Medicaid-only patients.

▲ Treatment

Children with HIV disease should be seen by an expert physician at least once every three months. They must be monitored for growth and development and for signs of thrush (candidiasis), swollen glands, and enlarged organs.

HIV-infected children with relatively minor symptoms may be in the process of developing major infections. Fevers, coughs, failure to eat, failure to gain weight, excessive crying, and apathy are all possible danger signs and should lead to prompt consultation with a physician.

PCP tends to be more severe in children than in adults, perhaps because it is a primary infection rather than a reactivation. Most cases develop in the first year of life and the median age of diagnosis of PCP is 3 to 6 months. PCP prophylaxis is particularly important for HIV-infected children and should be started by one month if indicated. PCP prophylaxis should be started on the basis of age-appropriate T4 cell counts, even if no HIV diagnosis has been definitively made. In an infant less than 1 year of age, PCP prophylaxis should be started if T4 cell counts fall below 1,500.

Opportunistic infections are generally treated with the same medications as those used in adults.

Children with LIP who develop significant deficiency of oxygen in the blood (*hypoxemia*) are treated with corticosteroids.

While all patients are likely to be undermedicated for pain, infants and young children may be particularly vulnerable to undermedication because they are inarticulate. If you are caring for an HIV-infected child, make sure the child is adequately treated for pain. Newborns and infants feel pain just as much as older children and adults. Drugs that can be used to control pain include aspirin, acetaminophen, codeine, ibuprofen,

Normal Age-Appropriate Absolute T4 Count, T4 Percent of Total Lymphocytes, and T4:T8 Ratio
(MMWR, 3/15/91, 40:RR–2)

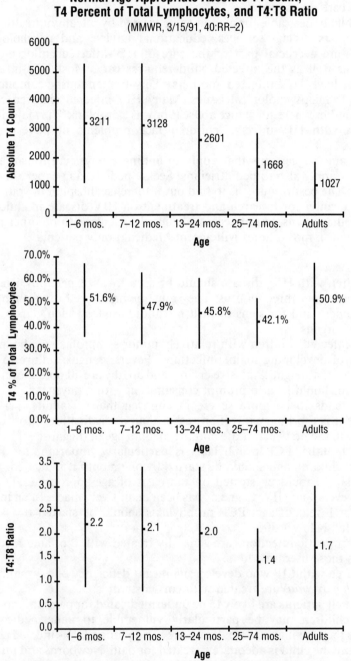

(Vertical bars indicate range; tick marks and labels indicate median values.)

morphine, and methadone. Consult your physician about which pain medication to use.

▲ Immunizations and Immune Globulin

HIV-infected children should receive the immunizations listed in the chart below. With a few exceptions (inactivated polio vaccine instead of live oral polio vaccine, and the addition of pneumococcal and influenza vaccine), they are the same as vaccinations for non-HIV-infected children. Anyone living in a household with an HIV-infected child should receive the killed-virus polio vaccine (Salk, IPV) rather than live oral polio vaccine (OPV): recipients of OPV may shed polio virus, posing a hazard to the infected child.

ROUTINE IMMUNOLOGIC INTERVENTIONS FOR HIV-INFECTED CHILDREN

Intervention	Recommendation
Measles, mumps, rubella (MMR)	Recommended for asymptomatic children; probably indicated for all HIV-infected children.
Intramuscular immune globulin	Recommended after exposure to measles
Serum intravenous immune globulin (IVIG)	Recommended after exposure to measles if child does not have adequate level of protection from measles vaccination (as measured by poor specific antibody response) or has had a significant recent decline in immune functioning. Needs to be given within 6 days of exposure. Also recommended on a regular basis if child has recurrent life-threatening infections.
Inactivated polio vaccine (IPV)	Recommended for all children; use instead of oral polio vaccine
Influenza vaccine	Recommended for all HIV-infected children once each year in November
Haemophilus influenzae b vaccine (HbCV)	Recommended for all HIV-infected children 6 months or older except those with allergies to eggs
Pneumococcal polysaccharide vaccine	Recommended for HIV-infected children at 2 years or older
Varicella zoster (chicken pox) immune globulin (VZIG)	Recommended for children exposed to varicella zoster (chicken pox)

HIV-infected children have difficulty in developing adequate protection from vaccination. This is particularly a problem because measles can be life-threatening. Measles antibody levels should be tested at least once a year. Those who do not have adequate levels of protection should be considered for treatment with serum intravenous immune globulins (IVIG). Varicella zoster immune globulin (VZIG) is also indicated after exposure to chicken pox (which is caused by the virus *varicella zoster*).

Intravenous immune globulin is sometimes given on a monthly basis to deal with impaired antibody formation caused by B-cell defects. It is used for children who have recurrent life-threatening bacterial infections.

▲ Antiviral Treatment

AZT and ddI are approved for use in children with HIV infection and have been shown to be effective. AZT helps children with HIV-related neurological disorders, sometimes quite dramatically. As with adults, loss of red and white blood cells are the most common side effects. Studies are under way on the use in children of different doses of AZT, ddI, and ddC. AZT is available in a syrup form for children. The standard dose is based on the estimated area of the child's skin surface: 180 mg per m^2 every six hours. This is comparable to the higher dose that used to be given to adults. Studies are under way to look at the efficacy of smaller doses. However, because children with neurological disturbances may respond better to higher doses, the higher dose may continue to be standard.

Drugs have been approved even more slowly for children with HIV disease than for adults. It is, therefore, sometimes a good idea to get access to new medication for a child through entry into clinical trials. Call 1-800-TRIALS-A for information about the nature and location of clinical trials for HIV-infected children.

▲ Education

According to the Centers for Disease Control, children with HIV disease do not present a risk to other children or adults in a school setting. HIV-infected children (especially very young ones) may be more susceptible to opportunistic and childhood infections in a nursery or daycare setting but at the same time would benefit from the care and stimulation provided by such settings. Decisions about schooling will depend on the individual child's health and social situation. Generally speaking, there is no reason for an HIV-infected child to stay out of school unless there is outbreak of measles or chicken pox.

RACE AND ETHNICITY

The incidence of AIDS is dramatically higher among blacks and Latinos. Of the reported cases of people with AIDS in the United States, 55 percent were whites, 27 percent were blacks, and 16 percent were Latinos. Blacks and Latinos represent only 12 percent and 6 percent, respectively, of the U.S. population, and are therefore overrepresented among people with AIDS.

Nationwide, the incidence of AIDS among black or Latina women is about a dozen times higher than the incidence of AIDS among white women. Among black children the incidence of AIDS is fifteen times higher than among white children. In New York City 93 percent of children with AIDS are black or Latino.

Individuals are not at higher risk for AIDS because of their race or ethnicity. Rather, the disproportion of AIDS among black and Latino people occurs in cases that were transmitted by needle sharing. The high incidence of IV drug use and needle sharing in some black and Hispanic communities is due to the combined impact of underlying social and economic factors including poverty, racism, unequal schooling, and unequal opportunity for employment. Further, black and Latino communities are concentrated in large urban areas, which have a high incidence of HIV infection.

The spread of HIV infection among black and Latino needle sharers has continued essentially unchecked: AIDS education and prevention has largely been targeted toward a white middle-class population and has only recently begun to address the issues relevant to needle sharers.

Certain opportunistic infections are more common among African-American and Latino people with AIDS than among whites. These infections include: *endocarditis,* an inflammation of the heart common among intravenous drug users; tuberculosis, a disease that has been associated with poverty; and vaginal candidiasis, which is more common among racial and ethnic minorities with AIDS because these groups contain proportionately more women.

White people with AIDS have a **life expectancy from time of diagnosis** that is two to three times longer than that for black people with AIDS. This is due to differences in general health because of economic privation and to the fact that some HIV-infected people get much better care than others. Survival differences are probably not attributable to biological factors. Poverty increases the likelihood of previous illness, which increases vulnerability to the complications of HIV disease. Intravenous drug use is associated with greater exposure to a wide variety of infectious organisms that may worsen the course of illness.

Poverty, intravenous drug use, and racism may all cause alienation from and lack of access to health care. This in turn may cause members of minorities to avoid health care. Late presentation for diagnosis and treatment hurts treatment response and survival.

Response to antivirals: Because of a great variety of factors (including many of those mentioned above), clinical trials of antiviral drugs have had relatively few subjects who were African-American or Latino. This has raised the question of whether the benefits reported for antivirals such as AZT hold true for racial and ethnic minorities. Preliminary results from one study were widely interpreted in the popular press to mean that AZT worked less well in certain racial and ethnic groups than in others. Two recent authoritative analyses contradict this interpretation and confirm that AZT's effect is similar whether you are African-American, Latino, white, male, or female (Lagakos, Easterbrook).

The nature and availability of health care in the United States differs greatly depending on economic status. **Although as a biological factor, race does not affect the course of HIV disease, in our society rac*ism* certainly influences economic status and access to health care and thereby directly reduces the survival of minority people with AIDS.**

Chapter 9
Learning About Experimental Treatments

GETTING INFORMATION ABOUT TREATMENT

This book is intended to give you the basic information you need to get the best possible care for HIV disease. However, part of being well informed about HIV disease is keeping up-to-date. Because new developments occur fairly frequently, you need to become part of a network that will give you information about the current state of knowledge. How do you become part of this information network? How do you sort out wild rumors from promising possibilities?

Individuals have different psychological and learning styles. If you have some background in science it will make it easier for you to read technical material. On the other hand, some people with *no* prior science background find that they can learn scientific material and in fact find it very interesting.

Psychological issues affect what you will want to learn about HIV disease. At one end of the scale, some HIV-infected people feel worse when they get information about HIV disease. They feel it focuses their attention too much on the disease and increases their anxiety or depression. Such people may decide even to avoid reading articles about AIDS in the daily newspaper. At the other end of the scale, many other people feel better when they learn a lot about HIV disease. They feel better able to make rational decisions, more in control, and less anxious and depressed. They may read widely about HIV disease, attend lectures and conferences, and become experts who teach others, or activists in the AIDS treatment movement.

You have to ask yourself where you fall on this scale. If you have the impulse to avoid all mention of AIDS, make sure this is not interfering with your treatment. Your lack of information leaves you more reliant on the decisions of your doctor. Most people fall somewhere in the middle. They need to discover a strategy for keeping relatively knowledgeable while not being overwhelmed with anxiety.

There are several ways (in addition to discussion with your doctor) to keep current on developments in AIDS treatment. First, find out what kind of informational forums are available in your community and get on the mailing lists of the organizations that run them. AIDS service organizations, medical centers, organizations of people with AIDS, and political groups such as ACT UP (the AIDS Coalition To Unleash Power) run such forums.

A large amount of information is shared on an informal basis among people who are HIV infected. If you remain isolated from others with HIV disease, you will have less access to new information. If you have friends who are HIV positive, if you belong to a support group, if you do AIDS service or political work, you will be more likely to hear of new developments.

AIDS service organizations are nonprofit groups that have been formed throughout the country to provide a variety of services related to AIDS and HIV disease. Many of these organizations have telephone hotlines that provide information. They also conduct educational programs and distribute written material. They often provide direct services for people with AIDS: psychological and financial counseling, free legal services, assistance to people who are homebound and need help with chores or companionship. (See the appendices for a list of local AIDS service organizations; you can also call the National AIDS Clearing House at 800-342-AIDS or 800-342-2437. This is a hotline run by the Centers for Disease Control that will give you information about AIDS service organizations in your area.)

Another source of information and help are groups specifically run by and for people with AIDS (PWAs). These groups function both locally and nationally. These groups also sometimes provide opportunities to socialize with other people with AIDS. Contact the National Association of People with AIDS (NAPWA) at 202-898-0414 for information about a group in your area. (See the appendices for listings of groups in New York and San Francisco.)

A number of AIDS service and PWA organizations and hospitals sponsor support groups for people with HIV disease. These groups meet regularly on either a short- or long-term basis. The meetings are conducted as discussions and are intended to provide both information and psychological support. People usually talk about their emotional reactions to dealing with HIV disease. Some groups have facilitators, others are leaderless. Some are restricted to people with an AIDS diagnosis, others accept any HIV-infected person. In New York City, contact the organization Body Positive at 212-633-1782.

ACT UP is the major direct political action group. They do political organizing and protest to fight for improved treatment and access to treatment for people with HIV disease. Branches exist in many cities, including New York (212-564-2437); San Francisco (415-563-0742); and Los Angeles (213-669-7301).

You should subscribe to at least two newsletters that provide information specifically designed for people who are HIV infected. Such newsletters are generally free or cheap and discuss both new drugs and evaluation of treatment strategies currently in use. Following is subscription information for five newsletters that provide information:

Treatment Issues is published by the Gay Men's Health Crisis, a large and prestigious AIDS service organization in New York City. Call 212-337-1950 for subscription.

Notes from the Underground is published by the People with AIDS (PWA) Health Group, an organization that imports and distributes drugs not available in this country. Such organizations are often called *buyer's clubs.* Call 212-255-0520 for subscription.

Project Inform, a pioneering AIDS information organization, publishes fact sheets on particular drugs, a newsletter called *PI Perspectives,* and periodic *PI Briefing Papers.* Project Inform also runs a treatment information hotline. For subscriptions, fact sheets, or drug information, call either 800-822-7422 from outside California, 800-334-7422 from inside California, or 415-558-9051 from San Francisco.

BETA (Bulletin of Experimental Treatments for AIDS) is published by the San Francisco AIDS Foundation. Call the San Francisco AIDS Foundation Hotline at 415-863-AIDS for subscription.

Another newsletter that many people find useful is *AIDS Treatment News,* published by John James. *AIDS Treatment News,* in contrast to the other newsletters listed above, discusses many substances for which no scientific data are available. Therefore, it should be read with a particular care and sophistication. Call 415-255-0588 for subscription.

CRITERIA FOR CONSIDERING UNPROVEN TREATMENT

Taking any substance that has not been shown to be safe through large-scale controlled clinical trials means taking a risk. Any drug may have adverse side effects, particularly in people with impaired immune systems. Given the gravity of the prognosis for seriously symptomatic HIV infection, some people have decided to risk taking untested (and possibly useless) medications. The problem is complex; there are no definitive answers about the effectiveness or dangers of using these drugs. The following principles may help you to decide whether to take a drug not yet proven safe or effective in the HIV setting.

- Is there some theoretical basis for hoping that the drug may be effective against AIDS or HIV infection? Are test-tube studies encouraging?
- Is there a body of anecdotal evidence from clinicians or HIV-infected people in the AIDS treatment movement supporting the use of the drug?
- Is the drug known to have adverse side effects or to be toxic? Evidence suggesting that a drug is safe for use against HIV may be

based on experience with the drug in other settings. Some experimental therapies tried against HIV infection are FDA-approved for other uses.

- Is the drug known to interfere with any effective therapy you are currently taking? Your physician can help you answer this question.
- Is the drug so expensive that you will not be able to afford standard medical care?

Your physician cannot recommend unproven treatments but may be willing to advise you about the efficacy and safety of treatments you yourself suggest.

It is unfortunate but true that treatment for HIV infection will probably advance in small increments, rather than through discovery of one "wonder drug." If someone tries to sell you a total "cure" for AIDS, watch out: people who face serious illness make easy targets for fraud. Fraud of this type has been reported. Derek Hodel, of the People With AIDS Health Group, a ground-breaking buyer's club in New York City, urges that you be skeptical if:

- The benefits of the treatment are not measurable by standard medical methods
- The proposed treatment is very expensive and the only supporters of the treatment are those who stand to profit from it
- You must travel far away or outside of the United States to obtain the treatment
- The credibility of the treatment depends upon an implausible massive conspiracy to suppress information

ACCESS TO UNPROVEN TREATMENT

There are two major ways of getting access to unproven treatments. These are by enrolling as a subject in a clinical trial or by purchasing the drug through a buyer's club (underground treatment supply organization).

INFORMATION ON EXPERIMENTAL DRUG TRIALS

Specific information about current trials that you might wish to enter is available through a variety of sources. To get information about clinical trials in your area that are open for enrollment, call 800-TRIALS-A (800-854-2572). Call Monday to Friday, 9:00 A.M. to 7:00 P.M. EST. This is an information service sponsored by the Centers for Disease Control (CDC). Information is available in both Spanish and English. You will get to speak to someone in person who will give you information about government-approved clinical trials and also about specific drugs, both antivirals and those for opportunistic infections. They will do computer searches for you. Services are free.

You can also get written information on drug trials from the American Foundation for AIDS Research at 212-682-7440. Local AIDS organizations may have information on clinical trials that are recruiting subjects in your area.

If you are interested in becoming an experimental subject, please see Chapter 19: Understanding Clinical Trials.

BUYER'S CLUBS

Buyer's clubs are community organizations that were developed to gain access to unapproved drugs for people with HIV disease. These organizations usually provide both medication and information about medication. They obtain drugs from foreign countries and other sources. Some drugs they provide require a prescription from your doctor. Some drugs that are in wide use by expert physicians (such as itraconazole) are available only through buyer's clubs.

In some cases the clubs are stretching the law to provide medication that is otherwise unavailable: the directors of these clubs are in some cases risking jail to provide this valuable service to HIV-infected people. You, however, are not taking any legal risk: it is absolutely legal to *purchase* unapproved drugs from these clubs.

Buyer's clubs vary. Some are trustworthy sources of information and have been run by people who are pioneers in seeking better treatments for HIV disease. Others seem to be run with less care than might be desired, and a few are actually profit-making ventures. Two of the most reliable are: the People With AIDS Health Group, 150 W. 26th Street, New York, NY 10001, tel. 212-255-0520; and the Healing Alternatives Foundation, 1748 Market Street, Suite 204, San Francisco, CA 94102, tel. 415-626-2316. Call these two clubs for information about the reliability of buyer's clubs in your area.

Part Two
Managing Complications

This part of the book is designed to give you some technical information about many of the complications that more commonly occur in later stages of HIV infection, say when T4 counts drop below 200. Of course, this book cannot substitute for a physician expert in the diagnosis and treatment of HIV disease, but it may give you an outline of some of the issues that arise in the management of secondary illnesses. This part of the book tells you which illnesses are relevant at various stages of immune deficiency, whether they are preventable, and what decisions you may be called upon to make during diagnosis and treatment.

For ease of reference, this part of the book organizes illnesses in two basic ways: by location (or *organ system*); and by disease. Some medical problems may be caused by any of a variety of disease organisms. For example, pneumonia in the lungs may be due either to *Pneumocystis carinii* or to one of a number of bacteria or fungi. Also, one disease organism may cause a variety of medical problems. For example, cytomegalovirus can cause problems in the gut, the eyes, or the lungs.

Chapter 10: Organ System Complications provides detailed information about the specific diseases and their causes, organized by the part of the body that is affected. Chapter 11: Infections, and Chapter 12: Cancers, describe specific diseases.

Chapter 13: Procedures and Tests, is devoted to descriptions of procedures and tests that you may undergo during diagnosis and treatment of the illnesses described here.

Chapter 14: The Experience of Hospitalization is devoted to the circumstances under which more severe illness happens, is detected, and is treated. This chapter describes the outline of basic events that usually happen in the course of being hospitalized. It will also give you some idea of what it is like to use the emergency room.

This part of the book contains descriptions of many potentially unpleasant or frightening things. Only a few of these may ever be relevant to your situation. We suggest that you read only those pieces that are relevant and skip the others.

Chapter 10
Organ System Complications

We experience disease in particular locations in our bodies. It is therefore natural to group the problems that arise in HIV disease by anatomical location, or *organ system.* For each organ system that follows we have listed some of the problems that may occur later in HIV disease. These problems are described very briefly here—a more complete description of the causative disease is given in the following chapters.

MOUTH PROBLEMS

Most HIV-related problems that affect the mouth, or *oral cavity,* are not life-threatening. However, since we use the mouth for (among other things) eating, speaking, and having sex, even minor mouth problems can be unpleasant and bothersome. These activities are not only biologically important, but are part of the pleasures and reassurances of daily life. Many of the problems described below can be treated, so it is worth attending to even minor symptoms.

Common problems of the mouth in people with HIV infection are:

- Herpes simplex (cold sores)
- Candidiasis (thrush)
- Human papillomavirus lesions (warts)
- Hairy leukoplakia
- Gingivitis (gum disease)
- Periodontitis (disease of the tissues that support the teeth, including the gums)
- Oral or aphthous ulcers (canker sores)

▲ Herpes Simplex

Herpes simplex is a disease affecting skin and mucous membranes that is caused by the herpes virus. There are two kinds of herpes: Type I, or oral herpes; and Type II, or genital herpes. Type I usually causes sores on the edge of the lips, the nostrils, or in the mouth, on the gums or hard palate. Oral herpes, often referred to as "cold sores," are common in people without HIV infection, but people with HIV infection tend to have episodes that may be more frequent, more severe, or of longer duration. The sores may tingle or be painful. Herpes sores may disappear in a few days and can be helped by oral or topical acyclovir. In an

HIV-infected person with an impaired immune system, herpes may become a chronic problem. (See also the section on herpes simplex virus in Chapter 11: Infections, pp. 232–34.)

▲ Oral Candidiasis (Thrush)

Candidiasis is one of the most frequent oral problems of people with HIV infection and occurs at some point to almost all people with AIDS. It is caused by the fungus *Candida albicans.* Candidiasis may be referred to simply as candida or *thrush.* The symptoms of the most common kind of thrush are creamy white patches of material on the membrane of the mouth and the upper throat. It is important to have thrush diagnosed because it can usually be treated effectively. Maintenance therapy is necessary. (See also the section on *Candida albicans* in Chapter 11: Infections, pp. 275–77.)

▲ Human Papillomavirus Lesions

Human papillomavirus can cause warts in the mouth. They appear to be more common in HIV-infected people. They can be treated with surgery but may recur.

▲ Hairy Leukoplakia (HL)

Hairy leukoplakia (HL) is a tongue condition of viral origin. It looks like irregular white patches on the tongue with small projections that look like tiny hairs. Hairy leukoplakia often looks much like thrush. However, it usually occurs only on the sides of the tongue and cannot be scraped off. HL does not cause pain or discomfort. Diagnosis can be made by examination of the tongue. Hairy leukoplakia does not necessarily require treatment, but will disappear with high doses of acyclovir. Sometimes thrush is found at the same site as hairy leukoplakia and may require treatment.

▲ Gum (Periodontal) Disease

Gum disease, such as gingivitis and periodontitis, is more frequent in HIV-infected people. These diseases cause redness and swelling of the gums, loss of tissue and bone, and sometimes ulcers, bleeding, or pain. See a dentist experienced in HIV care promptly: these problems may progress rapidly but they do respond to treatment.

▲ Aphthous Ulcers

HIV-infected people may develop ulcers (sores) in the mouth. They are referred to as *recurrent aphthous ulcers* (RAU) or, in everyday language, canker sores or cold sores. (Some people also call herpes sores *canker sores* or *cold sores.*) They can appear as individual sores or in clusters that may be painful. The cause of these ulcers is unknown. They often respond to topical treatment with a liquid suspension of tetracycline or with steroid solutions. Your pharmacist may be able to prepare tetracycline suspension if no commercial source is available. If tetracycline suspension is not used, a second choice would be to use a suspension of Decadron: two teaspoons, four times per day, swish around and spit out.

▲ Neoplasms (Cancers)

Kaposi's sarcoma (KS) may cause symptoms in the mouth. The most common manifestations are red, blue, or purple lesions (color may vary depending on natural pigmentation), usually on the hard palate. Diagnosis is made by biopsy and microscopic examination of the affected tissue. If bulky lesions interfere with eating or speaking, they can be treated with radiation therapy, chemotherapy, or laser surgery. See also the section on Kaposi's sarcoma in Chapter 12: Cancers, pp. 280–89.

Lymphoma, or cancer of lymphatic cells, can also occur in the oral cavity. It usually appears as firm swelling, sometimes with ulceration. Lymphoma is diagnosed with microscopic examination of tissue. See also the section on lymphomas in Chapter 12: Cancers, pp. 289–92.

SKIN PROBLEMS

In general, mild skin problems are common in HIV-infected people, affecting about 90 percent at some point. Most of these problems also appear in people who are not HIV infected. While the immune system is not severely impaired these skin problems are often mild and treatable. Because they often recur they may require continuing treatment to control. In people with more advanced HIV disease, skin problems may be more severe and harder to treat.

HIV-related skin problems are divided into four categories: infections, hypersensitivity (allergic) reactions, scaly or bumpy skin *(papulosquamous* disorders), and cancers.

▲ Infections

Skin infections may be caused by bacteria, fungi and yeast, or by viruses.

▲ Bacterial Infections

Infections of the skin may be caused by staphylococcus or syphilis bacteria.

Staphylococcus aureus (colloquially, *staph*) infection of the skin can appear in a variety of forms: folliculitis, bullous impetigo, ecthyma, or abscesses (which may require draining).

Folliculitis is inflammation of the *follicles,* the sac-like depressions from which hairs grow. Folliculitis is the most common of the various manifestations of staphylococcus infection. It generally occurs on the armpits, groin, or face and appears as pustules (small pus-containing lesions). Folliculitis is caused by *Staphylococcus aureus* in about one-third to one-half of cases. It can also be caused by fungi. Other causes of folliculitis are not currently understood.

In **bullous impetigo,** staph infection causes blisters (fluid-containing elevated lesions). These blisters are often located in the groin or armpits. They are superficial blisters that break easily and do not itch. Bullous impetigo is more common in hot humid weather and should be treated with antibiotics.

Staphylococcus can cause "punched out" or eroded ulcers with pus and a crust. These sores, called *ecthyma,* are usually found on the lower legs and occur on top of an existing inflammation of the skin (dermatitis).

Treatment of staph infections: All these manifestations of staphylococcus can be treated with a course of a systemic *anti-staphylococcal* antibiotic, such as dicloxacillin or other *penicillinase-resistant* antibiotics. These antibiotics are generally taken in pill form for ten to fourteen days.

Topical antibiotic creams may be used in addition to systemic antibiotics. Washing the infected area with an antibacterial substance (Hibiclens, Betadine, benzoyl peroxide) may also be helpful. This may lead to dry skin, so moisturizing cream or skin lotion should be used.

Bacterial infections can also occur in more severe forms such as abscesses with pus or cellulitis (a serious tissue inflammation). Abscesses may need to be drained and cellulitis may require hospitalization.

Syphilis causes a variety of skin problems in HIV-infected people. See the complete discussion of syphilis in Chapter 11: Infections, pp. 269–71.

▲ Fungal and Yeast Infections

Fungal infections of the skin are generally caused by *Candida albicans* and tinea.

Candida albicans is the fungus that causes oral thrush. In addition to thrush, candida sometimes causes skin problems. Candida infection appears as red eroded eruptions, often in folds of the skin, sometimes with a white coating. Candidiasis of the skin is most often found in the groin, armpit, and below the breasts. In men candida can appear on the scrotum or around the anus. Candida lesions are itchy and sometimes cause a burning feeling. Topical treatment with an imidazole cream is usually sufficient: clotrimazole (Lotrimin), miconazole (Monistat), or ketoconazole (Nizoral). Oral ketoconazole is often sufficient by itself. If relapses are frequent, periodic preventive treatment can be used. Candida can also affect the fingernails, especially for people who frequently have their hands in water. This condition is also treated with topical imidazole. See also the section on *Candida albicans* in Chapter 11: Infections, pp. 275–77.

Tinea is an infection similar to candida, but it may spread to the lower abdomen and buttocks, groin, thighs, or feet. In the groin it is called *jock itch,* while on the feet it is called *athlete's foot.* It is less moist than candida. Tinea can also affect hands, feet, and nails. Like candida, tinea is treated with topical imidazole such as Nizoral or Lotrimin. It is likely to be persistent, especially on toenails, so ongoing use of antifungal cream or systemic treatment may be indicated.

▲ Viral Infections

Viral infections of the skin may be due to herpes simplex, herpes zoster (shingles), the molluscum virus, the wart virus, or HIV itself.

Herpes simplex may cause lesions on the skin of the genitals, fingers, mouth or face. See also the section on herpes simplex virus in Chapter 11: Infections, pp. 232–34.

Herpes zoster (shingles) may cause lesions on any part of the skin in HIV-infected people, but does not affect other tissues or internal organs. If you do not know your HIV status, are under 65, and develop shingles, you should be tested for HIV infection, since shingles is not common in younger healthy individuals.

Molluscum contagiosum is a skin condition that appears as small (2 mm to 3 mm), solid, raised, pearly or waxy-looking bumps that may be indented in the middle ("umbilicated papules"). They may be found on the genitals and the face. *Molluscum contagiosum* is common in symptomatic HIV-infected patients with low T4 cell counts: perhaps 10 percent of such patients have this problem. The condition spreads. Treatment should be done with curettage (scraping or cutting) or liquid nitrogen cryotherapy (freezing). *Molluscum contagiosum* is contagious.

Human papillomavirus (HPV) infection occurs with increased frequency in HIV-infected persons. It may cause warts that are widespread and hard to eradicate. Typically, warts cause only cosmetic problems, but they can spread. An exception: if warts occur on the bottom of the feet (*plantar warts*) they may be painful or interfere with walking. Warts are usually removed by freezing them with liquid nitrogen. This treatment is only slightly painful and usually leaves no scar. Topical antiwart medication sometimes works: pedophilin, or tridilon acetic acid. Relapses are to be expected.

One type of human papillomavirus is transmitted sexually, and is referred to as *condyloma acuminata,* or genital warts. Most warts are caused by the reactivation of previously acquired infections. Genital warts may appear on the cervix, vagina, penis, in the urethra, or in or around the anus. Condyloma on the cervix are associated with increased disorders of the cervix (*cervical dysplasia*) and possibly with cervical cancer. Anal condyloma may be associated with increased rates of anorectal cancer. Exterior genital warts should probably be surgically removed.

At the time of initial infection an **acute HIV rash** frequently appears, perhaps in as many as half of cases. A light reddish rash resembling

187

roseola is widely distributed over the trunk and limbs and can occur on the palms of hands and soles of feet. Acute HIV rash lasts one to two weeks. Other viral infections can also cause this reaction; it is not specific.

▲ Hypersensitivity

Hypersensitivity reactions include drug reactions, photosensitivity, and insect bite reactions.

Reactions to medication are more frequent in HIV-infected patients. These reactions are frequent with penicillins, sulfa drugs, ciprofloxacin (Cipro), and phenytoin (Dilantin). The most common manifestation of drug hypersensitivity is a stable elevated red rash (referred to as a *maculopapular rash*). Drug reactions can also cause hives (*urticaria,* itchy bumps that appear and disappear in different places) or an elevated red rash with blisters that blanch under pressure (*erythema multiforme,* which can be severe).

The reaction typically occurs eight to fourteen days after starting medication. Most hypersensitivity reactions to drugs stop after the discontinuation of the drug. If the reaction is mild, sometimes you can continue the drug.

A common example of a hypersensitivity reaction to a drug is the elevated red rash (maculopapular) that is an allergic reaction to Bactrim (TMP/SMX), a sulfa drug used to treat respiratory infections and commonly used as PCP prophylaxis. Although the rash caused by this drug may be severe, some people can be desensitized to the drug by starting with small doses and building up gradually. Dapsone, another sulfa drug used for PCP prophylaxis, probably causes fewer reactions than Bactrim. Desensitization to dapsone is easier than to Bactrim.

Other than sulfa drugs, most drugs commonly used against HIV disease rarely cause skin problems (including AZT and acyclovir). AZT can occasionally cause a reversible increase in nail pigmentation in dark-skinned persons, particularly some Hispanics and African-Americans. This appears as blue-black longitudinal streaks on the nails and goes away when AZT is stopped.

Drug reaction rashes may be itchy, uncomfortable, or accompanied by fever, but they are rarely dangerous. Minor drug reactions may be treated with Benadryl (diphenhydramine). In rare occasions, drug reactions with dermatological manifestations can be very serious and even life-threatening (*Stevens-Johnson syndrome*). This is particularly true for drugs that persist in the body long after the drug is stopped—drugs that have a long *half-life.* Some deaths have been reported due to reactions to Fansidar (sometimes used to prevent PCP and toxoplasmosis) and other drugs. These serious drug reactions may be controlled if they are treated quickly with Benadryl and steroids.

Be aware of the possibility of drug reactions whenever you begin taking a new medication. Ask your physician whether you are likely to experience rashes, fevers, or other symptoms in response to a new drug. For virtually all drugs these reactions are not life-threatening, but for your own peace of mind you should ask whether such reactions should be a cause for alarm. Get explicit instructions from your physician about what to do if you experience a drug reaction.

People who are HIV infected, especially those who are taking certain medications—such as sulfa drugs, nonsteroidal antiinflammatory drugs, or doxycycline—can have **heightened sensitivity to the sun** (photosensitivity). This shows itself as bad sunburn, or itchy, scaly patches. It may spread to areas of the skin that have not been exposed to the sun. It is caused by shortwave ultraviolet radiation (UVA).

If you are HIV infected, use sunscreen and protective clothing to avoid bad sunburns. This is desirable also because ultraviolet radiation increases the activity of HIV, at least in the test tube. If you are photosensitive and exposure to sunlight is inevitable, consult with your physician about suspending the use of medications that contribute to photosensitivity. A medium- or high-potency topical steroid (such as hydrocortisone cream) will reduce symptoms of bad sunburn and encourage quicker healing.

Insect bite reaction: Mosquito bites, flea bites, or scabies can cause exaggerated reactions in HIV-infected people. The bites will tend to be larger, longer lasting, and very itchy. Bites will be caused by the insects that are common in your geographical area (for example, fleas in San Francisco, mosquitoes in the east). The best way to avoid this problem is to try to avoid insect bites. Use antiinsect devices (insecticides, bug lights, candles, mosquito netting) in the environment if possible. Apply insect repellents that contain DEET (diethyltoluamide) on the body (Avon Skin-So-Soft™ is one such product). If you do have bad reactions to insect bites you can also use Benadryl or other oral antihistamines that will prevent the reaction (e.g., hydroxyzine or terfenadine). Long-lasting, itchy bites can be treated with medium- or high-potency topical steroids available through prescription: over-the-counter steroid creams are not as effective.

Some skin reactions in HIV-infected people closely resemble insect bites.

▲ Scaly Skin (Papulosquamous Disorders)

A certain category of skin problems is characterized by patches of scaly skin: technically they are referred to as *papulosquamous disorders.* There can be several causes of this problem. People who are HIV infected often have problems with dryness of the skin, which causes scaly patches, redness, and itching. This condition tends to be worse in winter. It can be alleviated by use of moisturizing lotion or cream.

Seborrheic dermatitis is a skin condition that is very common in people with symptomatic HIV infection. Its cause is not understood. Generally the symptoms are faint pinkish patches that can be slightly swollen and have greasy scales. It is found in hairy areas: the scalp, and also the central face, chest, back, and groin. The condition can be itchy when on the scalp or trunk. Seborrheic dermatitis is best treated with a combination of topical imidazole and topical steroids. Affected areas on the scalp can be treated with dandruff shampoo, tar shampoo, or medium-potency topical steroids. If the condition is very severe, you can use oral ketoconazole or ultraviolet-light therapy. Because the condition is likely to recur, long-term treatment may be necessary.

Eosinophilic pustular folliculitis is a very itchy rash that resembles folliculitis but is not caused by infectious agents. It usually appears on the torso and extremities. The condition seems to respond best to ultraviolet (UV) light therapy (this short-term therapy poses little risk in terms of HIV activation).

Psoriasis is a common skin condition. If you already have psoriasis, it may get worse with HIV infection. It is similar in appearance to seborrheic dermatitis, but with more scaling, and is more likely to affect armpits, groin, elbows, knees, and lower back. It is treated with medium- to high-potency topical steroids. If this is not effective, other treatments are available. Consult a dermatologist expert in HIV-related problems. Severe cases sometimes improve (at least for a period of time) when anti-HIV medication is started.

▲ Cancers

Kaposi's sarcoma (KS) can cause skin problems in HIV-infected people. Please refer to the full discussion of Kaposi's sarcoma that follows in Chapter 12.

GUT PROBLEMS AND WEIGHT LOSS

Problems that affect the gastrointestinal (GI) tract are very common in HIV disease (50 percent to 93 percent of AIDS patients experience GI symptoms at some point in the illness). Diarrhea, loose stools, and abdominal cramping are the most common symptoms. Other problems are weight loss, malnutrition, pain on swallowing, and abdominal pain.

There are many causes for these symptoms, most often some kind of infection. Occasionally lymphoma and possibly HIV itself may cause these symptoms. It is important to have these symptoms diagnosed because in many cases accurate diagnosis can lead to effective treatment. This can reduce pain and suffering and alleviate the weight loss and general weakening that can often accompany GI problems. An example of this is that both cryptosporidium and *Isospora belli* cause severe diarrhea that can lead to rapid weight loss. Isospora can usually be treated quickly and effectively with medications that are not the same as those used for cryptosporidium—accurate diagnosis is important. You may be tempted to ignore GI symptoms and hope they will go away because evaluation of these symptoms may seem time-consuming, unpleasant, or embarrassing. Proper treatment, however, can make a major difference in your general well-being and functioning.

Your doctor will often not be able to make a diagnosis on the basis of symptoms alone. The same symptoms can be caused by different infections. Also, it is common to be infected with multiple organisms. Because of this it is important to sort out which organism is producing the symptoms.

People frequently develop gastrointestinal problems when they travel because they are exposed to new microorganisms. Chapter 6: General Health Care contains suggestions on how you can avoid infection with enteric pathogens while traveling.

▲ Diarrhea

Diarrhea is the most common GI symptom connected with HIV disease. It may loosely be defined as at least three or four liquid bowel movements per day lasting for more than a few days. Diarrhea is not a medical problem unless it is persistent; everyone has loose stools or frequent bowel movements now and then. Diarrhea is commonly caused by such things as transitory infections, reactions to food, or stress.

Diarrhea may be more common in people who are HIV infected for a number of reasons. It may be that reduced secretion of gastric acid and impairment of the mucous membrane lining of the intestine make it easier for organisms to create disease.

You should report diarrhea to your doctor if it persists more than several days, especially if it is severe or associated with pain, weakness, or weight loss. Severe diarrhea may result in dehydration and electrolyte imbalances (an imbalance of important chemicals dissolved in the blood).

Diarrhea can be caused by viruses, bacteria, and protozoa. The most common causes are cytomegalovirus (a virus), *Mycobacterium avium* complex (MAC, a bacterial disease), salmonella, *Escherichia coli* (bacteria), and cryptosporidium (a parasite). Other organisms that can cause diarrhea are *Isospora belli, Giardia lamblia, Entamoeba histolytica* (protozoans), shigella, microsporidium (*Enterocytozoan bienusi*), *Campylobacter jejuni, Clostridium difficile* (bacteria).

Some of these organisms also cause symptoms in those who are not HIV infected. However, HIV-infected people tend to develop them more frequently and more severely.

More than one organism at a time may cause diarrhea. A recent study showed that 25 percent to 40 percent of AIDS patients with diarrhea are infected by multiple organisms.

Diagnosis usually cannot be made by clinical symptoms alone because many different organisms cause the same symptoms. Location of the pain

Diagnostic Workup for Diarrhea

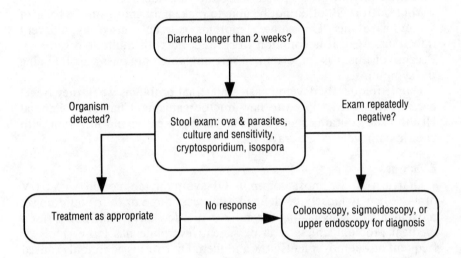

may help identify what part of the GI tract is being infected. This may narrow the diagnosis since various organisms tend to infect different specific parts of the GI tract.

The first step in a work-up for diarrhea is to **have a stool sample examined** in order to identify the organism that is causing the symptoms. You may need to get multiple stool sample examinations because these organisms can be hard to find. Stool exams are simple: they are described in Chapter 13: Procedures and Tests, pp. 299–310.

If no infection is found after multiple stool tests, **some physicians will treat diarrhea on a *presumptive* basis**—that is, without doing further tests to identify the organism causing diarrhea. Empiric treatment with metronidazole (Flagyl) or ciprofloxacin (Cipro) might be reasonable to treat symptoms in people with less severe immune suppression. However-er, in people with more advanced immune suppression, diarrhea may be a valuable warning sign of more serious illness that should be identified and treated. For immune-compromised people, further testing may be more useful than presumptive treatment. One study showed that a specific cause or specific causes could be found in 80 percent to 85 percent of AIDS patients with diarrhea.

If nothing is found in stool examinations or if diarrhea persists after presumptive treatment, then your physician will probably recommend further tests. These tests allow the physician to look at the GI tract and remove small samples of tissue (biopsy) using instruments inserted through one end or the other of the GI tract (that is, through the throat or the rectum). Such a test is called an **endoscopy, sigmoidoscopy,** or **colonoscopy,** depending on which portion of the GI tract is examined. CMV or MAC must be diagnosed by endoscopy or colonoscopy.

Treatment depends on the organism identified. Chronic treatment is often necessary because these infections may recur when treatment is stopped. In addition to treating the underlying cause, symptomatic relief can be obtained with antidiarrheal medication such as Lomotil, Imodium, opiates, octreotide acetate (Sandostatin), and Humatin. If you are dehydrated, drinking a lot of liquid is important—Gatorade is a good choice. Fluid replacement by intravenous method may be necessary if the diarrhea is very severe.

You do not need to stop eating when you have diarrhea. In fact, it is better to eat if you can. Foods containing lactose (dairy products) may make diarrhea worse. Bouillon, chicken soup, cereal, toast, and bananas are often good choices.

Frequent diarrhea may irritate the anus just as a runny nose can irritate the edges of the nostrils. To help prevent irritation, wash the area, dry thoroughly, and use xylocaine ointment.

▲ Pain and Difficulty Swallowing (Esophageal Problems)

Difficulty swallowing (*dysphagia*), a sensation of food sticking, and pain on swallowing (*odynophagia*) are common problems caused by infection of the esophagus. The esophagus is the part of the GI tract between the pharynx (back of the mouth, top of the throat) and the stomach.

The most frequent cause of these symptoms is esophageal candidiasis. This usually occurs along with oral candidiasis (thrush). Esophageal candidiasis can usually be treated effectively with oral medications. These medications may be needed on a regular basis to prevent recurrence of the candidiasis.

Esophageal problems may also have other causes. Herpes simplex virus (HSV) or cytomegalovirus (CMV) are possible causes. Problems in the esophagus may (rarely) be caused by Kaposi's sarcoma or lymphoma.

If you have oral candidiasis (thrush) and you develop difficulty or pain on swallowing, it is most likely due to esophageal candidiasis. Generally, the first approach is a trial of anti-candidial medication (such as ketoconazole). If this is not successful or if you do not have oral candidiasis, endoscopy is necessary for diagnosis.

▲ Nausea and Vomiting

Nausea and vomiting can be transitory symptoms in many illnesses. They can be caused by infection, medication, or central nervous system problems. Contact your doctor if vomiting is severe or persistent. If you have chronic nausea be assertive with your doctor in pursuing relief from the nausea. Nausea due to a new medication frequently lessens as you get used to the drug. Sometimes it may be possible to switch medication to one that causes less nausea. Various medications that can help reduce the symptoms of nausea include Compazine, Phenergan, and Reglan.

▲ Special Diets for Diarrhea, Nausea/Vomiting, and Mouth Pain

There are some special dietary suggestions that can help you maintain weight in the presence of certain gastrointestinal problems. Consult a nutritionist for detailed suggestions suited to your situation.

DIET ADVICE FOR DIARRHEA, NAUSEA, VOMITING, AND MOUTH PAIN

Problem	Advice
Diarrhea	Increase fluids Avoid coffee and alcohol Eat small, frequent meals Reduce roughage, dairy products, and fats
Nausea/vomiting	Eat small, frequent meals Remain upright after eating Avoid greasy or very sweet foods Drink plenty of fluids Contact your physician if you can't keep down liquids
Mouth pain or difficulty swallowing	Eat soft foods that do not need a lot of chewing Avoid very hot or very cold food Avoid spicy food and alcohol

▲ Weight Loss

Weight loss is a common symptom in HIV disease. Opportunistic infections, cancers, and HIV disease can lead to weight loss through a variety of mechanisms. Weight loss can be the result of one or a combination of:

- Nutrient malabsorption caused by disease of the small or large bowel. Examples of opportunistic infections that may lead to malabsorption are cryptosporidiosis, isosporiasis, giardiasis, amebiasis, candidiasis, shigellosis, salmonellosis, MAC, and CMV.
- Lack of adequate intake caused by vomiting, pain in the mouth or other parts of the GI tract, or lack of appetite due to feeling sick from other symptoms of HIV disease. Appetite may disappear with nausea or high fever. It can be difficult to eat if you are depressed or anxious. Hospital food is very often unappetizing. Lack of money can lead to poor diet.
- Wasting, or the loss of lean muscle mass. This condition is also

called protein energy malnutrition. This loss occurs in other chronic infections (such as tuberculosis) and cancers. Wasting causes many problems in the body, and very severe wasting can be fatal. In certain patients, maintaining and even increasing intake of food does not keep the person from losing weight and lean muscle mass. This problem is caused by some kind of dysfunction of metabolism in systemic disease. Current explanations are all speculative.

Specific investigation of weight loss is useful in many situations. If you are otherwise asymptomatic, get a thorough evaluation of weight loss: it may have an identifiable and treatable cause. If you develop diarrhea associated with disorders causing malabsorption, it is important to be evaluated and diagnosed, because many of these diseases can be successfully treated before severe weight loss occurs. Certain medications are useful in controlling severe diarrhea: Lomotil, Imodium, deodorized tincture of opium, or octreotide acetate (Sandostatin/Somatostatin) or Humatin. Some patients with excessive weight loss are helped with an appetite stimulant called Megace (megesterol actetate).

Sometimes a high-fat diet can be useful in excessive weight loss because it is high in calories. However, there are many problems that can occur with high-fat intake, such as diarrhea and problems with the liver and gallbladder.

Liquid supplements high in calories and protein can be used to maintain weight. Examples of commercially available supplements are Enrich, Ensure, Osmolite, Sustacal, and Nutrament. Individual products vary in composition. The choice of supplement will depend on your body's ability to digest lactose, fat, and protein. Vivonex TPN is used for those people with severe difficulty in absorbing nutrition. Some contain specially formulated fats that are better tolerated by people with HIV and therefore reduce diarrhea. Consult your physician about which is most appropriate for your particular clinical situation.

If necessary, nutrition via the mouth can be supplemented or temporarily replaced by intravenous feeding (also called *parenteral nutrition*), or by feeding through a small flexible tube placed through the nose into the stomach (nasogastric feeding, also called *enteral nutrition*). Intravenous feeding is useful to bypass a malfunctioning intestine, while nasogastric feeding is useful to bypass a malfunctioning mouth or esophagus.

Several centers are testing recombinant human growth hormone (Bio-Tropin) in AIDS wasting syndrome, as it appears to increase weight and lean body mass in HIV seropositive people. The side effects include rises in blood sugar and blood pressure. It must be taken with AZT as there is a theoretical risk that growth hormone may increase HIV growth in the absence of antiviral medication.

▲ Anorectal Disease

The most common cause of anorectal problems is herpes, which is by and large treatable. Other possibilities are condyloma accuminata (genital warts), and cytomegalovirus (CMV). Anorectal lesions should be cultured to determine their cause.

LUNG OR BREATHING PROBLEMS

Your body's metabolism, or energy-using system, is like a fire that needs oxygen to burn. Also like a fire, your metabolism will "smother" if carbon dioxide produced by the burning is not removed. The function of the lungs is to get oxygen into, and carbon dioxide out of, the blood. Physically, the lungs are two large structures in the chest that extend from the collarbone down to the diaphragm (the muscular wall that separates the chest cavity from the abdominal cavity).

Air containing oxygen enters the body through the mouth and nose during *inhalation.* Warmed and moistened, air then travels along the major airway (the *trachea*) through the throat and into the chest. A branching system of successively smaller tubes (the *bronchial* passages) carry air to millions of tiny sacs called *alveoli.* Oxygen diffuses through the thin walls separating alveoli from small blood vessels called *capillaries,* which then carry the oxygen-rich blood to the rest of the body. Carbon dioxide diffuses from blood cells in capillaries into alveoli and is expelled from the lungs during *exhalation.*

Some **respiratory symptoms** that may occur in the context of HIV disease are:

- Cough
- Shortness of breath (labored or difficult breathing, *dyspnea*)
- Pleuritic pain (pain on inhalation due to inflammation of the linings of the lung cavities, the *pleura*)
- Spitting of blood or bloodstained sputum
- Wheezing (a whistling quality to breathing, perhaps due to constriction or spasm of the airways)

These symptoms are, of course, also typical of many respiratory problems that are *not* related to HIV. Coughs and congestion are usually caused by colds or the flu. The odds are that a respiratory symptom is *not* serious and *not* caused by an opportunistic infection. However, it is better to check with your doctor if symptoms persist for three or more days, or immediately if accompanied by fever. With opportunistic respiratory infections there is usually but not always a period of systemic symptoms (fever, malaise, weight loss) for several weeks before respiratory symptoms develop.

The organisms that cause respiratory symptoms for HIV-infected people are *Pneumocystis carinii, Mycobacterium avium-intracellulare* (the organisms responsible for MAC), cytomegalovirus (CMV), *Mycobacterium tuberculosis,* pus-producing (*pyogenic*) bacterial infections (caused by organisms such as *Streptococcus pneumoniae,* or *Hemophilus influenza*), fungi, mycoplasma, and legionella. Kaposi's sarcoma may also cause problems in the lungs.

Your doctor should not necessarily assume that respiratory symptoms are HIV related simply because you are HIV infected. A physical exam is not usually adequate to establish a diagnosis of HIV-related opportunistic infection. **X rays and other diagnostic procedures may be needed.** For a more complete description, see Chapter 11: Infections, pp. 212–77. However, sometimes physical findings may be enough for your doctor to tell that your problem is *not* HIV related. A diagnostic work-up should begin with noninvasive tests such as chest X rays although additional tests are frequently needed. Tests used to diagnose respiratory problems are:

- Chest X ray
- Sputum examination
- Gallium scan (should be done in anyone with persistent respiratory symptoms and fever, even if X ray is negative)
- Pulmonary function tests (PFT)
- Bronchoalveolar lavage (BAL) and bronchoscopy (this test usually establishes diagnosis if previous tests have been inconclusive)
- Biopsy—transbronchial and open lung (both definitely last-choice diagnostic procedures done on an inpatient basis because of the risk of collapsed lung—*pneumothorax*)

These tests are described in Chapter 13: Procedures and Tests.

NEUROLOGICAL PROBLEMS

Neurological complications are frequent in patients with AIDS. Clinical studies show that probably 30 percent to 40 percent of AIDS patients eventually have signs or symptoms of neurological problems. Some of these patients have only minor problems of the nervous system that do not interfere with daily functioning. About 10 percent of people with AIDS have neurological problems as the first symptom of HIV disease. Problems of the central nervous system and peripheral nervous system are largely confined to the seriously immune-compromised stage of HIV disease (T4 count below 100). You are not likely to develop any serious neurological problems in earlier stages of HIV disease (T4 count above 100).

Neurological problems in HIV disease may be the result of a number of factors. They may be caused by opportunistic infections or other systemic disease, tumors, side effects of medication, psychological factors, or HIV itself.

Relatively trivial symptoms can occasionally be signs of an underlying disorder, and prompt diagnosis is important to maximize the success of treatment. Many neurological disorders can be treated successfully. Tell your doctor if you have any of the following symptoms:

- Headaches which are severe ("worst headache ever"), of unusual duration, that wake you up from sleep, or that are associated with nausea or vomiting
- Sudden change in vision, or aversion to light (*photophobia*)
- Loss of feeling or movement in part of the body (especially if it occurs on only one side of the body)
- Lowering chin to chest increases headache or causes back pain; stiff neck with headache may also be significant
- Marked change in memory or intellectual functioning

Although many of these problems can also be caused by anxiety, check with your physician.

▲ Neurological Versus Psychiatric Disorders

The discussion of the nervous system will cover both problems that manifest themselves as changes related to the physical body (pain, loss of sensation, loss of function) and problems that manifest themselves as changes related purely to mental state (memory, behavior, intellectual functioning, mood).

Neurologists, psychiatrists, and other mental health professionals treat symptoms depending on their specific nature. Symptoms may be caused by a neurological problem, in which case treatment is directed at the infection, cancer, tissue damage, or biochemical imbalance responsible. However, sometimes symptoms are of psychological origin. Categorizing a disorder as psychological simply means that it may respond to treatment designed to reduce anxiety or resolve conflict.

The purpose of distinguishing neurological from psychiatric disorders is:

- Symptom relief: Diagnosis helps determine what kind of treatment is most likely to relieve the symptoms. If symptoms are *known* to be the result of a brain dysfunction associated with a medical problem, the symptoms will often disappear when the problem is adequately treated.
- Discovering hidden problems: Some symptoms point to a hidden underlying disorder that needs treatment.

These categories are imprecise and the distinctions cloudy. The concepts change as understanding of the physical basis for mental disorders increases.

Neurological disorders can cause either physical or mental symptoms. *Organic physical disorders* involve pain, loss of sensation, or loss of function of a body part or sensory organ. Behavioral and cognitive symptoms (affecting knowing, perceiving, recognizing, and reasoning) with a known or presumed brain dysfunction are classified in the category of *organic mental disorders.* They can sometimes occur without other symptoms.

Mental disorders are called *functional* if a specific organic factor has not yet been identified or if the disorders are psychological or social in origin. **Functional psychiatric disorders** are mental disorders without a known physical basis.

▲ Anatomy of the Nervous System

The nervous system comprises the brain, spinal cord, and nerves throughout the body. The nervous system is divided into two parts, the **central nervous system (CNS)** and the peripheral nervous system (PNS). The CNS consists of the brain and the spinal cord. The PNS consists of the rest of the nerves of the body.

The **brain** consists of three major parts: the cerebrum, the cerebellum, and the brain stem.

The cerebrum is divided into lobes, each of which has a special function. The cerebrum performs many functions. It controls reflex activities such as breathing, heart rate, and blood pressure. It is responsible for cognition—that is, knowing, perceiving, recognizing, judging, sensing, reasoning, and imagining. Along with other parts of the nervous system, the cerebrum helps control motor movement, aspects of sensation, speech, vision, hearing, and behavior.

The cerebellum is important in the coordination of motor movement. The brain stem is that part of the brain that connects the cerebrum to the spinal cord.

The **spinal cord** is the continuation of the lower part of the brain stem. It descends inside the bony column of the backbone. The nerves of the peripheral nervous system emerge from it. Disorders of the spinal cord are referred to as *myelopathy.*

The **cerebrospinal fluid (CSF)** is a clear watery fluid that is produced in the brain. It circulates through the chambers and passages of the brain and the spinal cord and nerves. It supports the brain and provides it with its extracellular fluid. In healthy adults, the CSF has a typical chemical profile that can be measured in laboratory studies (typical amounts of protein, lymphocytes, glucose, etc.). Variations from these normal values suggest neurological problems. Particular illnesses have characteristic laboratory abnormalities of the CSF.

The **peripheral nervous system (PNS)** consists of thirty-one pairs of nerves that connect the spinal column to all the various parts of the body. Some of these nerves are referred to as cranial nerves. These are the nerves that, among other things, connect the sense organs to the brain and allow for smell, vision, taste, and hearing. Disturbances in the peripheral nervous system are referred to as *peripheral neuropathy.*

▲ **Some Terminology**

There are a number of different terms used to describe cerebral syndromes.

The *cranium* is the skull. Disorders of the brain are therefore referred to as *intracranial* **disorders.**

Disorders of the cerebrum are referred to as cerebral disorders. Areas of disturbance that occupy space in the brain are referred to as *cerebral mass lesions.* Primary lymphoma of the brain and toxoplasmosis both cause cerebral mass lesions.

A disease that causes inflammation of the brain is referred to as an **encephalitis.** For example, brain disease caused by *Toxoplasma gondii* is called toxoplasmosis encephalitis.

Meningitis is inflammation of the meninges, the three membranes covering the brain and spinal cord. The type that occurs in HIV disease is usually cryptococcal meningitis, caused by the fungus *Cryptococcus neoformans.* The most common symptom is a severe headache.

Encephalopathy refers to any degenerative brain disease. It is usually used to refer to generalized disorders of the brain. Encephalopathy is characterized by symptoms such as confusion, change of level of consciousness, coma, fever.

Dementia is a global impairment of intellectual functioning, a deficit in perceiving, thinking, and remembering. Dementia can occur as part of encephalopathy. It is a syndrome that has multiple symptoms and can range from very mild (problems with concentration) to very severe (global loss of ability to function). It can be transient or long-lasting, but tends to be chronically progressive. Thinking and movement tend to be slowed down. Both long-term and recent memory are impaired.

Consciousness (awakeness and alertness) remains intact in dementia. This is in contrast to **delirium,** in which consciousness is clouded. Many people with serious illness (such as high fever) can be in a delirious state. Delirium is often further distinguished from dementia by a more abrupt onset, a shorter duration, frequent hallucinations, disordered thinking, and, often, agitated behavior. It is usually transient and reversible.

Seizures are random electrical disturbances in the brain. People commonly have a frightening image of seizures as involving violent muscular convulsions, but only a minority of seizures manifest this way. A seizure may consist simply of a small muscle twitching, a brief blank spell or lapse of memory, or even the illusion of an odor or image. Seizures generally last thirty to sixty seconds.

Focal neurological disorders: Scientists have partially "mapped" the anatomy of the brain and the rest of the nervous system. That is to say, they have some understanding of which parts of the nervous system control activities and functions of other parts of the body. There is a direct anatomical connection between specific parts of the nervous system and other parts of the body.

If you stub your toe, you can expect your toe to hurt and perhaps not to function well for a period of time. However, sometimes when your toe hurts or doesn't function well it may not be the result of an injury to the tissue of the toe, but of some injury to the parts of the nervous system that control function or feeling in that toe. The injury may be to a peripheral nerve, or it may be in the spinal cord or brain.

This is important in terms of understanding disorders of the nervous system. A particular symptom (pain or loss of sensation or function) can often be connected to problems in a particular area of the brain or other parts of the nervous system. A neurologist diagnoses by "localizing" the disorder—that is, identifying what part of the brain or nervous system is affected.

Focal neurological deficits are problems caused by disturbance in a particular area of the brain. They cause loss of some specific sensory or motor function(s) rather than generalized confusion, dementia, or change in level of consciousness. Some examples of focal neurological deficits are irregularities of muscle coordination *(ataxia),* paralysis or weakness of part of the body *(hemiparesis),* loss of sensation in part of the body *(hemianesthesia),* or loss of an area of vision *(hemianopia).*

Physicians who suspect a neurological disorder will first perform a physical exam and ask questions. The next step may be the use of imaging techniques such as X rays, ultrasound, brain *computerized tomography* (CT) scan, or *magnetic resonance imaging* (MRI). These procedures are all painless and can be done on an out-patient basis. *Lumbar puncture* (LP, also known as a spinal tap) is another commonly used diagnostic procedure. A sample of cerebrospinal fluid is removed with a needle for laboratory examination. For more description of these techniques, refer to Chapter 13: Procedures and Tests.

▲ Neurological Symptoms of Initial HIV Infection Are Transitory

Immediate symptoms of HIV infection may resemble the flu. A variety of neurological disorders can also appear at this time. They include inflammation of the brain *(encephalitis),* inflammation of the linings of the brain and spinal cord *(meningitis),* irregularities of muscle coordination *(ataxia),* disease of the spinal cord *(myelopathy),* or peripheral neuropathy. Such symptoms are common in many viral illnesses.

Because at the time of HIV infection the immune system is still functioning well, most neurological symptoms are better within a few weeks. It is believed that HIV itself may directly cause damage.

HIV can be found in the brain after initial infection and before any neurological symptoms develop. However, HIV infection of the brain rarely causes noticeable neurological symptoms prior to the development of other physical symptoms serious enough to merit a diagnosis of AIDS. Severe dementia typically occurs only when T4 counts drop below 50.

▲ AIDS Dementia Complex (ADC)

AIDS dementia complex (ADC) is an organic mental disorder believed to be caused by HIV infection of the brain. ADC is the most common cause of dementia (a loss of intellectual functioning) in HIV disease. HIV does not seem to be able to cause neurological disease until there has been extensive suppression of the immune system.

ADC has been called by different names in the past: HIV encephalitis, subacute encephalitis or encephalopathy, and multifocal giant-cell encephalitis. ADC is the most frequently used term at this point and is becoming part of the standard psychiatric nomenclature.

There is some evidence of changes to the central nervous system early on in the course of HIV disease. This evidence consists of anecdotal case reports, early detection of cerebrospinal fluid (CSF) abnormalities, brain abnormalities on computerized tomography (CT) scans, magnetic resonance imaging (MRI), and electroencephalograms (EEG), studies showing the presence of abnormal cells in the subcortex, and some results of neuropsychological testing. None of these signs is necessarily associated with any appearance of symptoms or loss of functioning.

Neuropsychological tests are written or oral tests that attempt to measure an individual's cognitive functioning (knowing, perceiving, judging, sensing, reasoning). More than thirty studies have been done to assess early neuropsychological deficits in HIV disease. **The largest studies show no significant early impairment.** The neuropsychological impairments that appeared in some studies on tests in asymptomatic HIV-infected patients were minor difficulties. Other tests, including those that measure vocabulary and object naming, tend to remain normal even in advanced ADC.

There are many complications in understanding the results of these studies. Studies used different neuropsychological tests and different criteria in choosing subjects. A variety of statistical procedures were used to analyze the results, and this affects interpretation of results. Most significantly, a "neuropsychological deficit" only means a less-than-average performance on a neuropsychological test. Data on neuropsychological tests have not been correlated with dysfunction in daily living or vocational activities.

Any neurological changes that occur in most HIV-infected people prior to the development of other physical symptoms are subtle and not evident in vocational ability. **No neurological evidence supports the banning of normally behaving HIV-infected people from any job.**

The important thing to remember if you are HIV infected is that you are not likely to suffer from serious mental changes unless you become severely ill. AIDS dementia complex rarely appears prior to other symptoms and few HIV-infected persons have dementia as their first diagnosis.

Any marked cognitive difficulty should be investigated. It should not be presumed that symptoms are being caused by untreatable ADC. Problems may be related to depression or anxiety and may be treated with therapy or medication, or they may represent a specific treatable physical disease, such as toxoplasmosis, cryptococcal meningitis, and primary lymphoma of the brain.

Course of dementia: The incidence of ADC generally increases for patients with more advanced HIV disease. However, for some patients ADC does not get worse as other symptoms progress. Some patients have multiple opportunistic infections and never develop ADC. Other patients have progressive neurological disease with few opportunistic infections. Occasionally mental decline may be rapid but it is usually slow with periods of recovery. Although ADC tends to be progressive, some patients can improve.

ADC can cause cognitive, motor, and behavioral dysfunctions. Most prominent are cognitive dysfunctions such as the impairment of recent memory. Symptoms are characteristic but can vary a good deal. Some patients may have primarily cognitive symptoms and others may have primarily motor symptoms.

The **earliest cognitive symptoms** are difficulties with concentration and memory. People with early ADC may be forgetful and may lose track of their train of thought. Someone with ADC may feel that his or her thinking is slower, or that complicated tasks are harder to do. There may be an increased need to keep lists or a discovery that routine tasks take longer to perform. There may be a loss of precision. However, anxiety and depression can produce essentially the same symptoms.

Early in ADC these cognitive problems are subtle and do not present any serious interference with functioning. A *mental status exam*—the general test clinicians use to assess mental functioning—will not show any major changes. Psychological tests may show some minor changes. CT or MRI scan may be normal or may show nonspecific findings with some cerebral atrophy (shrinking of tissue of the cerebrum). These tests are useful to eliminate the possibility of cerebral mass lesions, which may present with similar symptoms and require different treatment. Sometimes in late ADC there can be global dementia. Patients will have seriously impaired cognitive functioning—that is, extensive and interfering with functioning in a major way—and require help with many activities of daily living.

Early on in the course of ADC, there may be some **motor performance symptoms,** primarily poor balance and clumsiness (doing things more slowly or less precisely). Additional difficulties are slowed movement, ataxia (failure of coordination), dropping things more often, or minor gait problems that can lead to tripping. Some signs may be seen on careful early neurological exam. Significant weakness or asymmetry of symptoms suggests a diagnosis other than ADC. Very late in the course of

ADC, there may be severely diminished motor activity, extreme weakness, or partial paralysis.

Behavioral and other symptoms: In some people with ADC, there may be a tendency toward apathy and loss of initiative or social withdrawal. This can be difficult to distinguish from depression. A small number of people with ADC become irritable and hyperactive, even manic or agitated or psychotic.

Treatment for ADC: High-dose AZT (10 to 12 pills per day) halts or reverses symptoms in some patients, at least partially. The largest controlled study done so far showed an improvement in neuropsychological tests in patients with ADC treated with AZT as compared to placebo. This may have to do either with direct effects of the AZT on the nervous system or the general improvement of health in those treated with AZT.

Psychotropic medications for anxiety and depression associated with ADC are being investigated. Antidepressants may be helpful, although it is possible that some—maprotaline (Ludiomil), and trazodone (Desyrel)—may be associated with increased incidence of anticholinergic side effects (dry mouth, constipation, sometimes more severe symptoms).

Patients who are suffering from ADC can be helped with structure in daily activities. In early ADC, lists and reminders will be helpful. In more severe ADC, devices to help with orientation (a clock, a calendar) are useful. A balance should be sought between over-stimulation and lack of stimulation. That is, people with ADC need contact and activity and conversation. However, they may feel worse with large groups of people at one time or with rapid changes in their environment.

▲ Neurologic Opportunistic Infections by Organism

See Chapter 11: Infections for more complete information on the diseases listed below.

Toxoplasmosis is the most common cause of neurological disease in AIDS patients (5 percent to 15 percent of AIDS patients). It can cause both focal symptoms and encephalopathy with confusion and clouding of consciousness. Common symptoms are headache, weakness, seizures (new onset), personality change, loss of movement, and loss of sensation: a CT scan can detect signs of toxoplasmosis.

Cryptococcus neoformans is a fungus that is the most common cause of meningitis. It causes both encephalopathy and focal dysfunction. Common symptoms are headache, fever, nausea, vomiting, and confusion.

Aseptic meningitis is meningitis in which no organism can be found in the cerebrospinal fluid (CSF). The major symptom is headache. Aseptic meningitis can be acute or chronic. Remission can be spontaneous, but relapse is frequent.

Progressive multifocal leukoencephalopathy (PML): is caused by a virus called the JC virus. It is progressive at a variable rate. Cognitive deficits appear first, followed by focal signs. Common symptoms are *hemiparesis* (weakness on one side of the body), *hemianopia* (disturbance of half of the visual field), and *ataxia* (muscular discoordination or irregularity).

Viral encephalitis is usually caused by the herpes simplex or varicella zoster virus (or possibly sometimes by CMV). These viruses can also cause focal disorders and meningitis. Herpes simplex virus (HSV) encephalitis is treated with acyclovir.

Fungal encephalitis: Cases reported have been caused by candidiasis, aspergillosis, coccidiomycosis, mucormycosis. Diagnosis is made by finding fungus in biopsied tissue.

Neurosyphilis: Late-stage syphilis can cause neurological problems, including dementia, meningitis, strokes, or peripheral neuropathy.

▲ Cancers of the Nervous System

Primary non-Hodgkin's lymphoma (NHL) of the brain can cause either focal dysfunction or encephalitis. NHL of the brain is treated with chemotherapy and radiation. Systemic lymphoma can also metastasize (spread) to the brain, although this is rare. For more information on lymphomas, refer to Chapter 12: Cancers, pp. 289–92.

▲ Complications of Systemic Disorders (Metabolic or Toxic Encephalopathy)

Any drug or disturbance of the metabolism that can cause serious systemic symptoms can also cause neurological problems. Neurological problems can be caused by drugs that affect the CNS or by drug overdoses. They can also be caused by various nonneurological diseases (such as pneumonia) that lead to lack of oxygen in the blood, sodium deficiency, low level of blood sugar, or organ failure. Patients with these conditions sometimes develop encephalitis.

Neuroleptic drugs (such as Thorazine, Stelazine, or Haldol) used to treat psychosis and delirium can cause *dystonic reactions* (problems with muscle tone that cause movement disorders) and possibly increased incidence of *neuroleptic malignant syndrome* (a serious syndrome that causes fever, lung problems, and sometimes kidney failure). These side effects probably occur at an increased rate in people who are HIV infected.

▲ Intracranial disorders

People with HIV disease get **headaches**—just like everyone else. They are usually caused by stress, caffeine withdrawal, sinus problems, and other causes that are not connected to any serious disease. Severe headaches might be caused by cryptococcal meningitis, toxoplasmosis, or progressive multifocal leukencephalopathy (PML). New, persistent, or severe headaches should be investigated with use of a CT scan, magnetic resonance imaging (MRI), and lumbar puncture (LP).

Focal neurological disorders in HIV disease usually develop slowly over a period of days or weeks. They can be caused by toxoplasmosis, progressive multifocal leukencephalopathy (PML), or central nervous system (CNS) lymphoma. The symptoms in all these diseases are generally the same. Sometimes focal symptoms may be accompanied by encephalitis with confusion and clouding of consciousness.

Cerebral mass lesions are growths that displace brain tissue. The most common cause of cerebral mass lesions is toxoplasmosis, followed by primary central nervous system (CNS) lymphoma. Toxoplasmosis typically has a sharper presentation and more frequent focal signs. The symptoms of cerebral mass lesions are altered level of consciousness, seizures, and paralysis or sensory loss in part of the body. If the cerebellum is also involved, loss of motor coordination (ataxia) or cranial nerve signs can be involved. Diagnosis is made with use of a CT scan or an MRI exam. Multiple lesions usually indicate toxoplasmosis, single lesions indicate primary lymphoma. Physicians usually make a trial effort to treat with antitoxoplasmosis drugs since this is the most likely cause and it is important to treat toxoplasmosis promptly. If there is no response to medication for toxoplasmosis after three weeks, confirmation of lymphoma can be made by CT-guided "skinny needle" brain biopsy (a diagnostic procedure under investigation). Alternatively, if other causes of cerebral mass lesions have been ruled out, some physicians consider whole-brain radiation therapy.

Meningitis is inflammation of the meninges, the three membranes covering the brain and spinal cord. The type that occurs in HIV disease is usually cryptococcal meningitis, caused by the fungus *Cryptococcus neoformans.* The most common symptom is a severe headache.

Seizures can be caused by any of the HIV-related CNS disorders. The most common causes are cerebral mass lesions, meningitis-causing diseases, encephalitic diseases, and AIDS dementia complex. Diagnosis is made with CT scan or magnetic resonance imaging (MRI), followed by a spinal tap (lumbar puncture, LP) if the CT scan or MRI is negative. In 20 percent of HIV-infected patients, no cause is found. In such cases seizures are probably caused either by HIV or cytomegalovirus (CMV). Seizures are usually treated successfully with phenobarbitol or phenytoin (Dilantin).

The first step in **diagnosis** is a careful neurological exam. This may include both physical examination (for example, tests of reflexes and sensation) and a mental status exam (verbal questions designed to elicit information about memory, concentration, and thinking). Classifying and locating the disorder will help the neurologist diagnose and treat. The state of the immune system strongly influences what disease is likely to develop and must be considered in establishing a diagnosis.

After the physical exam, the next step may be the use of imaging techniques such as X rays, ultrasound, brain CT scan, or MRI. These procedures are painless and can be done on an out-patient basis.

Lumbar puncture (LP, also known as a spinal tap) is another commonly used diagnostic procedure. A sample of cerebrospinal fluid is removed with a needle for laboratory examination.

In some instances a biopsy of the brain may be needed.

▲ Disorders of the Peripheral Nerves

Peripheral neuropathy means any disturbance of function or change in the cells of the peripheral nervous system. Peripheral neuropathy occurs with increased frequency in those with HIV disease as compared to the rest of the population of the United States. Peripheral neuropathy is diagnosed by neurological exam and electromyography (EMG).

The most common type of peripheral neuropathy in people with HIV disease is called **distal symmetric polyneuropathy.** Some studies show that it affects about 35 percent of hospitalized AIDS patients with systemic symptoms. Neuropathy can also be caused by some drugs such as alcohol, vincristine, isoniazid, ddI, and ddC. Other causes are unknown.

The symptoms are mainly sensory and consist of numbness or tingling of the hands and feet, weakness in the legs, arms, and hands, or a burning feeling on the soles of the feet and the ends of the fingers and toes. Loss of reflexes can occur. Usually the numbness and weakness are mild but the burning feeling in the feet may be quite painful and interfere with the ability to walk. Symptoms tend to be worse at night. The symptoms are symmetrical—that is, the same on both sides of the body. Peripheral neuropathies are diagnosed by neurological exam. Treatment may include a drug that affects neurotransmitter levels such as the tricyclic antidepressant Elavil.

Another type of peripheral neuropathy is called **chronic inflammatory neuropathy.** These types of neuropathies occur in otherwise asymptomatic HIV-positive individuals and in symptomatic people with relatively well-functioning immune systems. The symptoms are patchy motor and sensory defects. They may appear suddenly or slowly. A treatment recently tried with success is a type of blood filtering called *plasmapheresis.*

MYALGIA (MUSCLE PAIN) AND MYOPATHY (MUSCLE DISORDERS)

Myopathy means muscle disease. At times, people who are HIV-infected develop pain or weakness of muscles, particularly in the legs. Progressive weakness can develop. Both AZT and HIV itself can cause myopathy.

Myopathy caused by AZT does not occur until after at least 6 months of use. If myopathy does occur, it takes an average of about twelve months to appear. AZT causes myopathy by affecting reproduction of *mitochondria,* cellular components that make the cell's basic fuel.

Myopathy can be detected by testing blood serum for the level of an enzyme called *creatine kinase* (CK). Elevation of CK shows that muscle tissue is being broken down, and is usually transient. People who are very active physically also show elevation of CK.

Myopathy is rare among those with early HIV disease. Symptomatic myopathy may be treated by stopping or switching antiviral medication, by taking a short-term course of prednisone (40 to 60 mg per day), or by use of a nonsteroidal antiinflammatory drug.

SYSTEMIC PROBLEMS

Fevers, night sweats, *anorexia* (loss of appetite), weight loss, lethargy, and malaise are collectively described as *systemic* symptoms. They are also called *constitutional symptoms* or *B symptoms.* Systemic symptoms can result from many possible causes: opportunistic infections, malignancies, or from HIV itself. Because these symptoms are not specific, the work-up required for diagnosis is difficult to summarize.

Discuss with your doctor the pros and cons of pursuing a diagnosis in the presence of any persistent constitutional symptom. Balance the costs of diagnostic testing (pain, discomfort, money, inconvenience, stress, side effects) against the chance that accurate diagnosis will lead to helpful treatment. Some diseases are self-limiting: the cost of work-up may exceed the benefit. At other times, waiting can lead to more serious illness and even death. A work-up of systemic symptoms generally should begin with tests that do not require undue discomfort or financial cost to narrow down possibilities: history, physical, certain lab tests.

Fever is a common symptom of many illnesses. For this reason, the question of when a fever should be medically evaluated is complicated. If you are HIV-infected and in fairly good health, a fever for a few days is usually not a sign of any serious problem. The most common causes of fevers are colds and flu. You should always consult your physician if a fever lasts more than four days. A high fever (over 102 degrees F) is also a reason to consult your doctor. If you have an in-dwelling catheter (Hickman or Port-A-Cath) and develop a fever be particularly diligent about calling your doctor. The fever could be a sign of infection at the site of the catheter and should be treated promptly, generally in the hospital.

Blood tests are the central diagnostic tools of a fever evaluation. Routine blood tests assess the general state of your health. Cultures of blood (and possible other bodily fluids such as urine and cerebrospinal fluid) will look for a variety of infectious organisms. There may be a long wait for results from some of these tests, because cultures may take a long time to grow out. Your physician may begin to treat you for the most likely illness while waiting for test results to confirm the diagnosis (*presumptive treatment*).

EAR AND SINUS INFECTIONS

HIV-infected people have increased incidence of sinusitis (inflammation of the sinuses). It may be caused by a variety of organisms, some of which can be treated with antibiotics. One regime in use is the combination of an antibiotic (such as Ceclor) with an antihistamine (such as Entex). Bactrim may also be helpful and is under investigation. It may sometimes be associated with post-nasal drip, which can also be caused by allergies. When the cause is allergy, inhaled topical therapy (cromolyn solution, Nasalcrom) may be useful.

HEART PROBLEMS

When physicians perform certain heart tests on HIV-infected patients, they frequently find laboratory evidence of cardiac (heart) abnormalities. This is particularly true of patients with advanced AIDS. However, these abnormalities do not usually cause any significant symptoms. Some researchers estimate that fewer than 5 percent of AIDS patients have clinically apparent cardiac disease and this occurs only in advanced AIDS. However, as survival time with AIDS increases, cardiac abnormalities may eventually cause disease more often.

Cardiac problems probably occur most frequently among those who have shared needles for drug use.

The cause of cardiac abnormalities in AIDS patients is not clear. They may sometimes be caused by infections such as *Cryptococcus neoformans, Toxoplasma gondii,* or *Mycobacterium avium-intracellulare* (which causes MAC), and cytomegalovirus (CMV) but in most cases no specific organism can be found. Cardiac abnormalities may in fact be caused by HIV itself.

People with cardiac abnormalities often notice shortness of breath. A chest X ray may also show that the heart is enlarged. The most frequent test used to diagnose cardiac problems is a painless ultrasound procedure called an *echocardiogram.* Echocardiogram is recommended if a routine electrocardiogram (EKG) shows abnormalities or if there is shortness of breath that cannot be adequately explained by lung disease.

Intravenous pentamidine therapy may cause cardiac arrhythmias (heartbeat irregularities). If you receive IV pentamidine while hospitalized you will be given tests to check on the condition of your heart every few days (EKG, serum electrolytes).

KIDNEY PROBLEMS

The kidneys are twin fist-sized organs located in the back of the torso, just under the bottom of the ribcage. Kidneys filter blood, removing the waste products of metabolism in the form of urine. Kidneys also regulate the amount of various chemicals dissolved in the fluids outside cells, including hydrogen, sodium, potassium, phosphate, and others. This regulation assures that cells have the chemical environment they need to function.

▲ Causes

If kidney problems occur, it is generally because a person is already sick with an infection or malignancy. For example, diarrhea, vomiting, or lack of sufficient fluid consumption can lead to loss of adequate sodium or potassium, affecting the kidneys. Kidney problems occur more frequently among intravenous drug users and people taking nonsteroidal antiinflammatory drugs.

Other factors that can cause kidney problems for people with AIDS include dehydration, lack of adequate oxygen, and the side effects of drugs. Drugs that sometimes cause kidney problems include pentamidine, amikacin, foscarnet, and amphotericin-B.

HIV itself can sometimes cause kidney disease; this is referred to as HIV-*associated nephropathy* (HIVAN).

A complaint that sometimes occurs in advanced HIV disease is increased frequency of urination, especially at night. The cause is unknown.

▲ Treatment

Kidney problems can generally be treated. One of the purposes of frequent and repeated blood tests when you are severely ill is to make sure that your kidneys are working well. If blood tests show signs of any potential problems, treatment can begin promptly. Treatment often requires adjusting doses of certain medications, increasing fluid intake, and a special diet.

▲ Renal failure

Acute renal failure (ARF) is a critical loss of function of the kidneys that is seen only in those who are critically ill with an HIV-related opportunistic infection or malignancy. ARF is very dangerous since without working kidneys the body is swiftly poisoned by its own waste products. Mechanical filtering of the blood outside the body (called *hemodialysis*) should be considered for HIV-infected people with ARF: there is evidence that some people in this condition do regain kidney function.

ENDOCRINE PROBLEMS (ADRENAL INSUFFICIENCY)

The endocrine system is composed of organs, glands, and tissues in the body that secrete hormones that regulate the activities of certain cellular and body functions. Examples are the adrenal glands, the pituitary gland, the thyroid gland, and the pancreas.

A variety of endocrine problems arise as complications of HIV disease. The problem that has been studied the most is a decline in production of adrenal hormones, a condition called *adrenal insufficiency*.

The adrenal glands are paired structures located near the kidneys. The adrenal glands secrete several types of hormones, including those that maintain the crucial balance of sodium and potassium in the body. Adrenal insufficiency is a condition in which production of hormones by the adrenal glands is altered from its normal balance. The most common causes of adrenal insufficiency among HIV-infected patients are cytomegalovirus (CMV), *Mycobacterium avium* complex (MAC), and autoimmune disorders. Adrenal insufficiency can also be caused by Kaposi's sarcoma (KS) lesions, other infectious diseases (cryptococcosis, histoplasmosis, tuberculosis) and some drugs: ketoconazole (Nizoral), rifampin (RIF).

The signs and symptoms of adrenal insufficiency are vague and include the following: low blood pressure (*hypotension*), light headedness, loss of appetite, weight loss, low-grade fever, fatigue, and sometimes aches in muscles or joints. Laboratory indication of possible adrenal insufficiency is high levels of potassium in the blood (*hyperkalemia*) or low levels of sodium (*hyponatremia*). If severe, adrenal insufficiency can be life-threatening.

Adrenal insufficiency is usually diagnosed based on clinical findings. However, patients with symptomatic CMV disease may show adrenal insufficiency on routine blood tests (*serum electrolytes*): the condition can be confirmed by more complex laboratory measures of adrenal steroid hormones.

Treatment for adrenal insufficiency is the same for HIV-infected and non-HIV-infected patients—restoration of the balance of sodium and potassium and the administration of synthetic adrenal corticosteroids to replace the missing hormones. These must be used cautiously in HIV-infected patients because they are immunosuppressive.

Chapter 11
Infections

This chapter begins with some basic information about infections and the organisms that cause them. The rest of the chapter is devoted to some of the more significant infectious complications of HIV disease.

BASIC INFORMATION ABOUT INFECTIONS

Infection is the introduction of microscopic foreign entities (often called *microorganisms*) into the body. Once microorganisms are established in the tissues of the body they may increase in number by any of a variety of methods of reproduction.

Most infections are benign and cause no damage. Some infections are useful or in fact necessary to proper functioning of the body. An example of such a *symbiosis* (an infection that is mutually profitable to host and parasite) is the presence of dozens of species of bacteria in the human gut that aid digestion.

Some infections, however, cause tissue damage. Our perception of infections in general is colored by harmful infections because these are the infections of which the average person is conscious. Infections can cause damage in a variety of ways:

- By releasing harmful chemicals (*toxins*)
- By multiplying inside cells to the point where the cells cannot function or may even burst open
- By consuming nutrients or useful chemicals needed by body tissue
- By stimulating a disastrous immune response from the host that backfires and destroys the body's own tissues

▲ Causative Organisms

Disease-causing agents have many forms. Some are familiar (bacteria, viruses) and some are less familiar (fungi, retroviruses, mycoplasmas).

Historically, microorganisms have been categorized based on common characteristics observable with the microscope. These include:

- Size and shape
- Characteristics of the enclosing membrane or wall (if any)
- Presence or absence of interior compartments that allow chemical

reactions to occur in isolation from the rest of the cell. The most famous of these compartments is the *nucleus,* which contains the genetic material.

• Details of the reproductive cycle of the organism

In the twentieth century, information about the chemical and molecular basis of genetic material has also been used to characterize microorganisms.

These categories are human constructs, based on observation and experience. The categories are often useful but are not necessarily reflective of any absolute truth. *Pneumocystis carinii,* the organism that causes PCP, looks and behaves like a protozoan parasite but has genetic material that shows it to be related to the fungi. How should this organism then be categorized? Is it a protozoan parasite or a fungus?

Some people are unsettled by scientists' inability to provide a definite answer to such questions. The problem is not that scientists are ignorant but that no set of categories neatly partitions the exuberant variety of natural organisms.

Be careful when thinking about infectious disease. Your first instincts may not always be right. For instance, viruses and retroviruses do not comfortably fit into commonsense notions derived from daily life, such as the distinction between living and unliving (because they have no independent biological activity) or between self and other (since they may spend part of their life cycle simply as a genetic sequence hidden within the host cell's chromosomes).

Viruses are protein-shelled particles containing genetic material and sometimes enzymes. Viruses sometimes have an enclosing fatty (lipid) membrane. Viruses have no ability to reproduce on their own and are completely reliant upon the host cell for protein synthesis and replication. Classic viruses carry DNA or RNA, which is then used to make viral proteins, which are assembled into new virus particles (virions).

Retroviruses use RNA as their genetic material, but use an enzyme called reverse transcriptase to force the cell to make a DNA copy that is then incorporated into the cell's own native genetic material. The part of the host's DNA that encodes the retrovirus is called the *provirus.* If the host cell divides, the provirus divides right along with rest of the host DNA, and the retroviral infection is passed along to the daughter cells. A more detailed description of retroviral behavior is given in Chapter 17: HIV: Virology and Therapeutic Strategies, p. 342.

Viruses and retroviruses have been implicated in the development of at least some cancers.

Bacteria are single-celled organisms that lack a nucleus or any other membrane-bound organelles (specialized structures). Bacteria are mostly rigid-walled and are usually spiral, rod-shaped, or spherical.

A useful laboratory test called a Gram stain distinguishes among species of bacteria based on whether their cell walls retain a particular dye. Gram-negative bacteria lose this stain, indicating a more complex type of cell wall, and a more complex (and more dangerous) organism. Gram-positive bacteria retain the stain, and are simpler.

Protozoan parasites are single-celled, soft-walled organisms possessing a nucleus. Protozoa are often able to transport themselves using whiplike *flagella*, hairlike *cilia*, or tentaclelike *pseudopodia*. Protozoa may have several distinct developmental stages in their life cycle.

A **fungus** is a single-celled, usually rigid-walled organism possessing a nucleus. Fungi lack chlorophyll. Examples of fungi are yeasts, molds, and mushrooms. Fungi may have several distinct developmental stages in their life cycle.

Mycoplasma are single-celled organisms that resemble bacteria (having no nucleus) but have a soft membrane rather than a bacterium's rigid cell wall. A mycoplasma has been suggested as a possible co-factor for HIV disease, although clinical trials of antibiotics that suppress mycoplasma have not shown any beneficial effect on the clinical course of HIV.

MICROORGANISM CATEGORIES

Entity	Enclosure	Inclosures	Genetic material	Protein synthesis
Virus	Protein-shelled particle	None	DNA or RNA	Dependent on host
Retrovirus	Protein-shelled particle	None	RNA	Dependent on host. Uses RT enzyme to make DNA that becomes part of host's genes
Bacterium	Rigid cell wall (usually)	None	DNA	Independent
Protozoan	Non-rigid cell membrane (usually)	Nucleus, organelles	DNA	Independent
Fungus	Rigid cell wall (usually)	Nucleus, organelles	DNA	Independent
Mycoplasma	Membrane instead of rigid cell wall	None, like bacteria	DNA	Independent

▲ Epidemiology

Epidemiology is the study of how diseases occur within populations. The first question that epidemiology sets out to answer is, "How should observations of illness be categorized as disease?" The second question is, "What population(s) does a disease affect?" The third question is, "How does a disease progress in a given population?"

Observations of illness stem from *cases*. A case is the report of *signs* and *symptoms* in one patient. A *sign* is a measurement of some kind, such as pulse rate, temperature, or the results from a blood test. A *symptom* is anything the patient reports directly, such as abdominal pain, headache, or shortness of breath. If many cases are reported in which similar signs and symptoms appear with unknown cause, this set of cases is called a *syndrome*. The *prevalence* of a syndrome is the proportion of a given population identified to have the syndrome. The *incidence* of a syndrome is the number of new cases of the syndrome reported over a given period.

If a cause or agency exists without which a syndrome does not occur (the cause is *necessary)*, and that accounts for all the signs and symptoms of a syndrome (the cause is *sufficient),* then the syndrome is called a *disease*. A syndrome may not be identifiable as the result of a single physical disease acting in a population. Also, different syndromes may turn out to be aspects of the same disease (as in the great variety of presentations of syphilis).

The Centers for Disease Control (CDC) is the governmental agency responsible for tracking epidemics in this country. Physicians and other health care providers must report cases of certain syndromes and diseases to the CDC for inclusion in epidemiological statistics. Health care providers notify the CDC if they notice any unusual patterns of illness in their patients. The CDC collects case reports of unusual illnesses and attempts to identify causes.

In 1981 physicians around the nation began to report clusters of young homosexual men who had developed a then-rare pneumonia caused by the organism *Pneumocystis carinii*. These patients went on to develop numerous other rare complications, previously seen only in those with severely damaged immune systems. The patterns began to emerge as more and more cases were reported.

To track this new epidemic, the CDC named it *acquired immunodeficiency syndrome* and defined it with a formal set of symptom-based criteria. To be defined as having AIDS a patient had to have one or more of a specific list of diseases and have no other reason to be immune deficient. When HIV was identified as the cause of AIDS and the antibody test became available, the definition was changed to include a positive HIV test. Still later, the definition was widened to include HIV-infected people who had lost substantial amounts of lean body mass (*wasting syndrome*), or who had certain cognitive deficits (*AIDS dementia complex*). The definition of AIDS may be changed yet again: all HIV-infected people with T4 counts below 200 may be defined as having AIDS.

Activists have been very concerned with the formal definition of AIDS for several reasons. Before the inclusion of people with wasting or dementia, a substantial group of people with HIV disease were sick, unable to work, and yet not eligible for benefits because they did not fit the formal CDC definition of AIDS. In addition, policy decisions and the

215

allocation of resources were based on the official CDC statistics—narrower definitions of AIDS understated the dimensions of the epidemic. However, epidemiologists were reluctant to alter the definition because the case figures depended on it: it is much harder to interpret trends in figures whose definition is constantly changing. Accurate epidemiologic analysis cannot be performed on a moving target.

The word *syndrome* is part of the acronym AIDS because the cause was unknown when the term AIDS was coined. AIDS refers to an advanced stage of a viral illness. HIV *disease,* on the other hand, refers to the full range of illness caused by infection with this virus. HIV is necessary to cause AIDS: the full syndrome does not occur in the absence of HIV infection. HIV may well be sufficient to cause AIDS by itself. However, HIV-infected people develop AIDS at such different rates that many researchers have suspected the existence of a *co-factor* (such as co-infection with another organism) that accelerates the appearance of AIDS.

▲ Transmission

Many people have misconceptions about how infections are transmitted. Some misconceptions are listed here, together with explanations of why these ideas are incorrect.

Misconception: If you come into any kind of contact with an infectious organism, you inevitably become infected (exposure versus infection).

Correction: We are constantly exposed to a large variety of microorganisms, both from other animals and from the environment. Only some of these exposures result in actual infection, defined as the establishment and reproduction in the body of a significant colony of a particular microorganism. Many factors affect whether an exposure results in infection: the inherent transmissibility of the strain of the microorganism; the quantity or concentration of organisms involved in the exposure; and the susceptibility of the host, which itself depends on the host's genetic predisposition, history of infection, current state of health, and other factors.

Misconception: Once infected you inevitably develop symptoms and get sick (acute versus latent or subclinical illness).

Correction: Most infections cause no symptoms at all. Consequently, we are usually aware of only the few infections that cause noticeable symptoms. Even those species of microorganism that do cause illness usually make only some infected hosts sick. Those who do get sick experience widely varying severity of illness.

Misconception: If you have no symptoms, you are not infected and not able to transmit to those around you (latent versus noninfectious).

Correction: It is absolutely possible for a person to become infected by transmission of an infection from an infected person who is experiencing no symptoms. In fact, in many common infections, the period of greatest transmissibility occurs before noticeable illness.

Misconception: Once infected you are able to transmit the infection to those around you, perhaps simply by being near them (specificity of transmission routes; infectious versus contagious disease).
Correction: Infections are transmitted by very specific and very different routes.

Some organisms infect via the lungs, some via the gastrointestinal tract, some via the mucous membranes of the genitals, and some by direct introduction into the bloodstream.

Only those diseases transmitted through airborne droplets that are inhaled into the lungs are called *contagious.* Other diseases are merely *infectious.*

Some diseases require that cells from an infected person be brought into contact with certain mucous membranes of the potential host before transmission is possible. Such diseases are said to be *sexually transmitted,* because this type of cell-to-mucous-membrane contact most often occurs during vaginal or rectal intercourse. Some people imagine that sexually transmitted diseases are especially transmissible. Actually, the reverse is true: sexually transmitted infections, by their nature, are less transmissible than other diseases. Guilt about sexual activity may encourage misconceptions about sexually transmitted diseases. Sexually transmitted diseases vary in the ease with which they are transmitted, and may also vary in the risk associated with various sexual activities (e.g., oral-genital versus genital-genital sex, or penile-rectal versus penile-vaginal intercourse).

In some diseases, organisms may be present in the blood of an infected host. These *blood-borne* infections may be transmitted by the direct injection of infected blood into an uninfected host. Blood-borne infections are very often transmissible by other routes as well. HIV and hepatitis B, for instance, are both blood-borne and sexually transmitted.

An important route of transmission in some infectious diseases is from a pregnant woman to her fetus, either during pregnancy or delivery. This is called *perinatal* transmission.

▲ Course of Illness and Corresponding Interventions

Each infectious disease has a characteristic course of illness. Some diseases are very predictable and follow a rigid schedule of stages, severity, and duration. The course of other diseases may be more variable. Genetic susceptibility and general health play large roles in determining the course of illness in individuals.

Certain stages in the course of illness are common to many diseases. For each stage a medical intervention may be possible to control or limit the illness.

Primary infection is the initial entry into the body of the infectious organism and the establishment of a significant reproducing colony of that organism. The earliest stage of infection with most organisms is often silent and produces few noticeable symptoms. Within a few days to a few weeks of a new infection the body's immune system may react with a wide variety of symptoms. Inflammation, fever, flu-like symptoms, or skin changes are common reactions to infection, but are not always present.

Clearly, the best way to control an infectious organism is to **prevent the initial infection.** Public health measures to control infectious disease have a long history and have included vaccination programs, the regulation of water and food sources, and promotion of the use of condoms. Temporary quarantine or isolation of people with contagious airborne diseases such as tuberculosis and measles is also used in some cases.

Latency (monitoring and prophylaxis): Some organisms may enter a latent or dormant stage during which they reproduce at a lower rate, are less active in producing toxins, or otherwise curtail their activities. During latency the organism may cause few symptoms and yet persist in the body for months or years. Examples of organisms that often go through a latent or dormant phase are the syphilis spirochete, the hepatitis B virus, and HIV.

If an infection is detected during a latent phase when symptoms are few, immediate treatment may or may not be recommended. When treatment is prescribed in advance of serious symptoms, it is called *prophylaxis* or preventive treatment. Most people are not very aware of prophylaxis, except perhaps for the fluoridation of the water supply, done to reduce tooth decay and cavities. Until relatively recently, Western medical practice has focused on treating patients with active disease, rather than on intervening to keep the patient well to begin with.

Various *co-factors* can help reactivate a latent infection so that it causes symptoms. Co-factors include other concurrent infections, immune system decline due to age or other reasons, or exposure to environmental pollutants. Intervention to eliminate known co-factors can reduce the chance that a latent infection will reactivate and cause illness.

Treatment of acute illness: Either immediately after primary infection or after a period of latency, an organism may cause noticeable illness and symptoms. This is referred to as *active illness* or *acute illness* and corresponds to what most people call "getting sick." In most common infectious illnesses, the acute phase follows closely on the heels of the primary infection, taking perhaps a few days to a few weeks to appear. Some infections may never become acute: these are called *subclinical infections.* Some acute infections have symptoms so mild as to escape notice. And some infections have long latent periods before becoming acute—this is sometimes called an *incubation period.* Some infections may alternate episodes of acute illness with latent periods.

What we think of as medical treatment is virtually always treatment aimed at the acute phase of an illness. Treatment for infections is most often done with antibiotics or other drugs. Any treatment using drugs or chemicals might legitimately be called *chemotherapy,* but in ordinary nonmedical language most people reserve that term for anticancer drugs.

Drug therapy may be *oral*—that is, via the mouth in pill, tablet, capsule, or liquid form. Oral drug therapy is convenient for the patient, but some drugs may not survive stomach acid, may not be absorbed in sufficient concentration, or may cause unacceptable side effects when taken orally. Some drugs that cannot be given orally may be administered by injection *intravenously* or *intramuscularly.* Less commonly, drugs may be inhaled or delivered directly to the interior of the body in various other ways. Some drugs have both oral and intravenous forms: the intravenous forms may be used for rapid action or to achieve high drug concentrations in the blood.

After the acute phase of many illnesses secondary to HIV disease has been successfully treated, there remains an increased risk that the complication may recur. **To prevent recurrence, maintenance drug therapy is often recommended**—this is sometimes called *secondary prophylaxis.* The drugs and dosages used for maintenance therapy may be the same as or different from the regimen used for treatment of acute disease.

Maintenance therapy is usually continued indefinitely. As with primary prophylaxis, there is a worry that the organisms may become resistant to any drug used over the long term.

VIRAL INFECTIONS

The viruses we will discuss are:

- HIV
- Cytomegalovirus
- Herpes simplex virus
- Hepatitis B virus
- JC virus (causes progressive multifocal leukoencephalopathy)

ACUTE HIV INFECTION

Acute or primary HIV infection is an illness that sometimes appears at the time of infection with HIV. The symptoms are those of a viral illness resembling flu or mononucleosis. They include sore throat, fever, sweats, malaise, swollen glands, loss of appetite, nausea, and headaches. Neurological symptoms may also be present. A rash is present about 50 percent of the time. Total white blood count typically rises while the T4 count decreases.

It appears that people who develop acute HIV disease get symptoms within six days to six weeks of infection. It is not known what percentage of people who are HIV infected develop acute illness at the time of infection or whether these symptoms are in any way correlated with the later course of illness.

See sections on skin and neurology in Chapter 10: Organ System Complications, pp. 185–90 and pp. 197–207, for more descriptions of the symptoms of acute HIV infection.

CYTOMEGALOVIRUS (CMV)

Cytomegalovirus, or CMV, is a member of the herpes virus family. In the absence of HIV, it is a common viral infection not associated with serious illness. In HIV-infected people, however, CMV is a major cause of disease.

CMV can cause a variety of syndromes, some of which are blinding or life-threatening. In fact, CMV is the most common viral cause of life-threatening opportunistic infection in people with AIDS. Twenty-five to forty percent of people with AIDS experience life- or sight-threatening illness due to CMV. Nonetheless, treatment for CMV has improved. Adequate, up-to-date treatment will improve your chances of doing well.

▲ Transmission
The incidence of CMV infection among all adults in the United States is estimated to be about 50 percent. Among men who have sex with men and people who share needles for intravenous drug use the incidence is believed to be greater than 90 percent.

During primary CMV infection, virus is shed into body fluids. Shedding may also occur during reactivation of a latent CMV infection. CMV is transmitted sexually via intercourse and possibly from oral-anal contact (rimming). Virus in semen is probably the major source of transmission among men who have sex with other men. It can be transmitted in blood by transfusions or by needle sharing for drug use.

▲ Avoiding CMV Infection
Transmission can be prevented by using condoms during intercourse, using latex barriers for rimming, and sterilizing needles. Even if you are already infected with CMV it is worth taking measures to avoid repeat exposure. There is more than one strain of CMV and HIV-infected patients are often infected with more than one strain at the same time. This is another reason to continue safer sex even if you and your partner are HIV-infected. CMV is not readily transmitted person-to-person nonsexually even with prolonged exposure.

▲ Primary Infection

At the time of initial infection, referred to as primary infection, most people (about 90 percent) develop no symptoms. Other people get *CMV mononucleosis,* which resembles ordinary infectious mononucleosis caused by the Epstein-Barr virus (EBV). Symptoms are fever, sore throat, swollen glands, and fatigue. T4 lymphocyte counts decrease during primary CMV infection. They return to normal after convalescence.

▲ Latent Infection

After a primary infection—whether symptomatic or not—the virus remains present. With an adequately functioning immune system, such *latent* CMV infection does not cause illness, although virus particles may be shed in various body fluids. Latent infection is characteristic of herpes viruses. In people with immune deficiency (newborns, transplant recipients, those with HIV infection) CMV can reactivate and cause disease. In most people with HIV disease, symptoms of CMV infection are thus a reactivation of a latent infection.

▲ Preventing Reactivation of CMV

CMV-related symptoms are rarely the first sign of AIDS; they occur during more advanced stages of immune suppression, typically not until the T4 count is below 100 and usually below 50. The best hope for the future is either to maintain a T4 count above 50 or, if your T4 count drops below 50, to use medication to prevent reactivation of latent CMV. Preliminary studies have shown that high-dose acyclovir (Zovirax, Burroughs-Wellcome, 800 mg five times daily) may be helpful in preventing CMV disease. The eventual goal is to control or prevent CMV disease as PCP is prevented now.

▲ CMV Causes Disease in Severely Immune-Suppressed People

CMV can cause a variety of medical problems, depending on what organ it infects. The most common severe manifestations of CMV infection are *retinitis* (infection of the retina of the eye) and gastrointestinal disease. CMV also infects the lungs (where it may cause pneumonia) and the adrenal glands (causing adrenal insufficiency, which leads to a variety of symptoms, see pp. 196–97 in Chapter 10: Organ System Complications. CMV also causes other problems, but much more rarely—these will be discussed later in the chapter. Prompt treatment is important; otherwise CMV almost always progresses rapidly. CMV also can adversely affect mucous barriers in the body (such as in the lining of the intestine) and may increase the possibility of infection by other microorganisms.

▲ Diagnosis

Prior CMV infection is diagnosed by the presence in blood of antibodies to CMV. Since CMV infection is so common, your physician may or may not perform a CMV antibody test. A CMV-infected person may excrete particles of the virus in urine, semen, or cervical secretions without having any CMV-related illness. Diagnosis of CMV *disease* must be made by showing the presence of the virus itself in the affected organ and the absence of other disease-producing organisms. The diagnosis of CMV disease is made in several different ways, depending on the organ that the virus infects.

Eye exam: CMV retinitis has a characteristic appearance and can be diagnosed by a specialist in a careful examination of the eye.

Biopsy: Other CMV diseases need to be diagnosed by examination of tissue from a biopsy. The biopsied sample of tissue is examined under the microscope and has a typical appearance. Biopsies for CMV can be falsely negative because even if CMV is infecting the organ concerned and causing disease, the tissue sample may not include any infected cells. Because it is easy to miss CMV on biopsy, sometimes biopsies will be repeated.

Tissue culture: In addition to examination under a microscope, the biopsy specimen can be cultured for CMV. By standard techniques it takes four weeks or more to culture CMV from tissue. Positive results from tissue culture may be false, as the biopsy may have included infected cells that are not part of any active disease process in the organ of concern.

Blood and urine tests: levels of CMV itself can be measured in blood and urine. However, most patients with HIV disease will have some CMV in these fluids even when CMV is causing no disease. Positive blood and urine tests do not provide proof of a CMV diagnosis at a particular location, and they may be negative when the virus is not shedding but the disease is still active.

▲ CMV in the Eye: Retinitis

CMV infection of the eye is the most common form of disease caused by CMV. It is referred to as CMV *retinitis* or *chorioretinitis.* The retina is a layer of nerves on the inside of the eyeball that detects light and transmits visual information to the brain. CMV retinitis is the most severe eye complication of HIV disease and has been estimated to occur in 5 percent to 30 percent of patients with AIDS.

Symptoms and effects of CMV retinitis: A person with CMV retinitis may experience blurred or partially blocked vision, decreased visual *acuity* (clearness) or *scotoma* (a limited area of vision loss surrounded by an area of normal vision), *photophobia* (intolerance to light), flashes of light, sudden onset of floating spots, redness, or pain. There may be no symptoms.

The infection causes bleeding that damages the retina and its supporting blood vessels (the *perivascular* area). Also, CMV frequently damages the optic nerve (which carries information from the eye to the brain). If not controlled, damage to the retina, perivascular area, and/or optic nerve may result in blindness.

Even in those whose retinitis is controlled by medication, the retina may still separate from the underlying tissue of the eyeball (*retinal detachment*) and cause partial or total loss of eyesight.

In most cases CMV retinitis is not immediately sight-threatening. However, CMV retinitis progresses quickly and can involve the whole retina in a matter of a few weeks. **It is crucial that you report eye symptoms to your physician promptly,** so that any CMV retinitis may be diagnosed and treated without delay. Damage to the optic nerve or the *macula* (the central and most important part of the retina) can lead to loss of vision and blindness. Treatment of CMV retinitis that is not producing symptoms is debatable. Most experts argue that it is best to start treatment immediately since the retinitis will probably progress and smaller lesions are easier to treat than larger lesions. Some, however, argue that it is better to delay treatment in order to postpone drug- and infusion-related problems.

CMV retinitis is diagnosed with exams done by an *ophthalmologist* (a medical eye specialist). The eye examination is simple and painless. The ophthalmologist will use eye drops to widen (*dilate*) the pupils. This makes it easier to look at the retina using an instrument called an *indirect ophthalmoscope.* CMV appears as fluffy, white areas on the surface of the retina. The ophthalmologist must distinguish CMV from a harmless condition called *cotton-wool spots* that is common in the eyes of HIV-infected people. Other infections that occasionally cause damage similar to CMV are toxoplasmosis and herpes virus.

Treatment is crucial: without treatment CMV retinitis progresses in 90 percent of people. If untreated, both eyes usually become affected, leading to blindness. CMV retinitis is treated with ganciclovir (DHPG) or with foscarnet (see below). With treatment, CMV retinitis usually stabilizes or sometimes improves in ten to twenty days. Lifelong maintenance therapy is necessary.

While CMV retinitis is progressing, patients should have eye examinations every two weeks.

▲ CMV in the Gut

CMV infection can affect all areas of the gut (also called the *gastrointestinal tract,* or GI tract). Most people with CMV will eventually have some CMV-related problems in this area.

CMV causes most GI problems by inflaming the mucous lining of the gut. The virus may destroy layers of tissue, causing an *ulcer.* When we say that someone has an ulcer, we are commonly referring to a stomach ulcer (*peptic ulcer*), but ulcers can occur in other parts of the GI tract as well.

CMV infects various sites in the GI tract: the *colon* (the bottom part of the large intestine), the *esophagus* (the part from the throat to the stomach), the stomach, or the small bowel. Symptoms in the colon are referred to as CMV *colitis.* Symptoms in the esophagus are called CMV *esophagitis.* Symptoms in the stomach are called CMV *gastritis.* The symptoms vary depending on the location of the infection.

Esophagitis and gastritis: CMV can inflame the esophagus and cause ulcers there. A person with CMV esophagitis may have pain or difficulty in swallowing, or possibly discomfort in the upper part of the digestive tract, especially after eating. The symptoms of CMV gastritis may resemble peptic ulcer disease.

In the esophagus CMV usually produces either a single deep ulceration or a very large superficial ulceration.

Diagnosis and treatment: Esophagitis can be caused by CMV or, more often, by one of a variety of other organisms, including the fungus *Candida albicans,* herpes simplex virus, and HIV itself. Your physician will probably try various medications presumptively, guessing that the symptoms are *not* caused by CMV. Since candidiasis is the most common cause of esophagitis, the first treatments tried are antifungal medications such as ketoconazole (Nizoral) or fluconazole (Diflucan). If the symptoms do not get better, the next most common cause of esophagitis is suspected: herpes. Acyclovir (Zovirax) is used as presumptive treatment for herpes.

If neither antifungal drugs nor acyclovir relieve the symptoms, it is likely that CMV is the cause. Treatment for CMV esophagitis begins after the diagnosis is confirmed with a biopsy obtained by endoscopy (described in Chapter 13: Procedures and Tests, pp. 304–05).

CMV treatment requires a specific diagnosis (unlike candidiasis or herpes) for two reasons:

- The drugs currently available against CMV, ganciclovir (Cytovene, DHPG) and foscarnet (Foscavir), have potentially serious side effects.
- These drugs must be given intravenously (IV) over the long term. It is difficult to do this by injection. The type of temporary IV line that is used for short-term IV drug therapy must be changed every four to five days. One way to get the drugs into the blood on a long-term regular basis is through a *catheter.* A catheter is basically a tube: One end is surgically inserted into a large vein in your chest. The other end of the catheter remains outside your chest (*Hickman catheter*) or has an injectable port just under the skin (*Port-a-cath, Infusaport*), providing access to your bloodstream so that you can give yourself the drugs you need. See Chapter 13: Procedures and Tests, pp. 307–09, for a complete description.

Before these therapies are started a diagnostic procedure called an *endoscopy* should be done to look for CMV. An endoscopy is a visual inspection of the esophagus using a slim, flexible, fiber-optic tube inserted through the mouth and down the throat. If an ulcer or other evidence of infection is seen, a small tissue sample may be taken (*biopsied*) through the endoscope to confirm the presence of CMV.

Symptom relief while awaiting diagnosis: You can use standard medications during the process of diagnosis to relieve the discomfort of esophagitis. Stomach juices are acidic and can cause pain and inflammation in esophagitis. Medication can help you feel better either by reducing the amount of stomach acid or by neutralizing it. The medications are:

- H2-receptor antagonists: cimetidine (Tagamet), ranitidine (Zantac), or famotidine (Pepcid)
- Antacids (aluminum hydroxide gel or magnesium trisilicate gel, Maalox, Mylanta)
- Sucralfate (Carafate)
- Anticholinergic drugs (a broad class of drugs)
- Bismuth subsalicylate (Pepto-Bismol)

The colon is the most common gastrointestinal site of CMV infection. **CMV colitis** occurs in 5 to 10 percent of people with AIDS at some point in their illness. It may be the first disease to appear in AIDS; this makes accurate diagnosis of symptoms important. CMV infection of the colon—CMV *colitis*—can cause inflammation, ulceration, or (sometimes) perforation of the colon.

The **symptoms** are watery diarrhea, weight loss, loss of appetite, cramping, abdominal pain or discomfort, fever, or blood in the stool.

Treatment differs depending on the organism causing the symptoms, so **diagnosis** is important and cannot be based on symptoms or physical examination alone.

Also, colitis may often be caused by more than one organism, including many microorganisms common in HIV-infected patients: salmonella, shigella, *Campylobacter pylorides,* cryptosporidium, *Clostridium difficile, Mycobacterium avium,* various ova, *Giardia lamblia, Entamoeba hystolitica,* and HIV itself.

Diagnosis must be made with an endoscopic examination of the colon (a colonoscopy) and a biopsy. This procedure may need to be repeated in order to locate CMV lesions.

Up to one-third of cases of CMV colitis improve without specific therapy (Dieterich), but since the disease usually recurs or progresses, **treatment is essential.** CMV colitis is usually treated with ganciclovir (Cytovene) or, if this is ineffective or not tolerated, with foscarnet (Foscavir, see below).

Additionally, standard treatments may be used to reduce diarrhea and to relieve pain and discomfort. These include diphenoxylate (Lomotil), loperamide (Imodium), and deodorized tincture of opium (a liquid suspension of opium).

On occasion, CMV colitis can be severe enough to cause gastrointestinal perforation. This constitutes a medical emergency and procedures may need to be done (surgically or with an endoscope) to repair the perforation. There is an increased incidence of appendicitis (probably due to CMV infection) in HIV-infected patients.

Other gastrointestinal sites: CMV can also, although less commonly, infect and cause symptoms in other parts of the digestive system: the small bowel, the liver and/or spleen, the biliary tract, and the pancreas.

CMV PNEUMONIA

Pneumonia is the most common clinical manifestation of CMV in patients with AIDS. However, CMV is rarely the primary or sole cause of pneumonia. It usually occurs along with other disease-causing organisms —most often *Pneumocystis carinii*. It has been difficult to determine how much of the illness is caused by CMV. CMV pneumonia results from infection of the walls of the lung sacs (*alveoli*) and the spaces between them. Infection in this area is called *interstitial pneumonia.* The symptoms are shortness of breath or labored breathing on exertion, fever, a dry nonproductive cough (no phlegm), elevated heart and respiratory rates, and insufficient oxygen in the blood (*hypoxemia*). These are identical to the symptoms of PCP.

CMV pneumonia cannot be distinguished from other pneumonias (such as PCP) solely on the basis of an X ray. CMV pneumonia is diagnosed by a number of indications: clinical signs, positive X ray, presence of CMV in the lungs, and the absence of other disease-producing organisms. A bronchoscopy with biopsy is necessary. Diagnosis is complicated by the fact that CMV may be present without being responsible for disease. If both CMV and *Pneumocystis carinii* are found in the lungs, the PCP is treated first. Treatment for CMV is then added if the PCP treatment is ineffective.

Ganciclovir is used to treat CMV pneumonia but seems to be less effective than it is for CMV retinitis. Results of studies have been inconsistent.

▲ Central Nervous System Infection

CMV is not particularly likely to infect cells of the brain and the nervous system. CMV may sometimes produce a condition called *subacute encephalitis* (an inflammation of the brain), but this condition is more frequently caused by HIV itself. The signs and symptoms of encephalitis are fever, personality changes, altered mental states, difficulty in concentrating, headaches, and sleepiness. There is no standard diagnostic method for CMV encephalitis, but a sudden onset of acute mental status changes probably implicate CMV rather than HIV. CMV can usually be cultured from cerebrospinal fluid; however, because other disease-producing organisms are usually found at the same time, it is not clear what role the CMV plays in producing encephalitis. Encephalitis suggestive of CMV may possibly be treated with foscarnet (Foscavir).

▲ Treatment

Two drugs are currently used for the treatment of active CMV disease: ganciclovir (DHPG) and foscarnet. Both drugs are administered intravenously—no oral forms are yet available. Both drugs are administered starting with an induction phase at a high dose that is then lowered to the standard dose. An indefinite course of maintenance therapy is usually recommended for CMV retinitis, but not necessarily immediately for a first episode of CMV colitis. If maintenance therapy is required, an in-dwelling catheter must be surgically implanted to provide regular access to the bloodstream.

See the discussion of in-dwelling catheters in Chapter 13: Procedures and Tests, pp. 307–09.

▲ Ganciclovir

Ganciclovir is used for treating most forms of CMV disease. It is manufactured by Syntex under the brand name Cytovene. It is also called DHPG, the abbreviation of the drug's rather long chemical name: 9-[(1,3-dihydroxy-2-propoxy)methyl]guanine. It is an antiherpes virus drug related to acyclovir. Ganciclovir is much more effective against CMV than acyclovir.

Ganciclovir suppresses active CMV infection but does not cure latent infection. Therefore, disease can return when the drug is stopped. For some kinds of CMV disease, ganciclovir must be taken on a continuing, permanent basis.

Ganciclovir markedly delays progression of CMV disease and has been shown to prolong life after a CMV retinitis diagnosis. The drug has clear antiviral effects: elimination of the virus in blood, urine, and lung secretions. Evidence of CMV in the blood (viremia) ends about five days after beginning treatment with ganciclovir for the majority of patients.

Efficacy: Small controlled (comparative) studies on CMV retinitis have been completed and indicate that the drug helps stop destruction of the retina. Extensive noncontrolled studies unequivocally document the efficacy of ganciclovir for treating CMV retinitis. Controlled studies of ganciclovir have shown it is effective in treating CMV colitis. Patients who are suffering from severe weight loss secondary to CMV infection show improvement of this problem when treated with ganciclovir. Uncontrolled studies of ganciclovir show that it is effective in treating other gastrointestinal and pulmonary disease, with signs of clinical improvement and disease slowing. A study (Dieterich) of a group of patients with gastrointestinal disease showed that 75 percent of patients had a positive clinical response. The drug was equally effective regardless of the site of the CMV infection.

During an initial induction phase of ten to fourteen days, you will receive two infusions each day. After induction, the standard dose is one infusion per day. Clinical improvement may take as long as a month to appear. The effectiveness of ganciclovir appears to be dose-related.

More than 90 percent of patients with cytomegalovirus retinitis improve initially. The first signs of improvement usually occur 10 to 14 days after treatment begins. About 30–50 percent of patients have a recurrence of CMV retinitis while on maintenance therapy. This is treated with a repeat induction phase and an increased maintenance dose. Baseline photographs of the retina during the period of CMV inactivity will help in making treatment decisions by making it easier to detect changes.

Although ganciclovir may save both vision and life, it has several significant **problems associated with its use.** These difficulties are incomplete efficacy, major patient inconvenience, and significantly toxic side effects.

Drug failure: Sometimes CMV retinitis recurs despite the fact that the patient is continuing to take ganciclovir. The reasons for this are not clear but are believed generally to have to do with continued immunological deterioration rather than the development of resistance to the drug. However, some cases of ganciclovir-resistant CMV have now been reported. It is not known whether people on long-term maintenance therapy will be at greater risk for developing ganciclovir-resistant strains of CMV.

Long-term IV therapy: The second problem—patient inconvenience—is caused by the need for the drug to be administered intravenously, five to seven days a week, on a long-term basis. The drug cannot be taken in pill form because the body cannot absorb it in this form. Ganciclovir must go directly into the bloodstream by intravenous administration. First, the infusion is time-consuming. Second, such frequent infusion requires that a permanent in-dwelling catheter (also referred to as a *central venous access line*) be surgically inserted into a vein in the chest. Veins in the arm cannot tolerate so many intravenous treatments. One drawback is that catheters sometimes become infected and must be replaced. Studies are now in progress for the use of oral ganciclovir to suppress relatively inactive CMV retinitis.

About one-third of patients taking ganciclovir develop serious problems with side effects. The major toxic side effects from ganciclovir are hematologic—that is, the drug may cause disorders of the blood. One of the functions of white blood cells is to protect the body from disease-causing microorganisms. These white blood cells are produced in bone marrow. Ganciclovir is one of a number of drugs that suppresses bone-marrow production of the white blood cells called *neutrophils.* **Neutropenia** (neutrophil deficiency) may occur in up to one-third of patients taking ganciclovir.

Patients taking ganciclovir must therefore have regular blood tests for neutropenia. It typically occurs early in therapy and can be controlled by reducing dosage or discontinuing the drug. Patients on the induction phase of ganciclovir should have a complete blood count including white blood cell differential (*CBC with differential*) two to three times per week. During maintenance therapy it should be performed once or twice weekly. Ganciclovir must be discontinued if the absolute neutrophil count is below 500 per microliter. Serum creatinine levels should be measured monthly and the dose of ganciclovir reduced if estimated creatinine clearance is below 80 ml per minute.

Studies indicate that drugs called *granulocyte colony-stimulating factor* (G-CSF) and *granulocyte-macrophage colony-stimulating factor* (GM-CSF) may help reduce bone-marrow suppression and maintain a normal neutrophil count while continuing ganciclovir. G-CSF is preferred because it has fewer side effects.

AZT is another drug that frequently causes bone-marrow suppression leading to neutropenia. Consequently it is difficult for most patients to combine AZT and ganciclovir. One study of the two drugs used in combination (Hochster) showed that 82 percent of the subjects developed very severe hematological problems that required discontinuation of the medication. However, some patients are able to tolerate the combination of ganciclovir and low-dose AZT (300 mg per day) and this may be a useful combination. Patients on ganciclovir should begin on a low dose of AZT and increase gradually. Frequent monitoring of leukocytes and absolute neutrophil counts is crucial. DdI and ddC do not produce AZT's hematological side effects and therefore may be preferable in combination with ganciclovir.

Another blood disorder associated with the use of ganciclovir is a decrease in the number of platelets (**thrombocytopenia**). Platelets are formed elements in blood necessary for clotting. Low platelets can lead to serious bleeding disorders. About 5 percent of patients on ganciclovir develop thrombocytopenia. Platelets are monitored by a blood test known as the platelet count.

Other side effects: Ganciclovir can adversely affect the kidneys and lead to renal insufficiency. It is known to reduce testosterone levels, with a consequent decline in libido (sexual desire). In addition, patients taking ganciclovir may experience several very uncomfortable side effects, particularly nausea, vomiting, diarrhea, and rash. These side effects improve for many patients over a matter of weeks as they become accustomed to the drug.

Because of these medical, psychological, and practical problems associated with use of ganciclovir, patients who begin to use the drug must make a major adjustment. Nonetheless, ganciclovir is the most effective drug now available and many people taking it have been able to function relatively well.

▲ Foscarnet

More recently, another drug effective against CMV has been approved: foscarnet (Foscavir, trisodium phosphonoformate). Results are encouraging: the reported response rate is greater than 80 percent. Foscarnet also has some effect on HIV itself (studies show a decrease in HIV activity as measured by p24 antigen).

The dose must be regularly re-calculated depending on its effects on the kidneys as measured by lab tests *(creatinine clearance)* and the patient's weight. Other drugs that adversely affect the kidneys should be avoided (amphotericin-B, parenteral pentamidine).

Foscarnet crosses the blood-brain barrier and thus treats susceptible organisms in the brain. Foscarnet is compatible with AZT because it does not contribute to the suppression of the production of white blood cells often caused by using AZT. Foscarnet and AZT together appear more effective than either one alone at a higher dosage.

As with ganciclovir, foscarnet must be given as long-term maintenance therapy. Since oral absorption of foscarnet is poor, it must be given intravenously. To get the benefit of foscarnet you must have a permanent in-dwelling catheter implanted. During induction foscarnet is infused three times a day. During maintenance once daily is sufficient. The rate of infusion must be controlled by an infusion pump (as opposed to a free drip) so that the drug does not overwhelm the kidneys.

Foscarnet produces a number of serious side effects. The most frequent serious problems are **kidney (*renal*) problems.** Dehydration and sodium (salt) depletion may impair the passage of fluid through the kidneys causing decreased function and sometimes failure. These problems typically occur in the third week of treatment. In order to avoid dehydration, patients taking foscarnet also use intravenous saline solution (1 liter of saline at each treatment). Drink lots of fluids if you are taking foscarnet. Your physician will monitor for early signs of kidney problems with blood tests *(creatinine clearance)* and urine tests (lack of sodium, or *hyponatremia*). Look out for warning signs of kidney problems: decreased urination, increased thirst, or light-headedness after standing up *(orthostatic hypotension)*. Treatment is replacement of fluid and salt. It is important to get treated promptly. Dosage can be adjusted downward to attempt to avoid kidney dysfunction.

Too large a dosage of foscarnet at one time can also cause *hypocalcemia,* a lack of calcium in the blood. This can lead to changes in mental status, cardiac arrhythmias, and seizures.

Other side effects: Foscarnet may cause mild anemia (decrease in red blood cells), or imbalances of phosphate and calcium levels in the blood. Unlike ganciclovir, foscarnet does not cause low platelet count *(thrombocytopenia)* or related bleeding disorders. Rare or mild side effects include mild tremors, rash, nausea, diarrhea, seizures, fatigue, irritability, and central nervous system abnormalities. In addition, foscarnet excreted in urine may sometimes irritate the end of the penis, causing sores about two weeks after the beginning of therapy. If sores occur they will resolve even with the continuation of foscarnet therapy.

Tests to monitor side effects: Serum creatinine, calcium, magnesium, potassium, and hemoglobin values should be monitored two or three times per week during induction and weekly during maintenance therapy.

Foscarnet compared to ganciclovir: Because the side effects of the two drugs are different, there is no additional problem to using the drugs together. Because foscarnet alone allows concurrent use of AZT, foscarnet alone may offer survival benefits over ganciclovir alone. However, foscarnet is harder to tolerate than ganciclovir.

The combination of ganciclovir *and* foscarnet is promising. Two recent studies show that patients may benefit from a combination of ganciclovir and foscarnet. The benefits of the drugs in combination may be greater than the benefit of either alone.

▲ Drugs Under Investigation

Oral ganciclovir: It would be an important advance for patients to be treated orally for CMV rather than intravenously through a surgically installed catheter. This would eliminate the inconvenience, psychological trauma, and risk of infection now attached to ongoing treatment for CMV. One very small study showed that the drug given orally could reach therapeutic levels and caused few serious side effects. Other, larger studies of oral ganciclovir are under way but are not yet completed.

Some small trials have been done using **monoclonal and triclonal antibodies;** others are under way. Some preliminary results in bone marrow transplant patients with CMV pneumonia have been promising.

Only uncontrolled studies have been done on the use of **CMV immune globulins** derived from the blood of healthy CMV-infected donors. CMV immune globulins may increase the effectiveness of ganciclovir when used in combination. Toxicities are not known but may include a risk of infection with other organisms (from the donor).

For information on how to stay up-to-date on experimental treatments, refer to Chapter 9: Learning About Experimental Treatments.

▲ CMV as a Co-Factor

CMV infection is not a necessary co-factor for AIDS because some people get AIDS who are not infected with CMV. However, CMV is believed to make HIV disease worse. There are several ideas about how this may work. CMV is immunosuppressive, it infects white blood cells (lymphocytes, monocytes, and natural killer cells), and may facilitate subsequent infection by HIV or reactivate a latent HIV infection. It is also one of the viruses—along with HIV and Epstein-Barr virus (EBV)— known as *polyclonal activating viruses* that activates and exhausts white blood cells called *B lymphocytes,* leaving few to respond to new immuno-logical challenges. (See Chapter 16: Immunology, Pathogenesis, and Etiology, pp. 332–33.) Some researchers have speculated that CMV infection in the presence of HIV infection may cause Kaposi's sarcoma, but evidence for this hypothesis is incomplete.

HERPES SIMPLEX VIRUS (HSV)

▲ General

Herpes simplex is a disease that affects skin and mucous membranes. It is caused by one of two strains of herpes virus. Type I usually causes sores on the edges of the lips, the nostrils, or in the mouth, on the gums or hard palate. Type II generally causes sores in the genital and anal area. However, infection with either virus may occur at any site and treatment is the same. There are now antiviral agents that are effective in treating herpes in a majority of cases.

This viral infection is common among people throughout the world and affects both those infected with HIV and those who are not. In some populations (living in conditions with a lot of person-to-person contact) 80 percent to 100 percent of people may be infected. In immune-compromised patients, herpes infection can be severe and even life-threatening. The symptoms of herpes infection tend to be worse as the immune system declines. In immune-compromised patients, herpes can cause lesions in the esophagus and colon and at times in other organs such as the brain.

The herpes virus is transmitted from person to person by contact between infected fluid and mucous membranes or broken skin. Trans-mission of HSV-1 usually occurs in early childhood; later outbreaks are caused by reactivation of the virus. HSV-2 is typically transmitted during sexual activity. Transmission generally occurs only during an outbreak. Using condoms for intercourse will generally reduce transmission. Herpes can recur because after initial infection the virus remains in the body in latent form in cells of the nervous system. Certain factors seem to trigger recurring outbreaks: sunlight, fevers, menstruation, stress, and any condition that suppresses immune functioning. Once infected, people with HIV disease have an increased likelihood of recurrence.

Herpes can be diagnosed by clinical appearance or by smear, culture, or biopsy. The sample is taken by lightly scraping the affected area with a cotton swab.

▲ Oral Herpes Simplex

Oral herpes, often referred to as *cold sores,* are common in people without HIV infection, but people with HIV infection tend to have episodes that are more frequent, more severe, and of longer duration.

The symptoms will be the same in an uninfected person or an HIV-infected person: oral herpes appears as groups of small, fluid-filled blisters *(vesicles)*. The vesicles break and produce small crusted areas that take about seven to ten days to heal. The sores may be itchy or painful. In an HIV-infected person with an impaired immune system, herpes may become a chronic problem. The sores are larger (2 to 10 centimeters or larger in diameter), longer lasting (several weeks to months), and may cause ulceration or damage of tissue.

▲ Herpes Simplex of the Esophagus and Colon

Herpes simplex can cause sores in the esophagus; typically a small number of deep lesions. They are often very painful but respond well to acyclovir. Diagnosis is made by endoscopy of the esophagus with a biopsy. HSV can also cause sores in the colon and can lead to symptoms of diarrhea. Diagnosis is made by colonoscopy and biopsy.

▲ Genital and Anorectal Herpes

Genital and anorectal herpes are usually caused by HSV-2 although they can also be caused by HSV-1. Episodes are more likely to recur if caused by HSV-2. In either case, treatment is the same.

Herpes begins as small papules (bumps) on the genitals, around the anus and in the rectum, or on the buttocks or thighs that rapidly develop into painful vesicles (fluid-filled blisters). The area is often swollen and tender. The sores break and crust over. In those with adequately functioning immune systems, these sores take two to three weeks to resolve. Some people also have systemic symptoms of fever, headache, muscle ache, and malaise. In people who are immune compromised, the local infection may be more severe, the healing time longer, and the systemic symptoms worse. In some cases, this may lead to continuously ulcerated areas that can develop secondary bacterial or fungal infections. A woman with active herpes may transmit the infection to the infant during delivery. Such an infection is very dangerous.

HSV around the anus and in the rectum can cause a condition known as *anorectal proctitis.* Symptoms are pain, ulceration, constipation, and difficult or painful defecation or urination. Ulcers in this area should be cultured for accurate diagnosis.

▲ Treatment

Episodes of herpes simplex can be shortened by use of the antiviral drug acyclovir (Zovirax). It is available in intravenous, oral, and topical forms. Severe acute episodes that do not respond to oral medications can be treated by use of intravenous acyclovir. Chronic herpes outbreaks may be prevented with the use of long-term oral acyclovir. Some strains of herpes simplex have developed that are resistant to acyclovir; they can be treated with foscarnet (Foscavir).

▲ Maintenance

As mentioned above, long-term therapy with acyclovir may be required in those with chronic outbreaks of herpes.

HEPATITIS B VIRUS (HBV)

Hepatitis B is a viral disease that can cause serious and even fatal damage to the liver. Vaccination is now available that can prevent infection with hepatitis B. People who are HIV-infected should be screened to see if they are hepatitis B infected: if infected, they should be monitored (and treated, if possible) for chronic infection; if uninfected, they should be vaccinated against future infection.

Hepatitis is a broad term that means inflammation of the liver. The liver can be inflamed by exposure to drugs, chemicals, or a variety of infectious organisms. Hepatitis B is caused by the hepatitis B virus (HBV). Other forms of hepatitis caused by infectious agents are hepatitis A, hepatitis C, and delta hepatitis.

Acute hepatitis B describes the disease at or near the time of infection. Seventy percent of people infected with HBV have *subclinical* acute hepatitis B—which means they have no symptoms (or only very mild and temporary symptoms) at or near the time of infection. Thus, most people who get infected probably don't realize they have had hepatitis B.

The remainder (30 percent) of HBV-infected people develop symptoms within 30 to 180 days after infection. Their symptoms are uncomfortable but rarely life-threatening. They include jaundice, fatigue, loss of appetite, abdominal pain, malaise, nausea, vomiting, muscle and joint aches, or fever.

Some people get very sick right away: acute hepatitis B is fatal in 1.4 percent of cases.

If blood tests show that you have not had hepatitis B virus (and therefore have not developed immunity to it), it is important to be vaccinated because of the dangerous effects of chronic hepatitis B infection in the long term.

Most people get over their initial infection with hepatitis B and thereafter cannot transmit the virus. However, in some people HBV may continue to reproduce in the body for a long time after the initial infection, in which case the disease is known as **chronic hepatitis B infection.**

A small proportion of people who are infected with hepatitis B (about 6 percent to 10 percent) become *chronic carriers* of hepatitis B. This means they have a lifelong capability to transmit the virus to others although they may have no symptoms and may not require any treatment.

About 25 percent of these carriers eventually develop chronic liver inflammation and have an increased chance of developing cirrhosis of the liver or liver cancer. People with hepatitis B-related chronic liver inflammation have abnormal liver function as revealed by blood tests. In the United States, about 4,000 people die each year from hepatitis B-related cirrhosis and about 800 from hepatitis B-related cancer.

About 3 percent develop *chronic active hepatitis,* which can cause very serious life-threatening symptoms.

You can develop chronic hepatitis B whether or not you had any symptoms at the time of infection. If you are not yet immune, the purpose of vaccination against hepatitis B is primarily to prevent a disease that can, over the long term, produce serious life-threatening medical problems.

Transmission: In the United States 23,200 cases of hepatitis B were reported to the CDC in 1988. The actual number is many times higher because many cases were not reported; there are estimated to be 300,000 cases per year, mostly among young adults. In the United States, there is an estimated pool of 750,000 to 1 million infectious carriers. In this country hepatitis B is most often spread through contact with blood or sexual fluids. It occurs mainly among men who have sex with other men, those who share needles for drug use, and health care workers.

In other parts of the world (China, Southeast Asia, tropical Africa, most Pacific islands, parts of the Middle East, and the Amazon basin) hepatitis B is common and not typically confined to the risk groups described above. Liver cancer from hepatitis B is a serious problem in these areas, where as many as 300 million people may have chronic hepatitis B infection. In these areas it is most commonly transmitted from mother to fetus during pregnancy, in addition to the routes of transmission common in the United States.

Hepatitis B is spread only by certain specific routes:

Hepatitis B virus cannot pass through undamaged skin. **HBV can enter the body through the mucous membranes that line the vagina, rectum, urethra, and possibly the mouth.** Careful use of condoms for vaginal or rectal intercourse will prevent the transmission of HBV.

The blood supply in the United States is screened for hepatitis B so transmission by transfusion is rare. HBV can be transmitted to health care workers **through needle-stick injury or other exposure to blood.** HBV can be transmitted **through sharing of needles for drug use.**

Hepatitis B can be transmitted from **mother to infant** during birth through exposure to blood.

HBV is spread by exactly the same routes as HIV, the virus that causes AIDS. However, HBV is a more easily transmissible virus, which is why hepatitis B vaccination is recommended even if you are using condoms for intercourse.

Hepatitis B screening and vaccination are recommended for:

- Men who have sex with other men
- Health care workers
- Those who share needles for drug use
- People from China, Southeast Asia, tropical Africa, most Pacific Islands, parts of the Middle East, and the Amazon basin

Before you are vaccinated, your blood must be tested to see if you have ever had hepatitis B in the past (remember—you may have had hepatitis B without noticing it). If you have ever had hepatitis B, you have developed natural immunity, cannot be reinfected, and will not need the vaccine. The blood test determines if you've ever been infected by looking for evidence of your immune system's response to the hepatitis B virus (specifically, for antibodies to hepatitis B core antigen, or anti-HBcAg).

These blood tests also tell you if you are a chronic carrier or have chronic hepatitis. The presence of viral fragments (hepatitis B surface antigen, or HBsAg) for more than six months indicates that you are a chronic carrier and are capable of transmitting the virus to others.

If blood tests show that you have not been infected with hepatitis B virus, you will receive the vaccine in a series of three injections in the arm. You will get an initial vaccination, one a month later, and one six months later. The timing does not have to be exact. There are few side effects—you may have a sore arm for a day. This vaccine provides an effective level of immunity in 90 percent of cases.

Treatment: Alpha interferon in injections of 3 to 5 million units three times per week shows promise in eliminating or controlling chronic infection. See Chapter 9: Learning About Experimental Treatments for information on how to keep up with the status of experimental treatments.

Hepatitis B and HIV: If you are not yet immune because of prior infection or vaccination, you may become infected with hepatitis B. It is important that you get vaccinated against hepatitis B, because acute hepatitis B often produces severe symptoms in those who are HIV infected. Also, there is a higher risk of developing chronic hepatitis B if you are HIV infected. HIV-infected persons who develop hepatitis B are at a 19 percent to 37 percent risk of becoming chronic HIV carriers. The vaccine is somewhat less likely to "take"—that is, to provide an effective level of immunity—in those who are HIV infected, but it is effective in the majority of cases. One study indicated that at least 75 percent of asymptomatic patients developed a protective response to HBV.

You cannot become infected with HIV from the hepatitis B vaccine. There are two kinds of hepatitis B vaccine:

- *Heptavax* is made from human blood, and is heat-treated to kill HIV
- *Recombivax* is synthesized using recombinant DNA technology. Since it is not made from human blood there is no danger of contamination with HIV.

PROGRESSIVE MULTIFOCAL LEUKOENCEPHALOPATHY (PML)

Progressive multifocal leukoencephalopathy (PML) is an unusual subacute or chronic progressive neurological disorder. It occurs in advanced HIV disease and only with severe immune suppression. It has been estimated to occur in 2 percent to 4 percent of AIDS patients. This disease causes destruction of cells in the white matter of the brain and *demyelination,* the loss of the myelin sheath of nerve fibers.

The symptoms of PML are dementia (disturbances in intellectual functioning), disturbances in speech, partial paralysis, loss of vision, and motor discoordination.

PML is caused by the *JC virus,* which belongs to the family of *papova-viruses.* Most people probably become infected with JC virus as children. In most parts of the world, 75 percent of adults have antibodies to JC virus. The initial infection is asymptomatic, but the virus remains alive in the kidneys. In the presence of severe immunosuppression it is spread by a type of white blood cell called *B lymphocytes* through the blood and into the brain.

If symptoms are mild, PML may be hard to distinguish from AIDS dementia complex. Computerized tomography (CT) scans and magnetic resonance imaging (MRI) frequently show a typical pattern of change. **Diagnosis** is usually done by imaging alone: a brain biopsy may be necessary in atypical cases. Refer to Chapter 13: Procedures and Tests for descriptions of these procedures.

There is so far no successful **treatment.** A few cases have been reported which developed slowly or remitted spontaneously. There have been a few reports of success in treating PML with high-dose AZT.

PROTOZOAL INFECTIONS

The protozoan parasites we will discuss are:

- *Pneumocystis carinii*
- *Toxoplasma gondii*
- *Histoplasma capsulatum*
- Cryptosporidium and *Isospora belli*
- *Entamoeba histolytica* (amoebas)
- *Giardia lamblia*

PNEUMOCYSTIS CARINII PNEUMONIA (PCP)

Pneumocystis carinii is a common microorganism that exists in every continent throughout the world and is found in rats, guinea pigs, other rodents, monkeys, foxes, dogs, sheep, goats, humans, and other animals. Most people are infected with *Pneumocystis carinii* during childhood and develop no symptoms. In North America 65 percent to 100 percent of children have been infected with *Pneumocystis carinii* by the age of 4. The organism is probably transmitted through the air.

In people with adequately functioning immune systems, *Pneumocystis carinii* remains a harmless latent lifelong infection. *Pneumocystis carinii* causes disease only in people with impaired immune systems. Active PCP is caused by a **reactivation of latent infection** in an immune-suppressed person. Active PCP was first observed in infants after World War II who were immune suppressed due to malnutrition. It has also been seen occasionally in patients whose immune systems are suppressed by diseases such as leukemia, Hodgkin's disease, other cancers, or in patients using immune-suppressant drugs as part of organ transplantation or for other medical purposes. People who are immune suppressed due to HIV infection have been particularly vulnerable to PCP.

PCP is now a generally preventable disease for HIV-infected people. The correct kind of preventive treatment at the correct time will probably keep you from developing PCP. If such treatment is not instituted at the appropriate time, you have a significant risk of developing PCP.

It is usually necessary to begin this treatment prior to the development of any symptoms of illness. In Chapter 5: Preventing PCP and Other Complications we discussed PCP prophylaxis in detail. We will not repeat that material here.

Parasite or fungus?: *Pneumocystis carinii* cannot be grown in the laboratory. This has made it difficult to study the organism's life cycle. As a result, scientists disagree about whether *Pneumocystis carinii* should be classified as a protozoan parasite or as a fungus. This is not just an academic question: if more is learned about the organism's life cycle, it will help researchers develop better treatments.

Pathogenesis: In the immune-suppressed person, *Pneumocystis carinii* causes disease by growing and filling the *alveoli* of the lungs. Alveoli are small sacs in the lung that are lined with blood vessels. Oxygen inhaled into the lungs diffuses across the walls of alveoli into the tiny blood vessels that line each sac. Carbon dioxide is expelled from the blood by a similar mechanism. If a large proportion of alveoli are filled with microorganisms and the fluid by-products of inflammation, the blood can neither get enough oxygen nor get rid of excess carbon dioxide.

▲ Symptoms

Pneumocystis carinii pneumonia usually begins with mild but gradually worsening symptoms. Symptoms of *Pneumocystis carinii* pneumonia are:

- Dyspnea (shortness of breath) is the most common symptom. The shortness of breath is generally first noticed only during exertion but as the disease progresses it occurs even at rest.
- Cough associated with PCP usually produces no mucus or, in patients who smoke, only thin, clear mucus.
- Tachypnea (very rapid breathing)
- Fevers
- Chills
- Sweats
- Progressive, profound fatigue
- Cyanosis (bluish discoloration from lack of oxygen) around mouth, extremities (hands or feet), and mucous membranes.

Respiratory symptoms are not always the first or most prominent sign of PCP. Many people have a few weeks or months of fever, fatigue, and weight loss (constitutional symptoms) before respiratory symptoms develop. In PCP-infected people taking antivirals such as AZT and/or PCP prophylaxis, the symptoms of PCP may be mild constitutional symptoms. This is one of the reasons to report persistent symptoms such as low-grade fevers to your doctor.

In very rare cases *Pneumocystis carinii* has been reported in parts of the body other than the lungs: this is called *extrapulmonary* PCP. The CDC has reported only a few dozen cases of extrapulmonary infection out of many tens of thousands of cases of HIV-related *Pneumocystis carinii.*

▲ Diagnosis

If PCP is diagnosed and treated early, treatment will be safer and more effective. Early diagnosis and treatment can mean fewer symptoms and better survival rate. If you are diagnosed when your symptoms are very mild, you may be able to avoid hospitalization by taking oral medication on an out-patient basis.

Promptly report any shortness of breath to your physician. Although the symptom may be caused by many other problems—such as anxiety—it is important to rule out PCP or any other serious respiratory disease. You should also tell your doctor about any persistent cough, fever, weight loss, or fatigue.

Your physician will not be able to tell whether you have PCP just by hearing your symptoms, looking at you, or even giving you a full physical examination, because the symptoms of PCP are similar to the symptoms of many other diseases. However, diagnostic laboratory tests can be used to tell if you have PCP. Diagnostic methods that involve little discomfort or danger will usually be used first. If they do not yield conclusive results, your physician will order further tests. In any case, your physician is likely to use a combination of tests before making a conclusive diagnosis of PCP.

Several tests are commonly used to diagnose PCP.

There is a pattern of **chest X ray** that is typical of patients with PCP; this is seen in about 75 percent of patients. The typical picture is of infection of spaces between tissue in all areas of the lung rather evenly. However, many patients with PCP have other presentations on chest X ray and between 5 percent and 10 percent of patients with PCP have normal chest X rays. Relapses for PCP patients on aerosolized pentamidine prophylaxis are often located on X ray in the upper lobes of the lung.

Pulmonary function tests measure how efficiently the lungs are operating. The most notable finding for patients with PCP is on a test referred to as DL_{CO} ("single-breath diffusing capacity for carbon monoxide"). Other test results that show a decline in functioning of the lungs are an increase in LDH (lactate dehydrogenase) in the blood, and a test of arterial blood gas (ABG) that shows a decrease of oxygen in the blood.

Gallium scanning is a painless noninvasive imaging technique that is useful for distinguishing infectious processes from other disease processes in the lungs. Gallium scanning is described in detail in Chapter 13: Procedures and Tests, p. 303.

None of these tests alone (X ray, pulmonary function test, or gallium scan) is adequate in all cases to diagnose PCP. They all tend to be positive for people who have PCP but also are sometimes positive for people who do not have PCP. In combination the three tests can often give an accurate diagnosis. However, if these tests are not adequate for diagnosis, several other tests can be used.

In the **induced sputum test** a solution of salt and water (a *saline* solution) is turned into a mist that you inhale into the lungs. This causes you to cough up sputum that can then be examined for the *Pneumocystis carinii* organism. Studies indicate that when this test is done in a hospital lab where the personnel are experienced in performing it, a positive test indicates PCP. A negative test should be followed up by the tests described below. The advantage of the induced sputum test is that it causes you less pain and discomfort than bronchoscopy.

Bronchoscopy is the common description of one or both of two diagnostic procedures for PCP that use an instrument called a *fiber-optic bronchoscope*. The bronchoscope is a thin flexible tube which is inserted through the nose, down the windpipe, and into the lungs. The insertion of the bronchoscope is somewhat uncomfortable, but not usually painful.

In *bronchoalveolar lavage*, saline solution is introduced into the lungs through the bronchoscope. The saline loosens mucus that can then be sucked out through the instrument and examined for *Pneumocystis carinii* organisms.

In *transbronchial biopsy,* tiny samples of lung tissue are snipped out and removed through the bronchoscope. These samples are then examined for the *Pneumocystis carinii* organism. With biopsy there is some risk of hemorrhaging or a collapsed lung *(pneumothorax).* Both lavage and biopsy are separately quite predicative and particularly accurate when used together. In patients who have been taking aerosolized pentamidine, lavage alone may not yield enough organisms to produce an accurate result; biopsy should be done as well. Lavage and biopsy can be done during a single bronchoscopy and cause no additional pain.

One further test, an open-lung biopsy, can be used in certain very special circumstances: when disease is progressing and other diagnostic methods cannot be used or do not yield results. This test is very accurate, but is invasive and may be dangerous and should not generally be used.

These tests are described in more detail in Chapter 13: Procedures and Tests.

If you have respiratory symptoms, the first step is to have a chest X ray. If the X ray is normal, you should have pulmonary function tests and gallium scanning. If the X ray is abnormal, skip these tests and have an induced sputum test for PCP, mycobacteria, and CMV. If the induced sputum cannot be done or gives a negative result, then bronchoalveolar lavage and possibly transbronchial biopsy are indicated.

▲ Treatment

Survival has improved as there has been more experience with treatment of patients with PCP. At the present time there are several different treatment options.

The first choice for treatment is trimethoprim/sulfamethoxazole (TMP/SMX, brand names: **Bactrim,** Septra), given for fourteen to twenty-one days. Some patients are unable to tolerate a full course of Bactrim. Adverse side effects include severe itchy rash, elevation of liver function tests, nausea and vomiting, anemia, creatinine elevation, hyponatremia (depletion of salt in the blood), neutropenia (a deficiency of neutrophils, a type of white blood cells). Due to side effects, only 35 percent to 45 percent of patients with AIDS who begin Bactrim therapy for PCP are able to complete the full course.

Adverse side effects typically occur during the second week of therapy and can be reversed by stopping the drug. If the gastrointestinal tract is absorbing well (no vomiting, diarrhea, or malabsorption) Bactrim can be used orally as well as intravenously.

Bactrim may take five to seven days to produce clinical improvement. Even with clinical improvement the chest X ray indication may worsen during the first seven to ten days of therapy. If chest X ray continues to

Diagnostic Workup for PCP

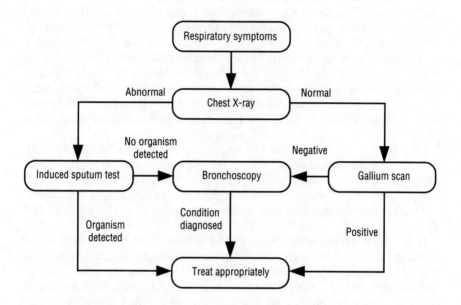

get worse after ten days of Bactrim therapy a different drug should be tried.

Twenty to 30 percent of patients with acute PCP do not respond to Bactrim and need to try an alternate drug, intravenous pentamidine. Unfortunately, many of these people also do not respond to pentamidine. Generally Bactrim is preferable to pentamidine because it is just as effective but better tolerated.

Pentamidine is used for patients who cannot tolerate Bactrim or fail to respond to the drug. **Intravenous pentamidine** should be given for 14 to 21 days. Aerosolized pentamidine is not recommended as therapy for active PCP because it may not be as effective.

The adverse side effects of pentamidine are anemia; creatinine elevation (a sign of kidney problems); liver function test elevation (LFT, a sign of liver problems); hyponatremia (a deficiency of sodium in the blood); pancreatitis, hypoglycemia (low serum glucose levels); diabetes; cardiac arrhythmias (heartbeat irregularities); and neutropenia (reduction in number of a type of white blood cells called neutrophils). About 45 percent of patients require a change of drugs because of adverse side effects.

Twenty to 30 percent of patients do not respond to pentamidine (although they can tolerate the drug).

Dapsone/trimethoprim is another promising drug for treating PCP. It is taken orally and thus permits more outpatient treatment than does Bactrim, which is initially taken intravenously. A 1990 study (Medina) indicated that dapsone was as effective as Bactrim for treating mild to moderate PCP but had fewer side effects. The side effects that it did cause—blood disorders, metheglobinemia (a type of disorder of hemoglobin) and hyperkalemia (an excess of potassium in the blood)—appeared to be dose related. Other side effects were nausea, vomiting, and rash. Further studies are under way.

Dapsone's side effects are less severe than those for Bactrim and pentamidine. These side effects generally do not require that patients discontinue the drug. Even though this is a sulfa-containing drug, patients who are allergic to Bactrim may not be allergic to dapsone.

A few other **experimental drugs** have been tried on a small scale with patients who do not respond to Bactrim, pentamidine, or dapsone. These drugs include difluoromethylornithine (DFMO), trimetrexate, and piritrexim. Data on success and intolerable side effects are limited for these drugs.

DFMO has been successful in some patients who have failed on other drugs. However, relapse appears to be frequent. Adverse side effects of DFMO are bone marrow suppression and gastrointestinal disturbances.

Trimetrexate and piritrexim are drugs that are similar to trimethoprim but more powerful. They are under investigation for patients who cannot take sulfa drugs or have not responded to therapy. They are used in combination with a drug named leucovorin, which acts to reduce the anemia caused by these drugs. They seem effective in mild to moderate cases of PCP but the relapse rate appears high. The main adverse side effects are neutropenia and thrombocytopenia (decrease in platelet count).

Other experimental treatments for active PCP are 566C80 and clindamycin/primaquine. 566C80 is an antiprotozoal drug from the family of drugs called hydroxynaphthoquinones. It has shown promising efficacy in animal studies. As of this writing, 566C80 is in phase II and phase III clinical trials. (See Chapter 19: Understanding Clinical Trials, pp. 359–66.)

In small clinical trials the combination of clindamycin and primaquine has been effective in treating acute PCP in those who do not respond to standard therapies. In the United States the use of primaquine is currently limited to people with acute malaria, due to a shortage of the drug's ingredients. Primaquine may be obtained through underground sources.

Refer to Chapter 9: Learning About Experimental Treatments for information on how to stay up to date on experimental treatments.

Adjunctive therapy with steroids: Adjunctive therapy refers to a medication used in addition to a primary medication. Corticosteroids have been used in combination with Bactrim or pentamidine for severe cases of PCP to reduce swelling of airways. This appears to be a helpful therapy, although the immunosuppressive effects of corticosteroids must be balanced against possible advantages. Corticosteroids are now used in moderate to severe cases of PCP, based on the amount of oxygen that is reaching the blood as measured by tests for arterial blood gases (ABG).

TOXOPLASMA GONDII

Toxoplasma gondii is a protozoan, a single-celled organism, that can cause mass lesions in the central nervous system (that is, lesions involving displacement of brain tissue) and consequent neurological problems. *Toxoplasma gondii* is a parasite that can survive only within cells. It belongs to the same class of protozoa as cryptosporidium and *Isospora belli,* the *coccidia.* It is the single major cause of neurological problems in people with AIDS, accounting for 25 percent to 30 percent of neurological disorders. The disease it causes is referred to as *toxoplasmosis.* Toxoplasmosis has been reported to occur in 3 percent to 40 percent of AIDS patients.

▲ Transmission
The parasite is transmitted either by ingestion or from mother to fetus *(perinatally).* Toxoplasma is not transmitted from person to person.

Toxoplasma gondii exists in three forms: tachyzoites, tissue cysts, and oocytes.

- *Tachyzoites* are larvae (an immature form of the parasite) and are not responsible for transmission of the infection. Tachyzoites invade tissue, multiply, and cause cell damage and acute illness.
- *Tissue cysts* are responsible for most disease transmission and are the "reservoir" of latent infection. They live in all kinds of body tissues but especially in the brain. Tissue cysts contain and release thousands of tachyzoites. **Toxoplasma gondii can infect people who eat undercooked meat** that contains live tissue cysts.
- *Oocytes* are a form of the protozoan that lives only in cats. They are excreted by cats in feces. In one to three weeks they take a form that can infect humans who accidentally ingest minute amounts of cat feces.

Perinatal transmission: Pregnant women may become infected from cysts in meat or oocytes in cat feces, and then transmit the infection to the fetus. Congenital toxoplasmosis can cause visual problems and retardation in the infant.

Avoiding toxoplasma infection: To prevent new infections with *Toxoplasma gondii,* avoid contact with cat feces. Use gloves to clean your cat's litter box or, better, have someone else do it. Cat litter should be cleaned daily. Do not eat raw or undercooked meat (especially pork and lamb) that may contain toxoplasma cysts. Meat should be heated to a temperature of 128 degrees F (60 degrees C) for at least ten minutes. Wash your hands after handling raw meat or unwashed vegetables. Wear gloves for gardening.

▲ Epidemiology

Toxoplasma gondii lives in many animals and millions of people without causing symptoms. It is present in all mammals, some birds, and some reptiles and insects.

The prevalence of infection among humans varies geographically. In the United States and Haiti, 50 percent of adults are infected. In other countries (such as El Salvador and France) over 90 percent of adults are infected. The difference is presumably due to different dietary patterns (such as a preference for rare meat) or differing exposure to cat feces. There is no significant difference in prevalence by sex.

▲ Course of Illness

An immune-impaired person can develop toxoplasmosis from a newly acquired infection or from reactivation of a previously acquired latent infection. Toxoplasmosis in people with AIDS is generally from reactivation of old infections.

Upon infection, *Toxoplasma gondii* enters the blood and lymphatic systems. The newly acquired infection may cause no symptoms or it may cause swollen glands (lymphadenopathy) and a mononucleosis-like syndrome (fever, fatigue).

In people with intact immune systems, the parasite is then contained. In people with impaired immune systems, the parasite can spread to other organs. In 90 percent of cases in immune-impaired people the parasite enters the central nervous system. Toxoplasma may also cause retinitis (diagnosable by an ophthalmologist). Toxoplasma also infects other tissues—such as the heart wall (myocardium), lungs, and skeletal muscles—but rarely causes disease in these sites.

In the brain, toxoplasma organisms multiply within cells, causing cysts. The immune system mounts a devastating and self-destructive response to these cysts, causing swelling and inflammation (encephalitis) that destroys brain tissue. The result is a variety of neurological problems referred to as *cerebral toxoplasmosis.* If sudden, intense encephalitis is not treated rapidly it can lead to coma and death. If untreated, even mild cerebral toxoplasmosis can lead to progressive, fatal disease.

▲ Signs and Symptoms

The symptoms of toxoplasmosis are often vague, nonspecific, and—unfortunately—may not be obvious enough to alert you to the need for medical care. The symptoms may be difficult to distinguish from those of many other HIV-related problems. Antibody testing for toxoplasma infection is therefore important so that this disease can be ruled in or ruled out as a cause of symptoms. Toxoplasma antibody testing should be part of your initial work-up for HIV disease.

Early diagnosis is very important, because prompt treatment increases survival and reduces serious aftereffects of neurological abnormalities. Generally, symptoms of neurological problems develop slowly over the course of a week or two. The most common symptoms are headaches, paralysis or weakness of half the body *(hemiparesis),* and seizures.

The typical **headache** is likely to be dull, persistent, and on both sides of the head *(bilateral).* Severe headaches may be present but are more likely to be caused by cryptococcal meningitis.

People are also likely early on to show **alterations in mental state** that may be subtle. These include impairment of recent memory, slowness to respond, and increased anxiety. These symptoms may be caused by HIV itself.

If not treated, toxoplasmosis can cause severe mental confusion and coma.

The *basal ganglia* of the brain are most likely to be affected. This area controls **motor coordination,** among other functions. Toxoplasmosis can cause failure of muscular coordination *(ataxia),* partial paralysis, and difficulty in walking. It can also cause disturbances in speaking and vision.

Toxoplasmosis is the most common cause of **seizures** in people with AIDS. Between 15 percent and 30 percent of people with toxoplasmosis have seizures. Seizures are random electrical disturbances in the brain. People commonly have a frightening image of seizures as involving violent muscular convulsions, but only a minority of seizures manifest this way. A seizure may consist simply of a small muscle twitching, a brief blank spell or lapse of memory, or even the illusion of an odor or image. Seizures generally last thirty to sixty seconds. All patients with cerebral mass lesions should be placed on medication to prevent seizures: phenobarbitol or phenytoin (Dilantin).

▲ Monitoring

Infection with *Toxoplasma gondii* can be detected by a blood test for antibodies to the organism. A positive antibody test shows infection but does not mean that the organism is necessarily causing disease.

All HIV-positive people should be tested for toxoplasma infection. Toxoplasma testing is useful for two reasons: patients who know they are infected with toxoplasma will be more vigilant for symptoms of toxoplasmosis; and physicians use a positive toxoplasmosis test to help diagnose neurological symptoms. Patients who know they are not infected with toxoplasma will have one less thing to worry about, and will also know to be careful about avoiding a new toxoplasma infection.

Physicians should do toxoplasma testing on all HIV-positive patients as baseline information.

▲ Prophylaxis

Typically, patients with low T4 count will already be started on Bactrim as preventive therapy against PCP. Bactrim may provide protection against toxoplasmosis also. Other possibilities under study include pyrimethamine either alone or in combination with sulfadiazine, clindamycin, azithromycin, Bactrim, or dapsone. Data are limited.

▲ Diagnosis

Diagnosis of toxoplasmosis is often difficult. Physical signs and symptoms lead to a suspicion of toxoplasmosis, but multiple tests are needed to confirm this. Because it is important to start treatment early in the course of an acute episode of toxoplasmosis, treatment will often begin when there are strong indications that toxoplasmosis is the likely cause of the illness. This is called a *presumptive diagnosis.* It is made on the basis of the presence of the symptoms described above, typical results of a CT (computerized tomography) scan or MRI (magnetic resonance imaging) scan, and a positive test of blood for antibodies to toxoplasma. A CT scan usually shows characteristic lesions in the brain. MRI may show lesions not apparent on the CT scan; an MRI scan should be done on patients with symptoms who are negative on CT scan. A lumbar puncture (LP) can help exclude other infectious agents as the cause of symptoms.

If a trial of antitoxoplasma medication produces no improvement, CT-guided "skinny needle" brain biopsy may be done to distinguish toxoplasmosis from lymphoma.

Refer to Chapter 13: Procedures and Tests for descriptions of these diagnostic procedures.

▲ Treatment and Maintenance

Most patients with toxoplasmosis respond to therapy. One study indicated an 80 percent response to the appropriate medication (Wong, Annals of Internal Medicine, 1984). Many people with toxoplasmosis also have other opportunistic infections at the same time.

Standard primary treatment is a combination of a sulfa (sulfonamide) drug (such as sulfadiazine) and pyrimethamine. Sulfa drugs and pyrimethamine interfere with the production of folic acid, a chemical necessary for the growth of the parasite. The two drugs must be used together to be effective. These drugs are used at a relatively high dosage, leading to a strong possibility of adverse side effects. There is some controversy about the amount of pyrimethamine that is necessary. These drugs cross the blood-brain barrier (enter the central nervous system) and can treat infection in the brain.

Many patients have allergic reactions to sulfa drugs, developing rashes and fevers. Other adverse side effects of sulfa drugs are suppression of a kind of white blood cells called neutrophils *(neutropenia),* fever, nausea, vomiting, and diarrhea. Kidney problems (interstitial nephritis) can also develop; the drug forms crystals in the kidneys, which can lead to blockage and kidney failure. Despite the many side effects, most patients do not have to discontinue treatment.

The major side effect of pyrimethamine is suppression of blood cells *(pancytopenia)*. This side effect can often be controlled by taking another drug called leucovorin (folinic acid—not folic acid), and this is usually given in combination with the sulfa drug and pyrimethamine. Other side effects are headache and gastrointestinal upset.

These drugs kill the form of the parasite that causes active disease (tachyzoites), but do not kill the form that is the reservoir of infection (tissue cysts). Consequently, these drugs do not eradicate latent infection; relapse occurs in 50 percent of patients who stop taking medication. For this reason it is important for patients to continue on maintenance medication, which is often a lower dose of the combination of pyrimethamine and a sulfa drug such as Bactrim.

Patients with toxoplasmosis generally require long-term suppressive therapy. Long-term use leads to many allergic side effects that may necessitate discontinuation of one or both drugs.

Only small studies have been done on suppressive maintenance therapy against toxoplasmosis, but these studies and clinical practice indicate that maintenance is effective.

For patients who are unable to tolerate sulfa drugs, **two alternative therapies have been used, pyrimethamine alone at a higher dosage and a combination of pyrimethamine and clindamycin (an antiparasitic drug).** Clindamycin has some side effects (nausea, vomiting, diarrhea, mild rash) and may not be effective in killing toxoplasma in the brain.

A large trial is under way in Europe comparing pyrimethamine and clindamycin with the standard treatment of pyrimethamine and sulfadiazine. Interim analysis of data shows no difference in survival or toxicity.

Other drugs: Spiramycin is a drug available in Europe and Canada (but not the United States) that has also been tried. This drug shows some promise but results so far are inconclusive and controversial. Other drugs that have been suggested as possible treatment and require further investigation are trimetrexate, Fansidar, gamma interferon, in vitro-stimulated macrophages, and Arprinocid (an animal antibiotic). Refer to Chapter 9: Learning About Experimental Treatments for information on how to stay up to date on experimental treatments.

A number of other drugs are used for treating symptoms of toxoplasmosis. They include decadron, for treating *edema* (swelling) surrounding toxoplasma lesions, and Dilantin or phenobarbitol for preventing seizures. The effect of AZT on the course of toxoplasmosis is not entirely clear but seems beneficial and without problems in combination with drugs for toxoplasmosis. Since AZT and the pyrimethamine/sulfadiazine combination both can cause neutropenia, regular monitoring for this side effect is important when using these drugs together.

Infections

HISTOPLASMA CAPSULATUM

▲ Epidemiology

Histoplasmosis is a disease caused by the fungus *Histoplasma capsulatum*. It currently accounts for less than 1 percent of AIDS cases, but it is becoming more frequent. This fungus is common only in people from certain geographical areas: central United States (the middle west, primarily the Mississippi and Ohio river valleys and the river valley areas of the east), the Caribbean (including Puerto Rico and the Dominican Republic), and South America. It also must be considered diagnostically in people who have visited these areas. Histoplasmosis occurs in up to 25 percent of people with AIDS in Indianapolis, Kansas City, and Memphis.

▲ Transmission

Histoplasma capsulatum lives in soil contaminated by bird or bat droppings. When the contaminated soil is disturbed, spores *(microconidia)* are spread and infection occurs when they are inhaled. The only advice relevant to avoiding a new histoplasma infection is to reduce contact with bird droppings, but it is not clear how to accomplish this other than avoiding caves, farms, and bird roosts. Wear gloves when handling pet birds or cleaning their cages. Histoplasma is not spread from person to person. Histoplasmosis in most AIDS patients is the result of a reactivation of a latent infection, not a new infection.

▲ Monitoring and Prophylaxis Unclear

We do not know the T4 threshold for histoplasmosis. Serologies to detect histoplasma infection in advance of disease are not routinely done. It is not known whether antifungals can prevent histoplasma disease.

▲ Course and symptoms

After the fungus is inhaled, spores sprout into a yeast form that can cause disease. In an immune-intact person, this will usually produce no symptoms or a time-limited flu-like illness. In people with impaired immune systems, including those with AIDS, the yeast-like organisms grow and are spread in the blood stream. This causes disseminated histoplasmosis, a systemic fungal infection that may affect multiple organs and produce a wide variety of symptoms that are particularly severe in people with AIDS.

The most common manifestations of histoplasmosis are fever; swollen glands (lymphadenopathy); weight loss; respiratory problems (including shortness of breath, cough); weakness, lethargy, and enlargement of the liver and spleen. Fairly commonly, histoplasmosis affects the bone marrow causing deficiencies of red blood cells (anemia); certain white blood cells (leukopenia) and platelets (thrombocytopenia); the skin; and central nervous system problems. Less frequently, it causes cardiac problems (pericarditis, myocarditis) and problems in the retina. In 10 percent to 20 percent of cases histoplasmosis leads to a syndrome resembling *sepsis,* an overwhelming infection of the blood. This can develop rapidly and lead to death. However, this can be avoided by early diagnosis and treatment.

▲ Diagnosis

Histoplasma capsulatum must be distinguished from several other organisms: *Cryptococcus neoformans, Pneumocystis carinii,* and candida. Histoplasmosis can be diagnosed by microscopic examination and culture of infected tissues (lung, bone marrow, and lymph nodes). Blood smears sometimes can indicate infection with *Histoplasma capsulatum* and thereby eliminate the need for more invasive procedures. Blood and urine can be cultured for fungus. Antibody tests of blood and skin tests are not reliable in immune-compromised patients. A recently developed antigen test may simplify diagnosis and the monitoring of response to treatment.

▲ Treatment

Amphotericin-B (Fungizone) is the current treatment of choice for acute histoplasmosis. (For more information on amphotericin-B, see p. 274 in this chapter). It can cause severe and unpleasant side effects: fevers; chills; kidney damage; and suppression of bone marrow production, which leads to various types of anemia. If the patient is unable to tolerate this drug or fails to respond, ketoconazole (Nizoral) has been used. Ketoconazole is definitely not the first-choice drug because it has been associated with treatment failures. In mild cases, treatment is sometimes attempted with fluconazole (Diflucan) or itraconazole (Sporanex). If untreated, histoplasmosis can be fatal.

▲ Maintenance Therapy Required

There is a high relapse rate of histoplasmosis in people with AIDS. Consequently, long-term maintenance treatment is necessary, either with ketoconazole or weekly or biweekly intravenous use of amphotericin-B (if there is central nervous system involvement). Fluconazole or itraconazole may be useful maintenance drugs against histoplasmosis but need to be studied.

▲ Experimental Drugs

A less toxic form of amphotericin-B called amphotericin-B lipid complex is under development. Refer to Chapter 9: Learning About Experimental Treatments for information on how to stay up to date on experimental treatments.

CRYPTOSPORIDIUM AND *ISOSPORA BELLI*

Both cryptosporidium and *Isospora belli* are protozoan (single-celled) parasites that infect the intestinal tract. They are the most common causes of chronic diarrhea in patients with AIDS. These parasites belong to the same family of organisms as *Toxoplasma gondii.*

Chronic diarrhea in HIV-infected people can be caused by a number of different diseases including salmonella, shigella, *Campylobacter pylorides,* cryptosporidium, *Clostridium difficile, Mycobacterium avium* complex, various ova, *Giardia lamblia, Entamoeba histolytica,* microsporidiosis, and HIV itself. In particular, the symptoms of cryptosporidium are indistinguishable from those of *Isospora belli.* Cryptosporidium is more common than *Isospora belli.*

Both cryptosporidium and *Isospora belli* can infect all parts of the lining of the gut (the *epithelium),* but particularly the small bowel. Physicians need to distinguish between the two organisms because *Isospora belli* responds quickly to appropriate treatment while cryptosporidium is generally unresponsive to treatment.

▲ Cryptosporidium

Cryptosporidium disease accounts for the initial AIDS diagnosis in 4 percent of patients. It is estimated that 15 percent of symptomatic AIDS patients in the United States are infected with this parasite.

Transmission: Cryptosporidium causes diarrhea in a wide variety of animals and can be transmitted both between species (for example, from animals to humans) and within species (for example, from human to human). An immature form of the organism (the *oocyte)* is excreted in the feces of an infected person or animal. Microscopic quantities of cryptosporidium-infected material can then be passed from one person to another directly or via inanimate objects. For example, tiny particles of fecal matter on inadequately washed hands can easily get in the mouth during a meal and spread infection. Medically this is referred to as the *fecal-oral* route of transmission. Cryptosporidium can also be spread through contaminated drinking water. *Isospora belli* is probably spread by the same routes as cryptosporidium.

Cryptosporidium and probably *Isospora belli* are highly infectious. Careful hygiene—particularly hand washing—can help keep the infection from spreading. The parasite is killed by a 5 percent solution of either ammonia or bleach. Sometimes this parasite can be spread in a hospital setting. Careful infection-control procedures in medical settings and laboratories are therefore important. Cryptosporidium is particularly common among men who have sex with men, perhaps because of oral-anal contact during sexual activity. The use of a flexible latex barrier between the mouth and anus will prevent transmission during oral-anal contact.

Cryptosporidiosis is common in many countries with inadequate water treatment or sewage control and is often the cause of so-called traveler's diarrhea in tourists who visit these countries. For this reason, HIV-infected travelers should take precautions to avoid infection (see the section on travel in Chapter 6: General Health Care, pp. 111–15).

Because the United States can afford a reasonably clean water supply, only about 4 percent of patients with AIDS have cryptosporidium, as compared with 50 percent of AIDS patients in Haiti and Africa. Severe weight loss caused by this and other gastrointestinal infections explains why AIDS is called *slim disease* in Africa.

Symptoms and course: Symptomatic infection with cryptosporidium is called *cryptosporidiosis.* In persons with intact immune systems, cryptosporidium frequently causes self-limiting diarrhea that lasts from four to twenty days and then stops even without treatment. Cryptosporidium is much more serious for people who are immune deficient due to HIV infection, because the diarrhea is usually chronic rather than limited to a few days. Severe chronic diarrhea causes serious medical problems.

In HIV-infected people, disease caused by cryptosporidium seems to appear primarily among those who are severely immune impaired (T4 count less than 100). Usually, people who develop symptoms of cryptosporidiosis have other secondary infections or advanced Kaposi's sarcoma.

The major symptom of cryptosporidiosis is watery, chronic, profuse diarrhea (six to twenty-six bowel movements per day). It is not known how cryptosporidium causes diarrhea or whether the organism directly interferes with the absorption of food (and thereby causes weight loss or wasting). In addition to diarrhea, abdominal pain is common. This pain is usually dull, crampy, and located in the upper part of the abdomen. The diarrhea and abdominal pain are often made worse by eating. Other common symptoms are cramping, malaise, flatulence (gas), low-grade fever, loss of appetite, weight loss, bloating, nausea, and vomiting.

Symptoms usually develop slowly and gradually. They tend to get worse as immune function decreases. The symptoms are usually chronic but some people may have periods of remission or even spontaneous cure, especially if they have a more adequately functioning immune system. Severity of the symptoms varies widely from person to person.

In 10 percent of patients with cryptosporidiosis there is involvement of the gallbladder (biliary tract). This causes symptoms of more severe nausea, vomiting, and abdominal pain (particularly on the upper right side).

Diagnosis of cryptosporidiosis can be made by a test done on a stool sample. This test is called an *acid-fast stained stool smear* and detects a stage of the parasite's life cycle in specimens examined under the microscope. This test can effectively distinguish cryptosporidium from *Isospora belli.* The test is somewhat complicated, so it should be done at a laboratory experienced in performing this procedure.

It can be complicated to diagnose the cause of chronic diarrhea in HIV-infected patients. Other gastrointestinal infections such as cytomegalovirus and *Giardia lamblia* can often be present at the same time as cryptosporidium. Several rounds of testing and treatment may be necessary, but it is worth the trouble. For instance, it is often necessary to repeat the stool-sample examination in order to detect cryptosporidium. This may be done up to four times in some cases.

There has been some progress in **treatment for cryptosporidiosis,** although much more research is needed. In addition, symptoms can be helped with various antidiarrhea treatments.

Dapsone has been used for treatment of cryptosporidiosis. Trials are under way on azithromycin (Zithromax). A drug called Letrazuril is also under study and may be better absorbed by the body.

Spiramycin, an antibiotic related to erythromycin, has been tried against cryptosporidiosis. Oral spiramycin showed little benefit in small trials and has had severe side effects. It is used widely in Canada and Europe but in the United States is only available in clinical research trials.

Much of current treatment focuses on relieving symptoms. Diarrhea, abdominal pain, and nausea can be lessened with opiates (tincture of opium), kaolin-pectin suspension (Kaopectate), loperamide (Imodium), antiemetics (Compazine, Phenergan), prostaglandin inhibitors, paromycin (Humatin) and antispasmodics. Drink a lot of fluids to avoid dehydration. Patients sometimes receive intravenous fluids to maintain adequate levels of fluid in the body. Serious weight loss may a problem: eat a high-calorie, low-fat diet. Some people may be unable to digest fat or milk and a dairy-free diet may be indicated. Nutrition may be supported with dietary supplements or intravenous feeding *(parenteral nutrition)*. (See the discussion of weight loss in Chapter 10: Organ System Complications, pp. 190–95.)

Currently there is no medication available that will prevent an initial infection with cryptosporidium or control the organism enough to avoid symptoms.

▲ Isospora Belli

Isospora belli is a protozoan parasite that causes symptoms very similar to those of cryptosporidium. Symptomatic infection with *Isospora belli* is sometimes called *coccidiosis.*

Transmission: As with cryptosporidium, *Isospora belli* is probably transmitted by the fecal-oral route; again, hand washing and use of a barrier method during oral-anal contact will help to avoid infection. Unlike cryptosporidium, *Isospora belli* seems to be transmitted only from person to person, and not from animal to human.

Isospora belli is less common than cryptosporidium, although its exact prevalence is unknown. It is found most commonly in tropical and sub-tropical climates and is extremely common in certain parts of South

America, Africa, and Southeast Asia. It has been implicated in outbreaks of diarrhea in institutional settings (such as prisons, hospitals, schools, the military).

In the United States probably at least 2 percent of patients with AIDS have symptomatic *Isospora belli* infection, while in Haiti 15 percent of AIDS patients are infected.

The **symptoms** of *Isospora belli* infection are generally indistinguishable from those caused by cryptosporidium, although the symptoms are often less severe.

Diagnosis: *Isospora belli* has been found only in the gut. If *Isospora belli* is detectable it is causing symptomatic disease. It is diagnosed by microscopic examination of a stool smear.

The most commonly used treatment is Bactrim (trimethoprim/sulfamethoxazole). Symptoms of *Isospora belli* respond quickly to medication —diarrhea is usually cured within two days of beginning treatment. For this reason, if a diagnosis cannot be made promptly to distinguish *Isospora belli* from cryptosporidium, a trial of Bactrim should begin. This drug is the first choice for treatment. *Isospora belli* can also treated with furazolidone (Furoxone), or Fansidar (pyrimethamine and sulfadoxine).

The most common side effect of Bactrim is itching. Many HIV-infected people develop sensitivity to Bactrim and other sulfa-containing drugs that may escalate into rash or fever but can be controlled by discontinuing the drug. Furazolidone is an antiprotozoal and antibacterial drug used to treat gastrointestinal problems including diarrhea. Fansidar may sometimes cause a severe uncontrollable allergic reaction. Patients who are already allergic to sulfa drugs have responded to pyrimethamine alone (Daraprim).

Maintenance: One study indicated that 50 percent of patients treated for *Isospora belli* developed symptoms again within two months of stopping treatment. Since symptoms are likely to recur after medication is stopped, ongoing maintenance treatment is necessary. Drugs for this purpose include Bactrim, possibly Fansidar, or—for those who are allergic to sulfa drugs—metronidazole (Flagyl) or pyrimethamine alone. As these are all available in pill form, maintenance therapy is relatively convenient. Flagyl can cause metallic taste, nausea, or depression as side effects.

ENTAMOEBA HISTOLYTICA (AMOEBAS)

Entamoeba histolytica is a protozoan parasite that can cause gastrointestinal symptoms, particularly diarrhea. The amoebas infect the colon, often without causing any noticeable symptoms. Amoebas cause symptoms when they invade the bowel wall. Symptomatic infection with *Entamoeba histolytica* is referred to as *amebiasis* or, colloquially, as "having amoebas."

Infection with this amoeba is common: perhaps 10 percent of the world's population is infected—especially impoverished people in Africa, Asia, and South America and travelers to these areas. The amoeba is transmitted via the *oral-fecal* route (ingestion of microscopic particles of feces). This occurs when food or water supplies are contaminated. Transmission can also occur during oral-anal sexual contact. Amoebas are usually transmitted by someone who does not have symptoms.

In the United States, this parasite is found more often among gay men than other people, probably because oral-anal sexual contact is practiced more often among gay men. *Entamoeba histolytica* is neither more common nor more severe among HIV-positive people than among HIV-negative people; treatment is the same without regard to HIV status.

Amoebas can cause **symptoms** ranging widely from none to severe. Usually people get frequent loose stools (occasionally constipation), increased gas, nausea, lower abdominal pain, or a bloated feeling. Diarrhea may be severe or bloody. Fatigue and weight loss may also occur.

Diagnosis is made by using a microscope to examine a fresh sample of stool. The amoeba exists in two forms, *cysts* and *trophozoites.*

The best way to test for amoebas is to get a lab test called a *purged stool sample* (described in Chapter 13: Procedures and Tests, p. 299. The next best way to test for amoebas is to examine an ordinary stool sample collected at home and then brought to the lab. This stool sample can be examined only for cysts, because the trophozoites die too quickly.

You can get a false-negative test through temporary suppression of the amoebas if:

- You are taking antibiotics, laxatives, or antacids that contain castor oil or magnesium hydroxide (milk of magnesia, Gelusil, Mylanta, Maalox),
- You are taking antidiarrheal medication containing bismuth or kaolin (Pepto-Bismol or Kaopectate)
- You have had a barium X ray procedure or an enema within two weeks.

If the stool test is negative and symptoms persist, it should be repeated three times before giving up the search for amoebas. It is best to be tested by a lab experienced in this procedure.

Treatment: Amoebas are treated with a combination of metronidazole (Flagyl) (dose: 750 mg three times a day for five to ten days) and Iodoquinol (emetine hydrochloride) (650 mg three times a day for twenty-one days). Flagyl can cause many side effects: a metallic taste in the mouth, dark urine, fatigue, depression, headaches, nausea, vomiting, and fever. It can cause a severe adverse reaction when taken in combination with alcohol or disulfiram (Antabuse). Flagyl is also used to treat

Giardia infection. Diarrhea may continue for several days to weeks after the amoebas are cured because of irritation to the colon or reaction to Flagyl. You should be retested twice after treatment to be sure you have been cured.

GIARDIA LAMBLIA

Giardia lamblia is a protozoan parasite that can cause gastrointestinal symptoms. Infection is often asymptomatic. If *Giardia* does cause symptoms, they are often self-limited, that is, the symptoms go away without treatment. However, effective treatment does exist and can lessen discomfort and inconvenience. Giardiasis is not more severe and not harder to treat in people with HIV disease.

Transmission: Like all parasites, *Giardia* assumes different forms during different stages of its life. The infection is transmitted when *Giardia* cysts from the feces of an infected individual are ingested by another person. This can occur when drinking water is contaminated by feces (generally in Third World countries and in the United States in communities that get drinking water from streams or rivers without a water filtration system). It can also be transmitted from person to person, for example during oral-anal sexual contact. Transmission can occur during the entire period of infection; you can transmit *Giardia* even when you are asymptomatic. Using a latex barrier for oral-anal contact (rimming) can prevent person-to-person transmission. Washing the anogenital area before sex can be helpful.

Symptoms and course: *Giardia lamblia* principally infects the upper small intestine and this causes inflammation of the intestine. Only when *Giardia* is very severe will it cause any damage to cells. If diarrhea is severe it can lead to fluid and electrolyte imbalance. It can cause malabsorption of fat and fat-soluble vitamins.

The symptoms of *Giardia* are foul watery flatulence, abdominal pain, malabsorption, and malodorous watery diarrhea. In the first few days diarrhea can be watery and explosive. This usually changes to loose bulky stools on an intermittent basis.

Infection with *Giardia* is diagnosed by a stool test. The most effective test is the *purged stool test* (see Chapter 13: Procedures and Tests, p. 299). This must be repeated up to five times if negative because it can be difficult to find the parasite even when infection is present.

Sexual partners should also be tested; household contacts should be tested if they are symptomatic.

Treatment: Because *Giardia* can be difficult to diagnose, if you have typical symptoms and a history of possible exposure you can begin treatment on a trial basis without waiting for results of the stool test. Drugs used are antiprotozoal: a commonly used drug is metronidazole (Flagyl). Another possible drug is quinacrine hydrochloride (Atabrine).

You should respond to medication within a few days. The drugs may

256

cause dizziness or light-headedness, a funny taste in the mouth, or gastrointestinal problems that are actually similar to the symptoms being treated. You can reduce side effects by taking medication along with food. While you are taking these drugs you should not drink alcohol, use alcohol-containing preparations, or take the drug disulfiram (Antabuse).

You should have stool retested three times, each several days apart, beginning one to two weeks following the treatment.

BACTERIAL INFECTIONS

The bacteria we will discuss are:

- *Mycobacterium avium*
- *Mycobacterium tuberculosis*
- Salmonella
- Shigella
- *Campylobacter jejuni*
- *Treponema pallidum* (syphilis)
- Encapsulated bacteria (bacterial pneumonia)

MYCOBACTERIA

Mycobacteria are a family of bacteria that can cause tuberculosis and various other diseases in HIV-infected people. Mycobacteria can remain dormant in the body for long periods of time.

Full treatment for mycobacterial disease typically takes months or years. Mycobacteria do not respond to medication when dormant because the relevant antibiotics interfere with cell-wall formation, a stage of the bacterial life cycle that doesn't take place during dormancy. To be effective, treatment must therefore catch the mycobacterium while it is reproducing.

An individual patient's strains of mycobacteria are often resistant to one or more antibiotics. Consequently several drugs must be used simultaneously to treat these organisms successfully.

In HIV-infected people maintenance therapy may be required indefinitely.

Mycobacterial diseases are primarily defended against by the cell-mediated branch of the immune system. Since cell-mediated immunity depends on T4 cells, HIV-infected patients whose T4 cells are depleted may have problems with mycobacteria.

Mycobacteria that cause disease in HIV-infected people include:

- *Mycobacterium avium* and *Mycobacterium intracellulare*
- *Mycobacterium tuberculosis*
- *Mycobacterium kansasii* (rare, not explicitly discussed here)
- *Mycobacterium hemophilum* (very rare, causes skin and joint

problems; must be diagnosed by special culture; not explicitly discussed here).

MYCOBACTERIUM AVIUM COMPLEX (MAC)

MAC Outside AIDS: Before the AIDS epidemic, *Mycobacterium avium* complex (MAC) was a rare disease that caused slowly progressing lung infection in patients with underlying chronic lung-disease problems. It does not generally cause disease in patients who are immunocompromised for reasons other than HIV disease. Now it is seen frequently in AIDS patients late in the course of HIV disease and causes a number of symptoms including fever, shaking, chills, malaise, anemia, and weight loss. Advances have recently been made in the treatment of MAC.

MAC was formerly called *"Mycobacterium avium-intracellulare* disease" (MAI) because it was not clear whether one or both of the organisms *Mycobacterium avium* and *Mycobacterium intracellulare* were responsible for the illness observed. **"MAC" has replaced "MAI" as the standard name for this disease.**

The prevalence of MAC is unclear. HIV-infected people in all parts of the United States frequently carry MAC, and the incidence of MAC is the same among all the various groups of HIV-infected people: men who have sex with men, needle sharers, transfusion recipients, etc. Autopsy studies of people who died from AIDS have shown that 21 percent to 50 percent were infected with MAC. MAC may not be diagnosed if it is hidden by other coexisting infections. Most people infected with MAC eventually develop some symptoms.

MAC is an organism found throughout the world in soil, water, or dust that has been contaminated by the excretions of birds or mammals. Although **routes of transmission** are not entirely understood, it appears that MAC is probably acquired from the environment and not transmitted from person to person. The organism is thought to be inhaled or ingested. It spreads in the body when the organism enters the bloodstream.

When MAC causes disease, it is usually in patients with a T4 count below 50 who have had prior opportunistic infections. Thus, **MAC is considered a "late" opportunistic infection.**

It mainly affects the *reticuloendothelial system,* a group of related cells in the body that include *macrophages*—white blood cells with complex disease-fighting and immune-regulatory functions. Macrophage dysfunction caused by HIV is probably a key factor in the development of MAC. See Chapter 16: Immunology, Pathogenesis, and Etiology, p. 328.

In people with advanced HIV disease MAC usually causes disseminated disease (disease spread widely through the body). MAC also sometimes causes localized disease (disease concentrated in a particular part of the body, such as the lungs or gut).

MAC is worth treating even though it isn't clear how it causes disease.

258

Initially, MAC was believed to affect extremely sick AIDS patients but not to cause additional disease. Although the role of MAC in causing organ dysfunction and constitutional symptoms is not entirely clear, it is now evident that MAC plays a significant role in contributing to disease and death.

Microscopic examination of the structure of tissue infected with MAC shows little evidence of inflammatory response or tissue destruction. The organism appears to be able to infect tissue without any damage. Although MAC may not often be a cause of specific organ failure it probably contributes to general disability.

Studies have been contradictory regarding the effect of MAC on death rates in people with AIDS. Some studies of people with PCP and MAC versus PCP alone show no difference in various indicators of clinical status and disease outcome, but other studies have disagreed. It is difficult to sort out because MAC occurs late in the course of AIDS, when other illnesses are present. However, retrospective studies suggest that disseminated MAC infection has a negative effect on a patient's condition and may contribute to discomfort and disability.

Clinicians now favor prompt treatment of MAC. Treatment tends to reduce symptoms and increase survival.

▲ Diagnosis

A presumptive diagnosis of MAC is made by isolation (culture of blood, tissue, or fluid in the laboratory for the bacteria). Testing that does not require invasive procedures should be done first. Treatment is often started at the physician's discretion if there is a high suspicion that MAC is causing disease.

Tissue biopsy: Sites that normally have no bacteria (bone marrow, liver, lymph nodes) may be biopsied and examined under the microscope for evidence of mycobacteria. This technique is quick but does not provide a definitive diagnosis of MAC. This method cannot distinguish MAC from tuberculosis (TB), so if mycobacteria are found, standard TB treatment should be started until a definitive diagnosis has been made.

Samples for cultures for MAC may be taken from blood or the tissues mentioned above. **Although cultures take longer than biopsy smears to produce results, cultures provide definitive diagnoses.**

Obtaining samples of blood is less invasive than biopsying the other tissues. Definitive diagnosis can be made by culturing the mycobacterium from blood. Patients with invasive MAC will almost always test positive on blood culture. It takes from 5 to 51 days to get results. Usually, treatment should begin on presumptive diagnosis (as from a sample examined under the microscope) without waiting for the results of the culture.

The organism can also be cultured from bone marrow, lymph node, and liver and these cultures may grow faster. The reliability of culture grown from stool is in dispute. Positive cultures from the respiratory tract (including sputum) do not necessarily mean that the organism is causing disease; they should be confirmed by blood or other cultures.

▲ Signs and Symptoms

Symptoms and signs of disseminated MAC infection are often difficult to sort out because patients generally have other opportunistic infections that may cause similar symptoms. Nonetheless, an effort to diagnose MAC should generally be made because early diagnosis and treatment appear to improve prognosis.

The signs and symptoms of MAC are often similar to the signs and symptoms of TB. Differences are that GI symptoms are more common in MAC and cough is much less common. Manifestations of disseminated MAC are:

- Chronic fever (often high)
- Weight loss (often quite dramatic and associated with anemia)
- Malaise (fatigue and weakness)
- Neutropenia (reduction in the number of neutrophils, a type of white blood cell needed to resist bacteria)
- Chills and night sweats
- Chronic diarrhea
- Abdominal pain caused by abdominal lymphadenopathy (swollen lymph nodes)
- Chronic malabsorption ("Whipples-like syndrome" of the small bowel)
- Enlargement of the liver and spleen *(hepatosplenomegaly)*
- Jaundice (very rare)

If there is bone marrow involvement there may be problems with a deficiency of certain types of blood cells (of red blood cells, causing *anemia;* of white blood cells, causing *leukopenia;* or of the blood-clotting elements called platelets, causing *thrombocytopenia).* Respiratory symptoms due to MAC are unusual and are hard to sort out because they usually occur when MAC is accompanied by PCP (*Pneumocystis carinii* pneumonia). Rarely, skin and oral lesions caused by MAC may occur. MAC has an unclear role in producing neurological symptoms.

▲ Monitoring and Prevention (Primary Prophylaxis)

A number of different medications are being tried for prevention (primary prophylaxis) and maintenance (secondary prophylaxis) of MAC. Some of the drugs being investigated are ethambutol (Myambutol), rifabutin (Ansamycin), clarithromycin (Biaxin), and azithromycin (Zithromax). There is no clear-cut answer at this point about the best drug or combination of drugs that should be used.

Maintenance therapy after an episode of MAC is now routine, even though it is not known which of the existing treatments is most effective.

Primary prophylaxis (prevention for those who are at risk for MAC but have not had an acute episode) is not yet routine practice. Some physicians, however, are putting their patients with T4 counts below 50 on clarithromycin, an experimental drug available through buyer's clubs (see p. 179 in Chapter 9: Learning About Experimental Treatments). The concern with this course of action is that long-term prophylaxis with clarithromycin might make the drug useless for the treatment of acute illness.

▲ Treatment

Treatment should begin upon diagnosis. If other infections have been ruled out and the physician has a high degree of suspicion that MAC is causing disease, treatment may begin presumptively (that is, without a confirmed diagnosis). At the present time there is no standard and universally effective therapy for MAC. MAC is related to tuberculosis: although it does not respond to any single antitubercular medication, it can respond to a combination of antitubercular medications. There has been some success in treating MAC with various combinations of drugs; usually three to five drugs are used. Multidrug therapy reduces mycobacterial colony counts in blood (a measure of the degree of infection) and leads to clinical improvement (especially reduction of fever).

Since medications against MAC are used in combination, it has been hard to sort out which drugs are more effective. Side effects are often additive and idiosyncratic, so it is difficult to predict in advance what combination of drugs will be tolerated.

Research published in September 1990 indicated that a combination of three antitubercular drugs—amikacin, ethambutol, rifampin—can reduce the amount of bacteria and symptoms in patients with disseminated MAC infection. Variations in response seem to depend on the state of the patient's general health and immune system, the strain of MAC, and the ability to tolerate a combination of medications. The addition of the drugs ciprofloxacin (Cipro) and clofazimine may improve this regimen even further.

The decision about what medication to take must partly be based on how sick you are and whether treatment has a chance of improving your quality of life. Those who have clinical symptoms but a relatively well-functioning liver and kidneys will respond best to treatment. Medication usually helps within two to four weeks. If it does work, ongoing suppressive maintenance therapy is necessary.

Possible treatments include various combinations of:

- Rifabutin (Ansamycin)—side effects: possible kidney and liver effects, bone marrow suppression

- Clofazimine—side effect: gradual skin discoloration, GI problems
- Ethambutol (Myambutol)
- Rifampin (various brands)
- Azithromycin (Zithromax)
- Clarithromycin (Biaxin)
- Ciprofloxacin (Cipro)
- Amikacin (Amikin)—dose-limiting toxicity usually occurs after a month; a new less toxic form is under study.

▲ Maintenance (Secondary Prophylaxis)

If you are treated for MAC, ongoing maintenance therapy is necessary. The exact composition of maintenance therapy is controversial. Some expert clinicians use the same multidrug therapy for maintenance as for treatment of acute MAC.

MYCOBACTERIUM TUBERCULOSIS

Tuberculosis is caused by the organism *Mycobacterium tuberculosis.* It is the most common cause of mycobacterial infection world wide.

Active TB is often the first HIV-associated illness to appear. It may occur very early in the course of HIV disease (T4 count below 400), before other opportunistic infections such as PCP.

If you are HIV-infected, you should be tested for TB infection even if you have no symptoms. If you have a positive *purified protein derivative* (PPD) skin test for TB (see "Detecting TB Infection," pp. 264–65), and you are under 35 years old, you should be treated with one to two years or longer of isoniazid (INH) to prevent active disease.

TB should be diagnosed and treated promptly because active TB is generally curable, and unlike almost all other complications of HIV disease, TB is contagious. Cases of drug-resistant TB seem to be increasing. The Centers for Disease Control identified about 200 cases of drug-resistant TB between 1990 and 1992. Ninety percent of these cases occurred in HIV-infected people.

▲ Epidemiology

Unlike most complications of HIV disease, TB is common even among people who are not HIV-infected. TB does not require immune suppression to cause disease.

TB has always been very common in poor and developing (Third World) countries because transmission is increased by crowded living conditions, inadequate hygiene, and lack of medical care.

One hundred years ago TB was the chief cause of death by infection in this country. However, there has been effective medication to treat TB since the 1950s. Before the AIDS epidemic, the prevalence of TB was steadily decreasing in the United States. TB has increased in the United States since 1985, primarily due to increased incidence among HIV-infected people. It is estimated that 10 million people in the United States are infected with *M. tuberculosis.*

TB is a disease of poverty. Crowding and lack of medical care leads to a higher incidence of TB. In the United States, groups with historically high rates of infection include immigrants from areas where TB is common, such as Haiti and some Latin American countries. The incidence of TB is high in the United States among African-Americans and Latinos. TB is particularly common among people who share needles for drug use (20 percent to 25 percent estimated prevalence among needle sharers). There has been a dramatic increase of TB among AIDS patients in this country: New York City, 5 percent; New Jersey, 10 percent; Florida 10 percent; Puerto Rico, 11 percent.

▲ Transmission and Prevention of Initial Infection

Transmission: *M. tuberculosis* infection is newly acquired by inhaling airborne droplets that have been coughed up by a TB-infected person. The droplets can also be spread through sneezing, singing, and even talking. Droplets can remain airborne for extended periods of time, then lodge in the lungs and cause infection. If not treated, the TB bacillus can be transmitted while the disease is active. HIV-positive TB patients (including those with AIDS) transmit TB infection in the same way as any other person with active TB—no more and no less readily.

All patients with active TB should be isolated during the first two weeks of effective treatment, whether HIV-infected or not. Without treatment, patients with active TB may be continuously contagious.

Isolation is not the same as quarantine; it means only that the infected person should sleep alone in a well-ventilated room, cover the mouth and nose when coughing or sneezing, or have visitors wear masks. (Masks may not be fully effective in preventing transmission of TB over extended contact such as that given by health care workers.)

Some medical procedures or therapies may provoke coughing. An example is the administration of aerosolized pentamidine as PCP prophylaxis. When done with patients with active or suspected TB, such procedures should be accompanied by measures to prevent TB transmission. In the case of aerosolized pentamidine, those in the same room might want to wear masks, or the inhalation should be done in a specialized booth.

Prevention: It may be easier for HIV-infected people to become newly infected and their illness may be severe. Consequently, HIV-infected people should take particular care to avoid exposure to TB. You are very unlikely to become infected while riding the subway or in other public places. If household members have symptoms that might be TB, they should be checked by a doctor. If you are a health care worker in a setting of high incidence of TB, discuss the dangers with your physician.

Bacille Calmette Guérin (BCG) vaccine may help prevent TB infection in certain cases, but carries some real risks in other cases. Recommendations are summarized in the section on routine immunizations in Chapter 6: General Health Care, p. 95.

▲ TB Activation Aided by Immune Deficiency

In HIV-infected people, active TB is usually the reactivation of an old latent infection, typically acquired during childhood.

Many people infected with the TB bacillus do not fall ill. An adequately functioning immune system may often be able to keep the tuberculosis bacillus under control so that it does not cause disease or even become noticeable.

A proportion of healthy HIV-uninfected people fall ill with TB disease after infection with the TB bacillus. People who are infected with TB during childhood may develop active disease later in life if medical problems such as malnutrition or HIV infection cause immune suppression. Immune suppression simply offers a previous TB infection that much more chance to reactivate, grow, and cause active TB disease.

▲ Detecting TB Infection

You can be infected with *M. tuberculosis* and have no symptoms. However, the infection may become active later and cause serious problems. Treatment can prevent the infection from developing into active disease so if you are HIV-antibody-positive, you should be tested to see if you are also TB infected.

Initial infection is usually not noticed by the patient but may leave some lung changes that can be observed on a chest X ray. In people with adequately functioning cell-mediated immunity, the immune system will usually halt growth of the organism three to eight weeks after infection and the TB bacillus will become latent in the body and not cause disease.

TB can be detected by a skin test that becomes positive a few weeks after infection. The test is performed in a doctor's office by inserting a small amount of tuberculin antigen (PPD, or purified protein derivative) under the skin. The TB skin test is often referred to as a "PPD."

If you have previously been infected with *M. tuberculosis* your cell-mediated immune system will "remember" and mount an allergic response, causing a small, hard, swollen area (an *induration*) to develop on your arm temporarily. If this occurs, you are considered positive on the PPD test.

If you have a positive skin test, a negative chest X ray, and you are coughing, your sputum should be cultured to see if you have active TB.

Because HIV-infected people may have weakened allergic responses even with a relatively high T4 cell count, special consideration must be given to interpreting the results of a PPD. In an HIV-infected person a PPD should be considered positive if the induration is greater than 5 millimeters in diameter (about a quarter of an inch across). In HIV-uninfected patients, larger induration is required for a positive PPD result.

Two years prior to AIDS diagnosis 70 percent of patients with TB are positive on the PPD test. After an AIDS diagnosis, only 40 percent of patients with TB are positive on the PPD. This reflects a loss of reaction to the PPD due to weakened allergic responses.

If you have significant immune suppression, it is also useful to test a part of your immune system called *cellular immunity,* or *cell-mediated immunity.* Cellular immunity is responsible for allergic responses in general. Cellular immune response may be measured with a set of skin tests referred to as an *anergy panel.* If the anergy panel shows that your immune system is not mounting allergic responses (called "being *anergic"*), then a negative PPD does not necessarily indicate that you are free of TB infection. If you are anergic and you have recently been exposed to infectious TB or have possible TB symptoms, you should get further testing for TB (see below, under Diagnosis).

▲ Prophylaxis for TB-Infected People and Contacts

If you have latent but inactive TB and you are under 35 years old you should be treated for at least one to two years with the medication isoniazid (INH) to keep the infection from causing active disease. If you are under 35 and cannot take isoniazid, you should be treated with rifampin (or rifampin and pyrazinamide).

This course of preventive medication is particularly important in HIV-infected patients because in the presence of HIV disease a latent TB infection is much more likely to become active.

Close household and sexual contacts of a TB patient who have been exposed to the patient during an active phase of TB should receive the same course of preventive medication.

▲ Diagnosis

Diagnostic criteria for TB in HIV-infected people differ depending on the degree of immune deficiency.

T4 count above 200: Your physician will suspect active TB if you have certain symptoms, including weight loss, fever, night sweats, or a cough. Of course, in the HIV-infected patient, these symptoms can be due to many causes other than TB.

A diagnosis of active TB can be made by a positive PPD, a positive smear of a sputum sample, and chest X rays typical of TB. Tests on sputum should be repeated (three times) if they are initially negative.

T4 count below 200: None of these criteria is as clear in patients with HIV disease and a significant degree of immune suppression (T4 count below 200 or an AIDS diagnosis). Both PPD and sputum smear may be negative despite the presence of active TB.

People with both AIDS and active pulmonary TB may have chest

X rays that are not typical of active TB. Chest X rays may in fact appear normal in more than 10 percent of such patients.

Diagnosis may require culture of one or more of the following: blood, sputum, bronchoscopy specimen, bone marrow, lymph nodes, brain tissue, central nervous system, urine, or stool. It will take one week for preliminary results of a culture and four weeks for definitive diagnosis.

In people who are HIV-infected, treatment should start as soon as a positive smear (examination of a sample under the microscope) is found, without waiting for culture.

▲ Extrapulmonary TB

When TB infection causes disease, it is usually in the lungs. TB can also sometimes spread via the blood and lymphatic systems and cause disease outside the lungs (extrapulmonary TB). Extrapulmonary TB in the presence of HIV infection is an AIDS-defining illness.

One-quarter to one-half of AIDS patients with TB have extrapulmonary TB. In TB patients who are not immunocompromised, this is less common—only about 20 percent have extrapulmonary involvement.

The most typical sites for extrapulmonary TB are peripheral lymph nodes, gastrointestinal mucosae, the urogenital tract, and bone marrow. TB can also infect other sites in the body. TB is infectious to others only if it appears in the lungs, larynx, or skin.

▲ Treatment

If disease does occur, it generally appears within the first six to twelve months after infection. If untreated, TB has a variable course, with periods of illness and periods of remission. If treated, it is almost always curable.

TB in HIV patients is usually treatable. Although the disease may be more rapidly progressive and more widely disseminated in people with AIDS, it responds just as well to drugs as in HIV-negative TB patients. Drugs are usually not toxic. Drug-resistant strains are unusual but are becoming more common. Severe toxicity is highly unusual.

The Centers for Disease Control (CDC) recommends that isoniazid (INH) and at least two additional anti-TB drugs be started simultaneously. Medication for TB is taken orally.

Following are the drugs generally used to treat active TB:

- Isoniazid (INH, 300 mg per day). INH interacts with ketoconazole and can reduce effectiveness of both drugs to subtherapeutic doses.
- Pyrazinamide (PZA, 20 to 30 mg per kg per day)
- Rifampin (RIF, 600 mg per day or 450 mg per day for patients weighing less than 50 kg). RIF interacts with ketoconazole, can reduce effectiveness of both drugs to subtherapeutic doses, re-

duces effectiveness of methadone, and may lead to withdrawal symptoms. RIF lowers serum dapsone levels, so the two drugs should not be used together.

The drug ethambutol (Myambutol 15 to 25 mg per kg per day) is used in addition to the above drugs under certain circumstances:

- If the patient's strain of TB is resistant to INH
- If the patient cannot tolerate INH or rifampin
- If the TB either infects the central nervous system or is disseminated

Pyrazinamide is taken for two months. There is controversy about how long the other drugs should be taken, with recommended times ranging from twelve months to indefinitely. At minimum treatment must continue for six months after you have a negative sputum culture for *M. tuberculosis.* If ethambutol is used, longer treatment may be needed. Isoniazid is sometimes continued indefinitely to prevent recurrence of active TB.

Drug-susceptibility tests should be obtained periodically and the medication changed if the infection develops resistance to a particular drug.

Side effects include liver toxicity, rash, kidney dysfunction, and eye disease (with ethambutol). These side effects are generally tolerable, except for liver toxicity, which may require adjustment of medications. Treatment for TB does not appear to cause cancer or other long-term adverse side effects.

It may be difficult to take multiple medications consistently over a period of many months, but compliance with TB treatment is important. TB is unlikely to recur if you take your medication faithfully.

▲ Maintenance

It is not yet clear whether lifelong maintenance therapy is necessary. Opinion leans toward continuing therapy indefinitely.

SALMONELLA

Nontyphoidal salmonella is a bacterium. Salmonellosis is caused by a newly-acquired salmonella infection: it is not a reactivation of latent infection. Salmonellosis is not a very frequent infection in AIDS patients. However, it is about twenty times more common in AIDS patients than in others who are not HIV-infected, due to the increased susceptibility of those who are immune compromised.

Transmission: Among people who are HIV-infected, salmonella is more common among needle sharers than among men who have sex with men. Salmonella is transmitted by ingesting infected food or traces of fecal matter found in food. The bacterium is most often found in milk, eggs, meat, and processed foods. It can also be transmitted from certain animals to people: chicken, fowl, livestock, domestic pets, and turtles. Salmonella is not transmitted via rectal or vaginal sexual intercourse.

To avoid salmonella, follow the nutritional and dietary recommendations in Chapter 6: General Health Care, pp. 100–03.

Symptoms and course: In nonimmune-compromised people, the infection usually causes mild to severe self-limited gastrointestinal symptoms. Symptoms tend to be much more severe in those who are immune compromised.

Gastrointestinal (GI) symptoms of salmonellosis include diarrhea, cramping, bloating, and nausea. The diarrhea may be severe and bloody. In people who are immune compromised other symptoms may include fever, chills, sweats, weight loss, loss of appetite *(anorexia),* and elevated blood pressure. The infection may affect any organ system.

Salmonella can also cause systemic and disseminated disease if the infection enters the bloodstream (bacteremia). This causes fever and other symptoms. Salmonella tends to recur in people who are immune compromised.

Diagnosis is established by stool culture (for GI symptoms) and blood culture.

Treatment: Ampicillin is the most frequently used medication. Depending on antimicrobial sensitivities, salmonella can also be treated with chloramphenicol (Chloromycetin), trimethoprim/sulfamethoxazole (Bactrim, Septra), or cephalosporin (Ceclor). Nonimmune-compromised hosts are not usually treated, but those who are immune-compromised should be. Symptoms can be treated with antidiarrheal agents.

Typical symptoms of **recurrence** are fever and chills. Chronic treatment may be necessary for those who have had one or more relapses. Ciprofloxacin (Cipro) may be useful for chronic treatment.

SHIGELLA

Shigella is a bacterium that can cause inflammation of the intestine with diarrhea and pain (*dysentery*).

Transmission: The organism is transmitted through oral-fecal contact —that is, swallowing of small amounts of feces. A typical route of transmission is via food washed in contaminated water. During oral-anal sex (rimming) use of latex barriers can prevent transmission.

Symptoms and course: Many people who are infected develop no symptoms. Infection has been prevalent among men who have sex with men. Shigella in HIV-infected people tends to last longer, and to be more severe. It tends to recur and require maintenance therapy. Symptoms include severe, often bloody diarrhea, cramping, nausea, and fever.

Shigella is **diagnosed by stool culture.** Results take twenty-four to forty-eight hours.

Treatment is with Bactrim, ampicillin, or tetracycline. Do not use opiate derivatives to control shigella diarrhea because they aggravate systemic symptoms.

CAMPYLOBACTER JEJUNI

Campylobacter jejuni is a bacterium that can cause diarrhea. It can be found in otherwise healthy people, but, like many other infections, it tends to be harder to treat successfully and more likely to recur in patients with HIV-related immune impairment. In those with AIDS it may occasionally cause *bacteremia,* infection of the bloodstream. It is sexually transmitted and common among men who have sex with other men. Use of barriers for oral-anal contact (rimming) can prevent transmission of campylobacter. Symptoms range from mild to severe diarrhea, abdominal pain, cramping, and fever. Diagnosis is done by culturing a stool sample. Treatment is with the antibiotic erythromycin, 500 mg four times a day for seven days.

TREPONEMA PALLIDUM (SYPHILIS)

Syphilis is a sexually transmitted disease caused by a spiral-shaped bacterium (*spirochete*) called *Treponema pallidum.* Using condoms for intercourse will prevent transmission. Syphilis caused severe disease and death until effective treatment was discovered in the twentieth century. In different stages the disease classically appears in very different forms, summarized in the following material. If syphilis is not treated in the early stages, it can go on to cause a bewildering variety of serious problems.

The first symptoms of syphilis appear 3 to 90 days after infection. It causes one or more painless but infectious genital lesions *(chancres).* Chancres usually appear as small, solid, elevated lesions that become ulcerated and hard. These sores usually heal in 3 to 6 weeks, even without therapy. Nearby lymph nodes may be swollen.

If syphilis is not treated adequately, the organisms (called *treponemes*) will continue to live in the body, although symptoms usually disappear for a period of time. This is called *latent syphilis.* Persistence of latent syphilis can lead to *secondary syphilis,* caused by growth and spread of the organism. It typically occurs from 2 to 12 weeks after infection. The most frequent symptom is body rash that usually involves the palms of the hands and soles of the feet. In the third, or *tertiary,* stage, syphilis is a generalized disease.

Syphilis of the central nervous system (*neurosyphilis*) can appear at any stage. Symptoms of neurosyphilis are serious but depend on the time from infection. This condition can be fatal.

CLASSICAL STAGES OF SYPHILIS

Stage	Time Frame	Incidence	Description
Primary	3–90 days after infection	—	Primary genital lesions (chancres): painless and infectious, these sores heal in 3–6 weeks even without therapy
Latent	Any	—	Treponemal infection without symptoms
Secondary	2–12 wks.	Occurs in 25 percent of untreated syphilis patients within 4 yrs.	Body rash usually involving the palms and soles of the feet Also: fever, reduced appetite, weight loss, malaise, multiform skin lesions (*syphilids*), iritis (inflammation of the iris of the eye), hair loss, mucus patches, severe pain in the head, joints, and periosteum (tissue covering bones), condyloma lata (flat lesions on mucous membrane), and generalized lymphadenopathy
Tertiary	10–25 yrs.	15 percent of untreated patients	Generalized disease which may appear in many parts of the body, including skin, bone, joints, cardiovascular and central nervous system
Neurosyphilis	May occur at any stage	5–10% of untreated patients	Potentially fatal, causes different symptoms at different stages: 5–10 yrs.　Menigitis, seizure, strokes 15–20 yrs.　Dementia, paralysis 25–30 yrs.　Spinal cord degeneration

If you are HIV-infected, you should be tested for syphilis. The two organisms are transmitted by the same route and thus there is an increased risk that an HIV-infected person has also been infected with syphilis.

The course of syphilis may be different in those who are HIV-infected. Anecdotal reports have indicated increased evidence of symptomatic neurosyphilis in patients who are HIV-infected, shorter latency period, and reduced response to treatment.

If you are being treated by a physician who is not experienced in diagnosing and treating syphilis in HIV-infected people, consider a consultation with a specialist (generally either a pathologist or an infectious-disease specialist).

Diagnosis should be based on history, clinical findings, direct examination of material from lesions, and serological tests for syphilis (blood tests for antigens and antibodies). It appears that in HIV-infected people syphilis may sometimes cause atypical symptoms.

Diagnosing neurosyphilis in HIV-infected people can be difficult and uncertain. Neurosyphilis can occur during any stage of syphilis. If you have clinical evidence suggestive of neurosyphilis (unexplained behavioral changes, psychological dysfunction, ocular, auditory, or neurological signs) your physician will do a spinal tap to test your cerebrospinal fluid. People who do not adequately respond to treatment or those who have had syphilis for a long time should also have a spinal tap. Some experts suggest spinal tap for *all* HIV-infected people with syphilis.

Treatment: Since the 1940s syphilis has been treated with penicillin. This led to a dramatic decline in the cases of neurosyphilis. Starting in 1956 the use of benzathine penicillin allowed single-dose treatment. The standard dosage was established in clinical practice, not through systematic studies.

Penicillin is the treatment of choice for all stages of syphilis. Primary and secondary syphilis are treated with intramuscular penicillin on an out-patient basis. Neurosyphilis requires intravenous penicillin treatment—this generally requires hospitalization. The CDC recommends that HIV patients receive penicillin regimens if possible, instead of alternative antibiotic treatment that may not treat neurosyphilis. If you are allergic to penicillin, desensitization is recommended. If pregnant, alternative antibiotic treatments must be used.

The dose of penicillin necessary to cure syphilis is still not known with certainty. In fact, the standard dose may not be adequate to cause eradication of the treponemes that cause syphilis, leaving open the possibility of recurrence or progression of the disease. Since 1985, there has been an increase in the incidence of syphilis and increasing reports of treatment failures, raising questions about the adequacy of the standard treatment. Case reports of treatment failures in HIV-infected individuals raise questions about the efficacy of standard treatment for this patient group. The studies necessary to answer questions of dosage have yet to be performed. As of this writing, if you are HIV-infected and are diagnosed with primary syphilis your doctor will probably treat you with a standard dose of penicillin. This may change. Your physician should check the Centers for Disease Control guidelines on treating syphilis.

Maintenance (secondary prophylaxis): Careful follow-up on treatment for syphilis is particularly important if you are HIV-infected. For a year following treatment your physician will want to do regular physical examinations and blood tests. Follow-up for neurosyphilis requires a spinal tap every six months. Treatment response in HIV-infected patients is not yet known. Treatment failure requires retreatment, possibly at higher levels of medication.

ENCAPSULATED BACTERIA

Pneumonia in the non-HIV-infected population is most commonly bacterial and caused by *Haemophilus influenzae* or *Streptococcus pneumonia.* If your doctor tells you that you have pneumonia, do not assume that you have *Pneumocystis carinii* pneumonia (PCP); ask whether the diagnosis is PCP or a pneumonia caused by some other organism. Special care needs to be taken in distinguishing bacterial pneumonia from PCP.

Bacterial pneumonias seem to occur with increased incidence in people with AIDS and probably with increased incidence in earlier stages of HIV infection. Symptoms and treatment of bacterial pneumonia are the same for HIV-infected people as for those who are not HIV-infected, although the rate of recurring infections is probably higher. Treatment is with antibiotics.

FUNGAL INFECTIONS

The fungi we will discuss are:

- *Cryptococcus neoformans*
- *Candida albicans*

CRYPTOCOCCUS NEOFORMANS

▲ Description
"Cryptococcosis" is the general name given to the diseases caused by the fungus *Cryptococcus neoformans.* This fungus has caused illness in 5 percent to 10 percent of people with AIDS. Most fungi tend to affect particular anatomical sites (places in the body). *Cryptococcus neoformans* typically infects the *meninges,* which are three layers of membranes that cover the brain and spinal cord. Inflammation of the meninges is known as *meningitis.* Cryptococcal meningitis is the most common and serious disease caused by *Cryptococcus neoformans.* It is often accompanied by inflammation of the brain (*encephalitis*). The two occurring together are sometimes referred to as *meningo-encephalitis.* Cryptococcus can also cause disease in other parts of the body, most commonly the lungs.

▲ Transmission and Epidemiology
Cryptococcus is a fungus that is found all over the world. It is found most often in soil that is contaminated by bird droppings. It is not transmitted from one human being to another. Because this fungus is common and widespread it is probably impossible to prevent exposure. However, HIV-infected people should avoid areas where birds roost and soil that may be heavily contaminated with bird droppings. Wear gloves when handling pet birds or cleaning their cages.

New infections are contracted through inhaling the fungus. Impaired immune function allows cryptococcus to grow, spread, and cause symptomatic disease. The disease is most common in people with HIV infection or other causes of immune dysfunction, but can occasionally occur in those with intact immune systems.

▲ Monitoring

The symptoms of illness caused by cryptococcus may initially be mild and subtle. It is not yet known how to predict who is at specific imminent risk for cryptococcosis, other than by reference to T4 counts. People who are HIV-positive are considered at risk for cryptococcal meningitis when T4 counts drop below 150. If you have symptoms of cryptococcal meningitis you should have a computerized tomography (CT) scan (to rule out cerebral mass lesions) and then a lumbar puncture to test your cerebrospinal fluid (even if blood tests for cryptococcus are negative).

▲ Prevention

Some fungal opportunistic infections can be prevented with antifungal drugs. It is not known whether medication can reduce the risk of developing an initial episode of cryptococcosis. Anticryptococcus drugs have not yet been shown safe and effective for primary prophylaxis. However, physicians often begin antifungal prophylaxis with fluconazole (Diflucan) after T4 count drops below 200.

▲ Signs, Symptoms, and Course

The first symptoms of cryptococcal meningitis are usually fever or severe headache (usually located in the forehead or temples). Other symptoms that sometimes occur are malaise, nausea, vomiting, stiff neck, blurred vision, mild confusion, or personality changes.

Cryptococcal meningitis is life-threatening and prompt treatment is crucial. **Untreated episodes of cryptococcal meningitis are often fatal.** Early diagnosis and treatment of cryptococcal meningitis dramatically improve the outcome of the disease. It is important to contact your physician immediately if you have severe, recurring, or unusual headaches. A false alarm is better than any delay in treatment.

▲ Diagnosis of Cryptococcosis

If you do have the illness it is crucial that you be treated promptly, so there is strong motivation to start treatment as soon as there is a suggestion of meningitis. But the traditional treatment for cryptococcal meningitis has serious side effects, so there is also strong motivation to diagnose the illness correctly before starting treatment.

There are a number of diagnostic tests that can be done to find out if you have this disease. The tests are done by examining specimens of blood or spinal fluid. Diagnosis of cryptococcal meningitis usually involves a lumbar puncture (spinal tap). Initial positive test results from the cerebrospinal fluid (CSF) obtained from the lumbar puncture are reason to begin treatment. Culture of cryptococcus from the CSF is used for confirmation. Tests are also used to see if you have responded to treatment. Consequently you are likely to have a variety of tests and to be tested more than once.

Refer to Chapter 13: Procedures and Tests for descriptions of specific diagnostic tests.

▲ Treatment of Acute Cryptococcal Meningitis

Amphotericin-B (Fungizone) has been widely used and shown effective for treatment of acute cryptococcal meningitis. This drug must be taken for a period of six to eight weeks or longer depending on the patient's response. It can only be given intravenously, therefore you need to be in the hospital while you are receiving treatment. The side effects of amphotericin-B can be severe: possible fevers; chills; kidney dysfunction; and suppression of bone marrow production, which leads to various types of anemia. The flu-like side effects can be substantially lessened by use of ibuprofen (Advil), acetominophen (Tylenol), diphenhydramine (Benadryl), or hydrocortisone one half-hour before use of amphotericin-B. Some clinicians administer meperidine (Demerol) both before treatment and during treatment in the same IV bag with amphotericin-B to reduce side effects.

Sometimes amphotericin-B is used in combination with the drug flucytosine (Ancobon, 5-fluorcytosine or 5FC). In people with AIDS, data on the efficacy of the combination are conflicting. However, the toxic effects of the two drugs are different: combining flucytosine and amphotericin-B allows for a lower dose of amphotericin-B for those who cannot tolerate the side effects of the drug at full dose.

A very promising development in the treatment and prevention of cryptococcal meningitis has occurred in the last two years. Disease caused by cryptococcus can now be treated with the drug **fluconazole** (Diflucan), one of a category of drugs known as *triazoles.* Fluconazole was initially approved in Britain for the treatment of vaginal candidiasis and has been in general use there for that purpose for several years. In the studies done so far, fluconazole is as effective as the standard drug, amphotericin-B, has relatively few side effects, is well absorbed by the body, and will treat infection in the brain. Fluconazole is taken orally rather than intravenously, as is amphotericin-B. Fluconazole can safely be taken with AZT. Because there are less data supporting the efficacy of fluconazole, some physicians still prefer to use amphotericin-B for the first two weeks of therapy, and only then switch to using fluconazole. The development of fluconazole is particularly important news for the many patients who cannot tolerate amphotericin-B.

▲ Experimental Drugs

Itraconazole (Sporanex) is in clinical trials for treatment of meningitis. Studies are also under way on Amphotericin-B lipid complex which may be as effective as amphotericin-B but less toxic. Refer to Chapter 9: Learning About Experimental Treatment for information on how to stay up to date on experimental treatments.

▲ Maintenance Therapy After Successful Treatment of Acute Illness

Although cryptococcal meningitis in people with HIV responds to treatment with amphotericin-B or fluconazole, the fungus probably cannot be entirely eliminated from the body. A majority of patients who do not receive prophylactic treatment will relapse. Therefore, as with many other infectious microorganisms in the context of HIV, the goal is to keep infection under control.

Fluconazole is currently the best maintenance medication. Studies so far indicate that fluconazole, taken orally, is as effective as amphotericin-B, is easy to use, and has few serious side effects. Maintenance therapy consists of 200 to 400 mg per day, continued indefinitely.

Fluconazole is very expensive. Pfizer, the manufacturer, has set up an assistance program for those who cannot get fluconazole prophylaxis paid for through insurance or government programs. You can call Pfizer at 800-869-9979 for information.

Intravenous amphotericin-B has been used effectively to prevent recurrence of cryptococcal meningitis. However, side effects are a problem and the patient must have a catheter implanted in the chest in order to receive long-term intravenous treatment. A controlled clinical trial published in 1992 (Powderly) found that fluconazole was superior to amphotericin-B for maintenance therapy after an initial episode of cryptococcal meningitis (97 percent on fluconazole had no relapse after one year compared to only 78 percent on amphotericin-B).

CANDIDA ALBICANS

Candidiasis is an infection caused by the fungus *Candida albicans,* a form of yeast. Most frequently, candidiasis affects the mucous membranes, particularly the oral cavity (the mouth). Oral candidiasis is also referred to as **thrush.** It also frequently causes vaginal infection and sometimes causes infection of the esophagus.

Candida is an organism that is present in most peoples' bodies most of the time. It can be found in normal samples from the vagina, intestine, and respiratory tract. Presence of candida in the body is not a sign of something abnormal. It is one of the "normal flora"—that is, bacteria and fungi that live in the body, generally without causing harm. Consequently, transmission is not an issue because candida is present in all people. Candida causes problems only when, for a variety of reasons, the balance of organisms in the body is disrupted and there is an overgrowth of candida leading to symptoms. Diabetes, pregnancy, and antibiotics may disrupt this balance as may diseases that impair the immune system.

Vaginal candidiasis, which causes itching and discharge, is a common problem among women who have no problems with their immune systems and tends to be more severe in those who are immune compromised. It is easy to infect the vaginal canal with candida from the gastrointestinal tract. (Refer to the discussion of vaginal candidiasis in

Chapter 8: Sex, Age, Race, and Ethnicity for more information.) Oral candidiasis (thrush) can also be seen in those with normal immune systems, generally after a period of antibiotic use. Oral candidiasis is a more common problem among those with impaired immune systems, particularly those who are HIV-infected. Candida can also cause infection of the skin in the groin and armpit or the fingernails. Candidal infection of the esophagus and colon is found only among those with immune impairment.

▲ Oral Candidiasis

Candidiasis is one of the most frequent oral problems of people with HIV infection and occurs at some point in almost all people with AIDS. The most common type of oral candidiasis is *pseudomembranous candidiasis,* usually referred to as *thrush.* The symptoms are creamy white patches of material on the membrane of the mouth and the upper throat. This white material is often described as looking like cottage cheese or curds. The white material can be scraped off and the areas around and underneath are reddish. If you have thrush you may have no noticeable symptoms or you may have a dry or burning mouth, sore throat, pain, problems in eating spicy foods, or changes in taste.

In addition to thrush, the two most common candidal infections of the oral area are *erythematous candidiasis* which produces red lesions on the palate and back of the throat and *angular chelitis* which causes redness and cracks in the corner of the mouth.

Generally **your physician can diagnose thrush** by looking at the affected area of your mouth. Sometimes it is necessary to scrape the area lightly with a wooden tongue depressor and look at the material under a microscope or culture for the fungus. This procedure is not painful.

Thrush and other forms of oral candidiasis are not life-threatening and can usually be treated effectively. Seeking treatment is important because thrush may be uncomfortable and interfere with eating. Treatment usually takes effect in under a week. If you are HIV-infected, it is likely that thrush will return at some time after an initial episode; repeat treatment will again clear up the problem. Maintenance treatment— continuing treatment over time—is usually necessary to avoid frequent episodes of thrush.

There are two types of **treatment for thrush:** topical and systemic. *Topical* means that the medication is applied directly to the infected area. This can be done with creams, liquids, or lozenges (sometimes called *troches*) that melt in the mouth. *Systemic* means that the medication reaches the entire body because it is distributed by the circulatory system—systemic medication is often taken orally, in pill form. This is the maintenance therapy of choice.

Systemic treatment has usually been done with ketoconazole (Nizoral). Taking Nizoral is more convenient than topical treatment because you only need to take one pill a day. However, you must have regular blood tests because Nizoral can damage your liver. More recently, candidiasis has been treated with oral fluconazole (Diflucan), which seems to be even more effective than Nizoral.

The most common topical treatment of thrush is with clotrimazole (Mycelex) or nystatin (Mycolog, Mycostatin, various others). There are no side effects. Both need to be used regularly several times a day and will be effective only if you follow directions carefully. It can be tedious to use the medication regularly. Nystatin comes in tablets or a liquid suspension that is meant to be swished around in the mouth and then swallowed. Nystatin may temporarily affect the sense of taste and thus decrease appetite. Clotrimazole (Mycelex) comes in troches, or lozenges, that are held in the mouth until they dissolve. Occasional side effects of clotrimazole include nausea, dizziness, diarrhea, and elevated liver enzymes.

▲ Esophageal Candidiasis

The major symptom of candidiasis of the esophagus is pain and difficulty swallowing (*dysphagia*). It almost always is accompanied by oral thrush and can be treated on a empirical basis with an antifungal agent. If this is not effective, an endoscopy may be necessary for diagnostic purposes. Symptoms often respond fairly quickly (within a few days) to medication.

Ketoconazole (Nizoral) and fluconazole (Diflucan) are used against esophageal candidiasis. Both ketoconazole and fluconazole have been proven effective in studies. Some cases that do not respond to these drugs (*refractory cases*) require treatment with amphotericin-B.

▲ Experimental Drugs

Itraconazole (Sporanex) is a promising new drug in the same family as fluconazole (the *triazoles*). There are less data available on the safety and efficacy of itraconazole and it is not yet formally approved, but it is likely to be considerably cheaper than fluconazole. Refer to Chapter 9: Learning About Experimental Treatment for information on how to stay up to date on experimental treatments.

Chapter 12
Cancers

This chapter begins with a description of some basic information about cancer. It then proceeds to discuss in detail the two main categories of malignancy relevant in HIV disease: Kaposi's sarcoma and non-Hodgkin's lymphoma. Although the incidence of Kaposi's sarcoma is declining, its importance as a cause of death continues to rise. In addition, certain lymphomas are rising in both incidence and as a cause of death. All told, malignancies now account for over 20 percent of in-hospital deaths from AIDS.

BASIC INFORMATION ABOUT CANCER

A *cancer* or *neoplasm* is the multiplication of abnormal cells derived from body tissue. Infections, in contrast, typically involve the multiplication of entities considered foreign to the body. Cancers and infections can sometimes be related: infections have been found that directly alter the genetic material of cells, causing them to become cancerous. Cancerous cells may form *tumors,* which are swollen growths or collections of cells. Tumors are sometimes also referred to as *lesions,* a more general term implying any interruption of normal tissue.

▲ Normal Cell Growth and Differentiation
The body contains an astonishing variety of cells that appear and function in many different ways. The appearance and behavior of a cell is determined by two factors:

- The pattern of activity of its genes
- The local environment that the cell experiences in the body

All cells in the body share the same basic genetic material. This material is divided into a very large number of *genes,* or functional subunits, which may be active or inactive in any individual cell. Active genes make proteins. Some proteins are used as building blocks for making static structures. Some complicated proteins become the tiny molecular machine-tools called *enzymes.* Some proteins act as messengers that communicate with other genes or other cells.

The interaction of messages turning genes on and off may cause a cell to change in appearance or behavior. The cell is said to mature or *develop.* Development is profoundly affected by the environment of the cell: other cells or structures nearby, nutrients, toxins, or other chemicals. Normally, an individual cell has a limited number of developmental paths open to its progeny. Cells may take different paths as they mature: this is called *differentiation.* Developmental stages of cells in the body vary: *precursor cells* are the ancestors of the fully differentiated cells of functional tissue. The normal developmental history of a population of cells is always forward: in the direction of differentiation.

▲ Cancerous Transformation

Cancer occurs when the normal growth and developmental pattern of a group of cells changes. Various events may transform normal cells into cancerous cells: environmental toxins called *carcinogens* may damage genes; radiation may cause genetic mutations; infections may alter or add genes; and sometimes inherited genes called *oncogenes* may spontaneously activate and cause cancer. The origin and function of oncogenes is not completely understood.

After transformation the normal checks on cell division may not operate. The original transformed cell divides and passes on to its daughter cells the tendency to divide without limit. A tumor forms from this population of dividing cancerous cells. Cell generations may move backward along developmental paths, becoming less rather than more differentiated, retreating to resemble primitive precursor cells with their capacity for growth and continued cell division.

Ordinarily cancer is more likely in tissue that is growing or regenerating. In such tissue cell division is happening at an increased rate and genetic errors are more likely. Some cancers nevertheless occur in other tissues also: both breast cancer and Kaposi's sarcoma occur in tissue that is not undergoing cell division.

Malignant tumors have three qualities: the cells have lost their differentiated quality (*anaplasia*), the cells enter and displace surrounding tissue (*invasiveness*), and the cells break away from the main tumor and spread to form tumors at other sites (*metastatis*). Benign tumors are not invasive, not metastic, and are less anaplastic than malignant tumors.

Cancers are divided into two categories: *carcinomas,* or tumors of epithelial tissue (tissue of linings and surfaces); and *sarcomas,* tumors of tissue resembling embryonic connective tissue. Despite its name, the cell of origin of Kaposi's sarcoma is not known.

▲ Treatment

Treatment for cancer in HIV disease can take many different forms: two that are frequently used are chemotherapy and radiation therapy (*radiotherapy*). Cancer therapies attempt to destroy cancerous cells while doing as little harm as possible to healthy cells.

Chemotherapy merely means treatment with medication and is used in describing drug treatment for cancer to distinguish it from radiation therapy. Chemotherapy has a reputation for serious and unpleasant side effects that is perhaps exaggerated, particularly in the case of chemotherapy for the malignancies that arise in HIV disease: many people receive chemotherapy and do not become nauseated. For some cancers that arise in HIV disease multiple chemotherapy drugs are used together. The advantage of this approach is that it is much more effective than the use of only one drug. The disadvantage is that the patient may develop multiple side effects.

KAPOSI'S SARCOMA

Kaposi's sarcoma (usually referred to as KS) is known by most for the purplish marks it sometimes causes on the skin. KS on the skin is visible but not necessarily harmful: serious problems are primarily caused by KS lesions on internal organs—particularly the lungs. KS lesions can occur at many sites on the body including both the skin and internal organs. Kaposi's sarcoma is usually described as a *neoplasm* or cancer, but some question this categorization.

▲ Patterns of Illness

Until the AIDS epidemic, KS in the United States was a relatively unusual disease that appeared among elderly men of Mediterranean heritage. The primary symptoms were nodules on the feet and legs. It had a slow course and was rarely fatal. (A different and more dangerous form was found in Africa.) KS is also seen in those who are immune suppressed due to medication. In such cases, when the immune-suppressive drug is withdrawn the KS goes away.

Since the start of the AIDS epidemic, there has been a tremendous increase in the incidence of KS. KS is 20,000 times more common among AIDS patients than among the population at large and 300 times more common among people with HIV as compared to other immune-suppressed persons. Unfortunately, KS in people with AIDS tends to be faster growing and more harmful than KS in HIV-negative patients.

There is an unusual pattern of prevalence of KS in people with AIDS. KS is overwhelmingly more common among gay men who are HIV-infected than among those who were HIV-infected through needle sharing. KS is even less common among other HIV-infected people (including women), although they too can occasionally develop KS.

KS was one of the first diseases recognized as part of AIDS. **The percentage of persons with AIDS who have KS has steadily declined over the course of the epidemic.**

The formal epidemiological definition of AIDS has been broadened several times in the past decade to include aspects of the syndrome not recognized initially, such as wasting and dementia. This may account for some but probably not all of the statistical decline in the incidence of KS among people with AIDS.

▲ Cause or Co-Factors

The cause of KS is not yet known. The declining incidence of KS in AIDS and the fact that KS is most prevalent among gay men with AIDS have led to a number of theories regarding co-factors in the development of KS. Possibilities that have been suggested are discussed below.

It is possible that KS develops only in immune-dysfunctional people who are also infected with some **unknown sexually transmitted disease.**

A KS agent may have been prevalent among men who have sex with men before the widespread use of condoms for intercourse. According to this theory, some of these men became immune suppressed due to HIV and then manifested KS. As condom use increased, fewer gay men were exposed to the KS agent, although some may still have been exposed to HIV. This may account for the decreased incidence of KS among gay people with AIDS.

This hypothesis is supported by the pre-HIV epidemiology of KS. Some elderly Mediterranean men get KS, either because they are genetically related (and therefore predisposed to similar illnesses) or because they have been exposed to the same environment (including infectious agents). A KS agent might have been transmitted commonly in certain geographical areas, but cause disease only in people with immune suppression due to old age.

Immune or cell-regulated disorders secondary to HIV. One KS co-factor theory hypothesizes that the healthy body has a mechanism for recognizing and eliminating certain cancers. In theory this "immune surveillance" system might ordinarily detect and destroy small naturally occurring KS lesions before they could cause noticeable disease. If HIV in some way interfered with such immune surveillance, KS lesions might be able to grow unchecked. By this theory, there is no new active agent that causes KS in AIDS.

In a similar vein, KS may not be a true malignancy but rather a condition referred to as *reversible vascular hyperplasia.* According to this theory, HIV induces cells to produce a chemical growth factor that makes lymphatic endothelial cells proliferate. Once started, this process cascades as each new KS cell makes more growth factor.

A related theory suggests that the product of one of HIV's genes (the *tat* gene, or *transactivator* gene) may be responsible for the development of KS. In this case, a drug that inhibits the activity of the *tat* gene could also be an effective treatment for KS. This theory does not explain why KS has appeared more frequently among gay men, however.

Chemical carcinogens: Inhaled nitrites ("poppers") were widely used as a recreational drug among gay men in the 1970s and early 1980s. Using poppers may increase the risk that an HIV-infected person will get KS, but epidemiologic studies have been inconsistent. No specific carcinogenic qualities have been found in these drugs, and using poppers does not in itself increase the risk of AIDS.

Known viral carcinogens: Infection with cytomegalovirus (CMV) was once considered a possible co-factor in the development of KS. There is an extremely high incidence of CMV among gay men, and *almost* 100 percent of AIDS patients studied have evidence of previous CMV exposure. Researchers currently discount the hypothesis that CMV is a co-factor for KS.

It is also possible that HIV itself might cause cancer.

▲ Course of Illness

KS can sometimes cause very serious symptoms, but it is **rarely the direct cause of death in AIDS.** In many cases, KS may remain a very minor problem for long periods of time.

KS is a disease which **affects both skin and internal organs.** It often causes visible marks on the skin that sometimes are disfiguring. As long as it is confined to the skin KS is not fatal and usually does not cause major medical problems. KS can also affect almost any internal organ, including the lymphatic system. When KS affects internal organs it can cause severe medical problems, particularly with lung involvement.

T4 cell counts and KS: KS can develop at any T4 cell count. However, it is not likely to be serious if the T4 cell count is high (T4 above 250). Prognosis is good if:

- Lesions are limited in number and not large
- There are no constitutional symptoms (fevers, night sweats, weight loss)
- There is no history of opportunistic infections

▲ Common Sites of KS

Most commonly, KS lesions first appear on the skin or oral cavity. Other common sites are in the gut, lymph nodes, or lungs.

On the **skin** KS frequently first appears on the head (tip of nose, eyelid), the neck, and the tip of the penis. The location of lesions is not significant in terms of predicting the course or severity of KS.

Generally, KS lesions on the skin look like small spindle-shaped bruises, although they do not blanch or change color when pressed (as bruises do). In lighter-skinned people, the lesions are pink, purple, or brownish. In darker-skinned people (such as African-Americans) they are brown or black.

KS lesions generally do not hurt or itch and rarely cause any break or damage of the skin. (In some cases, KS lesions that appear as flat patches on the thigh or soles of the feet may hurt.) Lesions can usually be felt as small solid lumps, 0.5 cm to 2.0 cm in diameter.

Typically, KS progresses over time. It is common for lesions to appear in multiple sites. As the disease advances, lesions become larger and more numerous. In more advanced KS, multiple small lesions may join together into one larger mass. Bulky lesions may become uncomfortable.

KS is unpredictable and, if untreated, lesions develop at various rates anywhere in or on the body. Lesions may disappear or decrease in number in one area even as they appear or increase in another. Some people have few lesions with no progression for a long time.

Limited KS of the skin is treated with radiation therapy, localized chemotherapy, or cryosurgery. More extensive lesions or rapidly progressive KS should be treated with systemic chemotherapy.

KS of the mouth usually develops on the palate (the roof of the mouth). It can also affect the pharynx (the back of the mouth or top of the throat). There is not much point in having an oral lesion biopsied if KS has already been diagnosed elsewhere. KS of the mouth usually does not cause symptoms but can cause soreness or teeth problems or—if it affects the pharynx—difficulty or pain in swallowing. Oral KS can be treated with radiation, surgery, laser surgery, or local or systemic chemotherapy.

It is very common for harmless KS lesions to occur in the **gastrointestinal tract.** Studies suggest that 40 percent of people with KS have some lesions in the GI tract (especially the stomach and duodenum). KS lesions in the gut rarely cause symptoms and usually do not require diagnosis or treatment. GI symptoms such as diarrhea are rarely caused by KS.

Pulmonary KS can cause problems in the lung—coughing, shortness of breath, and respiratory failure that may be fatal. It needs to be distinguished from PCP because the symptoms can be similar. Pulmonary KS is usually diagnosed if a gallium scan fails to reveal infectious disease that accounts for the symptoms. KS in the lungs is treated with aggressive systemic chemotherapy and medication to relieve the discomfort of symptoms.

Lesions that obstruct lymph vessels can cause swelling by blocking the drainage of lymph fluid from tissues. This swelling is referred to as *lymphedema.* It is unusual for lymphedema to be a problem until KS is advanced, with many lesions. When lymphedema develops it may cause pain or limit movement. Lymphedema may affect legs, feet, face, penis, or scrotum.

Lymphedema is treated with radiation therapy. Swelling in the legs can be helped both by elevating the legs and by wearing elastic stockings. *Diuretic* medication increases the production of urine, thereby reducing the amount of fluid and swelling in the body. However, the use of diuretics is controversial because diuretics may cause electrolyte abnormalities.

▲ Diagnosis

KS is usually first diagnosed when it is noticed on the skin. For this reason your doctor should examine your skin and mouth periodically. Report unusual changes or new marks on your skin to your doctor.

Psychological factors: Marks, bruises, and blemishes on the skin are common for many reasons. Any unexplained mark on the skin may worry you. Such marks are probably not KS, but knowing this may not keep you from worrying. Consult your physician if you are worried that you might have KS. It is perfectly legitimate for you to ask your physician to reassure you about even minor symptoms. It is more common for people to delay reporting possible KS symptoms than to visit their doctor too often. If you keep worrying despite repeated reassurances from your physician, talk to a psychotherapist about how to manage your anxiety.

Definitive diagnosis of KS: A physician with experience can make a tentative diagnosis by appearance but an initial lesion should always be biopsied and inspected under the microscope for confirmation. Skin biopsy can be done in the doctor's office and is relatively painless.

Lesions caused by a bacterial infection called ***cat-scratch disease* may look very similar to KS.** Cat-scratch disease is, as its name implies, spread by cat scratches and is successfully treated with antibiotics. Tell your physician if you develop a lesion, rash, or other skin problem after having been scratched or bitten by an animal or insect.

▲ Treatment

Options for treatment for KS are:

- No treatment other than the use of cosmetics—see pp. 288–89
- *Local* therapy: affects lesions on limited areas of the body
- *Systemic* chemotherapy: affects the entire body

People with KS often have some small number of lesions that do not necessarily require treatment for a long time. If KS is not causing serious medical problems, treatment may not be necessary or useful, except for psychological or cosmetic reasons. This is especially true if new KS patients have T4 cell counts over 500, no history of opportunistic infections, and no fever, weight loss, or night sweats. In this situation KS may progress quite slowly and cause no physical discomfort.

Choosing the correct treatment means weighing the benefits and costs of each treatment against the situation of the individual KS patient. If you have only limited KS and treatment is primarily for cosmetic purposes, it doesn't make sense to risk the possible side effects or immune suppression associated with systemic chemotherapy. Local treatment is what your physician will probably recommend in this case.

On the other hand, if the disease seems to be progressing rapidly (many new lesions appearing in multiple sites) immediate systemic chemotherapy makes good sense. The choice of exactly what type of chemotherapy depends on a number of factors. Some useful drugs may cause bone-marrow suppression as a side effect, and should be used only in those people who can tolerate it. Systemic chemotherapy used early in the course of KS is done with a single drug to avoid the side effects of using multiple drugs. It is worth combining several drugs for patients with more serious disease, especially pulmonary KS.

COSTS AND BENEFITS OF TREATMENT FOR KS

Benefits	Comment
Cosmetic improvement	Reduction or disguise of disfiguring lesions
Symptom relief	Reduction of lesions that are causing pain, discomfort, or impairment: lesions in the lung; lesions that cause lymphedema; painful lesions on the soles of the feet; lesions in the mouth or throat that may be uncomfortable or cause difficulty eating
Limitation of disease	Limitation of "aggressive" or quickly growing disease, particularly in the lungs
Costs	**Comment**
Pain, discomfort, and inconvenience	Some treatments may have unpleasant side effects
Bone-marrow suppression (*myelosuppression*)	Systemic chemotherapy with certain drugs may suppress bone-marrow production (especially neutrophil production)

▲ Local Therapy

Local therapy is used to destroy or remove limited lesions and includes:

- Radiation therapy
- Laser surgery
- Intralesional chemotherapy
- Cryotherapy
- Surgical excision

Radiation therapy is suitable for patients with a single or limited lesions that are causing problems. Radiation therapy is useful for cosmetic treatment of lesions on the face. It can also relieve swelling (edema) or remove painful lesions, such as lesions on the thighs and calves. Radiation has been used for oral lesions but can cause large painful mouth ulcers (known as *mucositis* or *stomatitis*).

Laser surgery is used for lesions in the mouth as an alternative to radiation therapy and may have fewer side effects. Laser surgery is usually done in one session under general anesthesia. Chemotherapy may be used in addition to laser surgery.

Intralesional chemotherapy (injection of medication directly into lesions) is useful for cosmetic purposes in small skin lesions. It is usually done with a drug called vinblastine (Velban). Repeated injections may be necessary. Side effects of intralesional chemotherapy are local pain and skin irritation.

Cryotherapy (freezing therapy) uses liquid nitrogen to treat small areas of KS. Freezing causes KS cells to die and lesions to fade. The cold hurts during the brief period in which the liquid nitrogen is applied. Cosmetic results of cryotherapy are good.

Surgical excision is used to remove small disfiguring lesions or lesions located where friction with clothing causes bleeding. A local anesthetic may be used to make surgical excision virtually painless.

Intralesional interferon is under investigation as a local therapy against KS. Anecdotal reports support the use of topical tretinoin cream (Retin-A). No hard data are available.

▲ Systemic Chemotherapy

Systemic chemotherapy is used to treat KS of some internal organs, widespread KS, or rapidly progressing KS.

Systemic chemotherapy must be closely monitored with blood tests to watch for dangerous side effects, particularly bone-marrow suppression. Experimental drugs (such as G-CSF or GM-CSF) may help counter the bone-marrow suppression that sometimes accompanies systemic chemotherapy.

If you have progressive KS and interrupt KS chemotherapy because it conflicts with treatment for another condition, resume chemotherapy as soon as practical.

The experience of chemotherapy: Most chemotherapy is received intravenously, during out-patient visits to your doctor's office. Injection or insertion of an intravenous line is not painful. Infusions are generally performed on a regular weekly schedule. It typically takes about ten minutes to complete the infusion. Chemotherapy for KS does not typically cause the side effects popularly associated with cancer chemotherapies (nausea, vomiting, fatigue, or hair loss), although adriamycin causes hair loss.

Drugs commonly used are listed below:

Vinblastine (Velban) may be used for systemic chemotherapy if KS is progressing. The drug's major side effect is *myelosuppression,* the suppression of bone marrow activity. Myelosuppression may lead to a decrease in certain white blood cells called *neutrophils* that are necessary for fighting bacterial infections. However, the myelosuppressive toxicity of vinblastine appears to be mild. G-CSF may correct myelosuppression and allow continued use of vinblastine.

Vincristine is sometimes used if the myelosuppression caused by vinblastine is not corrected by use of G-CSF. Its major side effect is reversible *peripheral neuropathy* (tingling or pain in the extremities). Vincristine and vinblastine may be used in alternating weeks to reduce *dose-limiting toxicity.* By alternating the drugs, you can use higher, more effective doses without suffering severe side effects.

If KS involves the lungs, is rapidly progressive, or does not respond to vinblastine, then the drugs **adriamycin (doxorubicin), bleomycin, and vincristine may be used together—a combination referred to as ABV.** ABV can produce rapid improvement. The major toxicity is myelosuppression.

Alpha-interferon (INF-alpha, INTRON, Roferon) is FDA-approved for use in KS patients with T4 counts over 200. To be effective against KS, alpha-interferon is given systemically by injection in high doses: 56 million units daily.

Unfortunately, the side effects of alpha-interferon can be so unpleasant as to limit the drug's usefulness. They include flu-like symptoms, anorexia, fatigue, low-grade fever, and weight loss. Side effects get worse with higher doses. Alpha-interferon does not cause bone-marrow suppression.

Alpha-interferon works best in patients with:

• T4 cell counts over 400
• No prior opportunistic infections
• No *constitutional symptoms:* sometimes called *B symptoms,* they include fever, night sweats, and weight loss

Low dose alpha-interferon is being tried in combination with AZT. This combination may be more effective (but may also have more side effects) than alpha-interferon alone.

The FDA-approved use of high-dose subcutaneous alpha-interferon against KS is different from the use of low-dose oral alpha-interferon

SUMMARY OF TREATMENT RECOMMENDATIONS FOR KS

Patient group	Recommendations for treatment	Comment
Minimal KS with or without constitutional symptoms	Observation, antivirals, local therapy, investigational drugs	Often has slow progression; treat for cosmetic reasons
Advanced cutaneous KS; rapidly progressive KS	Systemic chemotherapy with one of: Velban, Velban and bleomycin, Vepesid, Investigational drugs	Use systemic therapy to limit disease progression. Vepesid seems effective but causes total hair loss
Pulmonary KS	Systemic chemotherapy with: ABV (adriamycin, bleomycin, and vincristine) or Vepesid	Treat for symptom relief and limitation of disease. Bad prognosis motivates use of multiple drugs together
KS with neutropenia	Vincristine and/or bleomycin, Velban and G-CSF, Velban, bleomycin, and G-CSF	Avoids bone-marrow suppression due to velban; or use G-CSF to prevent neutropenia
Painful, bulky KS; lymphedema	Radiation therapy	Treat for symptom relief and limitation of disease

(such as Kemron). Studies show no benefit to KS patients from the use of Kemron or other low-dose alpha-interferon preparations.

Etoposide (VP-16 or Vepesid) is a drug that has shown effectiveness in preliminary studies for treatment of advanced skin KS. It is taken orally or intravenously. The difficulty is that Vepesid can cause total hair loss.

▲ Prospects for KS Treatments

For several years there have been glowing but unofficial reports of drugs that inhibit blood vessel development in KS tumors. Very little is publicly known about these drugs, presumably due to the intense commercial interest. The drug known as SP-PG, manufactured by Daiichi Pharmaceuticals in Japan, is associated with Robert Gallo, the National Cancer Institute researcher who shares credit with Luc Montagnier for the identification of HIV. As of this writing it is thought that basic studies are still in progress: human trials may start sometime in 1992. Another KS drug on the horizon is AGM-1470, manufactured by Taketa from a fungal derivative called fumagillin. Animal studies have shown promising efficacy with no side effects. AGM-1470 might also be useful against tumors other than those caused by KS.

▲ Using Cosmetics to Cover KS Lesions

Sometimes people with KS develop lesions on the face or other areas of the body that are visible when clothed. In some people, lesions may barely be visible while in others lesions may be disfiguring. If you develop KS that affects your appearance, you need to talk with someone about your experience. Your best source of advice and comfort is going to be other people with KS.

In our culture much emphasis is placed upon an idealized appearance. KS lesions can be a visible sign of illness that may make other people aware of your HIV disease. People react in various ways to any difference in appearance: some may stare or look away. You may be confronted with other people's uncontrolled emotional responses to the charged issues that surround AIDS, such as illness, sex, or stigmatized behavior. In addition, your own state of mind and resilience may be affected by your appearance. Lesions may make you feel less attractive or desirable. Even sympathetic reactions from others may contribute to a sense of rejection or isolation.

For these or other reasons you may decide to use cosmetics to cover KS lesions. Used correctly, makeup can help hide KS lesions.

Makeup is a skill that many women spend years learning. If you develop KS and are not familiar with makeup, get advice from an expert. The appendices provide contact information for a professional makeup artist who teaches people with KS how to use makeup effectively. Your local AIDS organization may also be able to refer you to a volunteer makeup artist in your area.

Here are some general rules for using makeup to cover KS lesions on the face.

The basic elements are *foundation makeup* and *face powder*. Foundation makeup is a pigmented liquid or cream. Face powder is used on top of foundation to *set* the foundation and make it last. Foundation comes in bottles or tubes, while face powder comes loose or in a small case called a *compact*. Both foundation and face powder are available in many shades. Cheap makeup works just as well as expensive makeup.

Choosing the right shade is the key to getting makeup that works. Sometimes this takes trial and error. If you have a close girlfriend who uses cosmetics, you might experiment with hers. Inexpensive makeup is often cheap enough to try several shades. If you live in a large city, consider going to a theatrical makeup store. They have the largest variety of shades (especially of powder). In addition, because the theater industry has been so hard hit by HIV disease, salespeople in theatrical makeup stores are often helpful and familiar with this use of makeup.

You can cover your whole face or just the area affected by KS. Apply foundation first, then powder. Use a *cosmetic sponge* to apply foundation to large areas. For small areas, you may use your fingers. Cover very dark lesions with Max Factor stick makeup in yellow or orange *before* using foundation. As lesions improve with treatment they may get lighter, therefore you may need to switch to lighter shades of makeup. Black skin tends to *hyperpigment,* that is, affected areas get darker—you can use makeup to lighten the area. Use moisturizer if your skin tends to be dry. If you use moisturizer under foundation, you may need a darker shade of foundation.

NON-HODGKIN'S LYMPHOMAS (NHL)

Non-Hodgkin's lymphomas (NHL) are a category of cancers that have become increasingly common in AIDS patients. As treatment improves, HIV-infected people are living longer with severe immune suppression. Because of this, NHL is becoming more common.

A lymphoma is any abnormal, uncontrolled growth of lymphocytes. Lymphocytes are a type of white blood cell that play an important role in immune function. The lymphatic system is part of the circulatory system of the body and helps drain tissue of fluid. It consists of lymph vessels and lymph nodes, areas where multiple lymph vessels enter and larger ones emerge. Lymphocytes migrate to all parts of the body and every part of the body has lymph nodes or lymphocytes. Thus, lymphomas can occur in a wide variety of different parts of the body.

NHL is categorized according to the location or spread of the lymphoma and the type of cell affected. These categories help in deciding on treatment and estimating prognosis. However, they were developed in people who were not HIV infected. Treatment and prognosis of lymphomas may be different in people who have AIDS.

In NHL the majority of the lymphomas are of B-lymphocyte origin; a minority are of T-lymphocyte origin. The aggressiveness of NHL is described as low grade, intermediate grade, or high grade. Paradoxically, higher-grade lymphoma is both more aggressive and more responsive to treatment. Low-grade NHL progresses slowly, but may be more difficult to treat successfully.

Non-Hodgkin's lymphomas are associated with various immunodeficiency disorders, both congenital and acquired. The cause of NHL is uncertain. They may be associated with infection by Epstein-Barr virus (EBV). However, EBV is not always present and is not found in half of HIV-related lymphoma patients. There is probably no single cause of lymphomas.

As of 1989, non-Hodgkin's lymphoma (NHL) was sixty times more common in AIDS patients than in the total United States population. One recent study (Beral) indicated that about 3 percent of AIDS patients had NHL.

▲ Risk Factors

As people with HIV disease are living longer, the incidence of HIV-related NHL is increasing. Some hypotheses have been advanced to explain this:

- Profound immunodeficiency late in HIV disease may compromise normal immune surveillance that otherwise would eliminate spontaneous lymphomas
- Immune deficiency may allow new viral infections that directly cause lymphomas
- Reactivation of existing latent viral infections may directly cause lymphomas

Certain factors are statistically associated with development of NHL: prior diagnosis of Kaposi's sarcoma or oral hairy leukoplakia (caused by Epstein-Barr virus). It should not be assumed that factors statistically associated with NHL directly cause NHL—these factors and NHL may both be the result of prolonged immunodeficiency. Some people have attributed the rise in the incidence of NHL to the use of AZT; however, use of AZT does *not* seem to increase the risk of NHL.

▲ Sites of NHL

Outside the HIV setting, NHL is usually located in one of the lymph nodes. In HIV-infected people, however, studies show that over 85 percent of patients have NHL outside of lymph nodes (*extranodal involvement*). Lymphomas can occur in multiple parts of the body at the same time. NHL is usually widely disseminated by the time it is detected in an HIV-infected person. The most common sites of NHL in HIV-infected people are central nervous system or CNS (42 percent), bone marrow (33 percent), gastrointestinal tract, meninges (linings of the brain and spinal cord), and liver. When lymphoma first appears in the central nervous system, it is referred to as *primary CNS lymphoma.*

▲ Symptoms

The symptoms of NHL vary depending on the location of the lymphoma.

Common symptoms are unexplained fevers, enlarged lymph nodes, enlarged spleen (organ on the upper left side of the abdomen), unexplained weight loss, or drenching night sweats.

Physicians do not generally biopsy swollen lymph nodes in HIV patients with generalized lymphadenopathy unless there are persistent constitutional symptoms (fevers, night sweats, etc.) or if the nodes are asymmetrical, rapidly enlarging, or bulky.

The most frequent **symptoms of CNS lymphoma** are confusion, lethargy, and memory loss. Other symptoms of CNS lymphoma are hemiparesis (weakness or paralysis of half of the body), aphasia (loss of ability to speak or comprehend speech), seizures, and headaches. Less than half of patients with CNS lymphoma have focal neurological abnormalities. The symptoms of CNS lymphoma are similar to those of toxoplasmosis.

▲ Diagnosis

Diagnostic procedures depend on the suspected location of the lymphoma.

Diagnosis of NHL outside the central nervous system: Diagnosis typically involves one or more X ray studies and biopsies. Multiple tests may be needed to locate all the lymphomas. Some blood tests are useful in indicating the possible presence of NHL. These are *lactate dehydrogenase* (LDH) elevation or *uric acid* elevation. The work-up should be done quickly because disease can progress rapidly.

Cranial imaging—computerized tomography (CT) scan or magnetic resonance imaging (MRI)—and lumbar puncture are used for **diagnosis of central nervous system NHL.** It is hard to distinguish between CNS lymphoma and abscesses caused by other microorganisms such as toxoplasma. The symptoms are the same and the focal CNS lesions appear the same on X ray. You should be treated for toxoplasmosis while blood tests for toxoplasmosis infection are being done. If the tests are positive, toxoplasmosis treatment should be continued. If your symptoms do not improve on three to four weeks of antitoxoplasmosis therapy, or if the lesions grow larger, a biopsy of the brain is necessary to confirm NHL.

▲ Treatment

Treatment for HIV-related NHL is changing as experience is growing. Although the prognosis for this illness has been grim, it is likely that it will improve as treatment is refined. This has been the case for NHL when it is not related to HIV. It is best to be treated by a doctor or facility that is experienced in treating NHL and connected to clinical trials.

Modality: Cranial irradiation (radiation therapy of the head) is the treatment of choice for primary CNS lymphoma. Lymphoma in other areas of the body is treated with chemotherapy.

The drugs used for chemotherapy of NHL are often immunosuppressive. The risk of further immunosuppression and increased incidence of opportunistic infections in HIV-infected people must be balanced against the benefits of treating the lymphoma. Modified regimes using smaller doses of medication are probably more appropriate in people who are immunodeficient. Some studies have shown that the use of highly aggressive chemotherapy regimens may be less effective. Recent small studies of reduced medication seem to be very promising.

PCP prophylaxis is important for patients undergoing chemotherapy for NHL. Many past deaths during chemotherapy for NHL were caused by PCP which followed increased immunosuppression.

The experience of chemotherapy: You will generally receive the drugs for treating NHL intravenously. This does not usually require hospitalization. You will go to the doctor's office and remain for the period of time it takes to receive the drugs, anywhere from a few minutes to a few hours. There should be a health care provider present to monitor your temperature and discomfort. You should be offered antianxiety medication (such as Ativan), and antinausea medication (such as Compazine) as needed. Chemotherapy for NHL is usually done periodically, for example once every two weeks for approximately six months.

Prognosis: Over half of patients with HIV-associated NHL have a complete response to an initial course of combination chemotherapy. Half of these subsequently relapse and must be retreated.

Prognosis is associated with previous HIV-related diagnosis. Previously asymptomatic people with T4 cell counts of over 100 have the best prognosis.

Balance side effects and efficacy: Patient and physician must make some difficult decisions about the benefits and costs of treatment for NHL.

A number of different drug combinations are used to treat non-Hodgkin's lymphoma in HIV-infected people. Some regimes have relatively few side effects. Some have very unpleasant side effects but may be more effective in certain situations.

Side effects vary widely. Some drug combinations can cause nausea, vomiting, hair loss, mouth sores, mucositis (inflammation of oral mucous membranes, causing pain, foul taste, and loss of taste), fever, chills, weight loss, loss of appetite, anemia, increased risk of infection, kidney and liver problems, neurological symptoms, or bleeding.

There may be no ideal combination of drugs for any single individual's situation. Treatment strategies for this complication are subject to change as experience increases. If you are diagnosed with NHL discuss chemotherapy options in detail with your oncologist.

Chapter 13
Procedures and Tests

This chapter describes some of the procedures and tests that you may undergo in the course of HIV disease. It begins with a general discussion of the circumstances under which procedures may be performed, together with everyone's favorite question: Will it hurt? The chapter proceeds to explain the common tests that are performed on bodily fluids such as blood and urine, the imaging procedures that give your physician indirect information about the inside of your body, and finally those procedures —called *invasive procedures*—in which instruments of various types actually enter your body.

WHAT TO EXPECT AND HOW TO PLAN

Almost all the procedures described below can be performed on an *out-patient basis,* that is, without being formally admitted to a hospital. Out-patient procedures may be done in a doctor's office, a commercial laboratory or clinic, or possibly on hospital grounds but on an out-patient basis. Some procedures can only be done on an *in-patient basis,* that is, they require that you be formally admitted to a hospital for at least an overnight stay.

The cost of most procedures is usually covered by medical insurance. Check the provisions of your policy. You will probably have to fill out separate insurance forms for reimbursement for various procedures.

For some out-patient procedures we specifically suggest that you bring a companion. It's generally a good idea for all but the simplest procedures. Having company can reduce boredom and anxiety. Afterward you can talk with your friend about the procedure. If the procedure requires anesthesia or medication that leaves you groggy after the procedure, you may need a companion to see that you get home safely.

Most of the procedures described in this section are not risky. Procedures rarely cause serious problems. If a physician you trust recommends the test, you can generally assume that any hazard is outweighed by the benefit of the test. Discuss the benefits and risks with your doctor thoroughly.

Make sure you ask what to expect following the procedure. For example, some procedures may be followed by soreness or a little bleeding. Contact your doctor if you experience severe pain or bleeding.

Ask how long you can expect to feel any side effects of the procedure: this will help you make realistic plans.

Ask your physician when you can expect test results. Preliminary results may be available at the time of the procedure. Many procedures are done to obtain fluid or tissue for laboratory testing. Some lab tests may require days or even weeks. If possible, work out a definite time that you will get the results back. If a technician is doing the test, he or she is not usually allowed to give you results at the time of the procedure.

MINIMIZING PAIN AND ANXIETY

The discomfort associated with procedures varies. Many of the procedures described here are painless. You will receive anesthesia for potentially painful procedures.

For example, a regular chest X ray is no more painful than having a photograph taken. Some painless procedures may be inconvenient or possibly embarrassing. You may have to travel to a special facility for a procedure and you usually spend time waiting. You may be embarrassed to provide urine or stool specimens, or embarrassed to disrobe.

Some of the procedures described in this section have bad reputations for causing pain and discomfort. This reputation is sometimes deserved and sometimes not. The amount of pain or discomfort associated with any procedure will vary depending on a number of factors: your physical and psychological state, the person performing the procedure, and the amount and kind of pain medication used. With good practitioners and good medication, procedures should not be very painful.

What can you do to control the pain? First, discuss the procedure and the associated discomfort with the person performing the test. For most people, more information means less anxiety. If you have no idea what is going to happen, the anticipation is likely to be much worse than the actual procedure.

Second, accept all the pain medication that is offered. This pain medication will often be an intravenous benzodiazepine (such as Valium). Used intravenously, these drugs work quickly and effectively to reduce pain and anxiety. Pain medication may make you feel groggy or tired afterward. Some people do not like the emotional feeling associated with pain medication. These disadvantages are usually small in comparison to effective pain relief. If you have had a procedure before and found it painful, be sure to mention this and to request extra pain medication.

Anxiety produces tension, and tension may increase pain in a variety of ways. Injections and other invasive procedures are less painful if muscles at the site are relaxed, not clenched or contracted. It may be difficult to relax muscles consciously. Some people are able to learn to relax muscles by deliberately tensing and releasing the muscle in alternation. Rhythmic, regular breathing can help you maintain relaxation.

Practice breathing while counting from one to eight: four slow counts breathing in, four slow counts breathing out.

Relaxation and breathing exercises will calm your mind as well as your body. Breathing and muscle control are the foundation of many meditation techniques such as yoga. Music or other recordings may help you to focus your attention on your breathing: physicians often play music during procedures, or you may be able to bring a Walkman. Learn from experience whether you feel better watching the procedure or looking away.

FLUID TESTING

The vast majority of medical tests are performed on three fluids: blood, urine, and stool (feces). Urine and stool can be excreted more or less at will and are therefore easy to collect for testing. Blood must be obtained by inserting a needle through the skin into a blood vessel and drawing out (aspirating) a small volume of fluid. Blood is usually taken from a vein rather than an artery: this procedure is therefore called *venipuncture.*

▲ Blood Tests

Blood is composed of almost equal volumes of *formed elements* and *plasma* that can be separated by spinning a test tube of blood at high speed in a centrifuge ("spinning down" blood). Formed elements are red blood cells, white blood cells, and platelets. Plasma is nine-tenths water. The remaining tenth of plasma is various dissolved substances: proteins, electrolytes (charged particles or *ions*), sugars, vitamins, minerals, hormones, and drugs. The nature and constituents of blood are described in detail in Chapter 18: Blood and Blood Cells, pp. 355–58.

There are two aspects to testing a sample of blood. One is to test the various formed elements of blood. These are referred to as *hematological tests.* The other is to test for substances carried in solution by blood plasma. These tests fall into three categories. *Blood chemistry* measures chemicals in the blood, including electrolytes and proteins. *Microbiology* tests for certain microorganisms in the blood. *Serology* tests for antibodies and antigens in the blood.

Most blood tests are recorded quantitatively. They are reported either as an absolute number per specified unit of blood or as a percentage per specified unit of blood. Results that are typical for a population of asymptomatic subjects are referred to as **reference values** and are given as a range. Not all laboratories use the same reference range.

You can ask your doctor to see a copy of your blood-test results. These records will list both your lab results and the reference range used by the particular laboratory. If possible, ask for help in understanding the results.

Different laboratories can get different results on the same sample of blood. If your physician changes laboratories or if you change to a physician who uses a different laboratory from your previous doctor, you should realize that your lab values may change somewhat. Laboratories can make mistakes (more frequently on some tests than others) and your physician may want to repeat certain tests if the change is sudden or dramatic.

It is also important to remember that lab values often need to be interpreted depending on your age, sex, and race. Generally a number of laboratory values need to be looked at together, along with your clinical picture, in order to develop a meaningful diagnosis. The tests described below are only a few of the most commonly performed tests out of dozens that can be done on blood.

▲ Hematology

The complete blood count (CBC), is one of the most common tests for diagnosis of illness and screening. It is a routine test to evaluate blood and general health. You should get a CBC done every 6 to 12 months if you are asymptomatic, every three to six months if you have serious symptoms of HIV disease, and more often if you are on AZT or have hematologic abnormalities. Your physician may want to order a CBC more often for special reasons. A CBC measures red blood cell count, hemoglobin level, red blood cell volume (mean corpuscular volume, MCV), hematocrit (percentage of blood that is formed elements), and white blood cell count (WBC).

Hemoglobin (the oxygen-transporting substance in red blood cells) is often low in HIV-infected people, even in those not on medication. MCV is a measure of the typical size and hemoglobin concentration of red cells. Red blood cells can become abnormally small or large during disease. The hematocrit is derived from the red blood cell count and mean red cell volume. It can also be referred to as the packed red cell volume. It is the percentage of the blood that is made up of cells (versus serum). The majority of cells are red blood cells. The hematocrit can be referred to instead of the hemoglobin.

A white blood cell (or *leukocyte*) **differential** count is often done along with a complete blood count. A test ordered this way is called a "CBC with differential." The leukocyte differential test tells you what proportions of the total leukocyte count are composed of the different types of white blood cells—neutrophils, lymphocytes, monocytes, eosinophils, and basophils—as well as the absolute number of each of these types of cells.

In the leukocyte differential, T lymphocytes and B lymphocytes are added together and expressed as a percentage of the white blood count. A lymphocyte count is not the same as a T4 cell count. T4 cells are one type of lymphocyte. The lymphocyte count can go up and down for reasons that have nothing to do with a change in the T4 count. A leukocyte differential test does not measure T4 lymphocytes; a T4 count must be ordered specially.

Platelets are central to the process of blood clotting. A low **platelet count** is called *thrombocytopenia.* HIV infection can lower the platelet count. This does not necessarily cause symptoms or indicate a general decline in the immune system.

A **reticulocyte count** measures new red blood corpuscles that have just entered the bloodstream. The success of treatment for anemia can be judged by measuring the increase in the proportion of reticulocytes in the blood.

▲ Blood Chemistry

Other common blood tests calculate the amount of certain chemicals in the body. There are literally dozens of these tests, and standard blood tests usually measure from six to twenty of these chemical levels. Measurements of these chemicals can indicate whether various body processes are working correctly. Chemical tests are especially useful to detect kidney or liver problems and toxic effects of drugs. Correcting chemical imbalances can sometimes be crucial.

Certain chemicals in the body (calcium, sodium, potassium, chloride, phosphorus, magnesium) are known as *electrolytes.* They play a crucial role in the operation of cells and the electrical activity of the heart. Monitoring electrolytes, and restoring balance if necessary, is a crucial part of medical care for any serious illness.

Other blood chemistry tests measure the amount of water in the body. Water accounts for about 60 percent of body weight, and both too little and too much water can lead to serious problems. Water in the body can be measured by two tests, *serum osmolality* and *serum sodium concentrate.*

Some other important blood chemistry tests measure:

- Fats—cholesterol, triglycerides
- Substances that indicate kidney function—creatinine and blood urea nitrogen (BUN)
- Iron
- Glucose (blood sugar)
- Liver enzymes (When the liver becomes inflamed or damaged, the level of liver enzymes in the blood increases.)

You can ask your doctor for information about these tests in order to understand the significance of any abnormal test or to understand which tests might be indication of some disorder or adverse side effect of medication. You should have blood chemistry tests done yearly if you are not on toxic medications and every two to four months if you are taking potentially toxic medication.

▲ Serology

Serologies measure the presence and levels of antibodies and antigens in the blood. The HIV antibody test is a serology. Other important serologies for HIV-infected people are:

- Hepatitis B—serology should be done once, followed by vaccination if needed. (See the discussion of hepatitis B in Chapter 6: General Health Care, pp. 94–95 and Chapter 11: Infections, pp. 234–37.)
- *Toxoplasma gondii*—a baseline test indicates past exposure: should be repeated yearly if unexposed
- Syphilis (VDRL or RPR)
- Cytomegalovirus (CMV)—very common infection, but useful to know about

SUMMARY OF HEMATOLOGIC BLOOD TESTS
(REFERENCE RANGES FROM HARVEY)

Test/Component	Normal Ref. Range
Complete blood count (CBC)	
Erythrocyte count (red blood cell count)	Men: 4.5–5.9 million/mm³ Women: 4.0–5.2 million/mm³
Hemoglobin (often low in HIV-infected people, even among those not taking medication)	Men: 13.9-16.3 g/dl Women: 12.0-15.0 g/dl
Hematocrit (percentage of blood that is formed elements)	Men: 41-53 percent Women: 36-46 percent
White blood cells (WBC)	4,500-11,000/mm³ range 8,000/mm³ mean
Differential count of white blood cells	
Neutrophils	31-76 percent
Lymphocytes	24-44 percent
Monocytes (macrophages)	2-11 percent
Eosinphils	0-5 percent
Basophils	0-2 percent
Platelet count	140,000-350,000/mm³
Reticulocyte count	10,000-75,000/mm³

mm³ = millimeter cubed, a measure of volume

g/dl = grams per deciliter

▲ Microbiology

Blood can be examined for the presence of many microorganisms (bacteria, viruses, fungi, and parasites). Blood can be directly examined under a microscope (often with the addition of a *stain*) for the presence of organisms that are large enough to be visible. Microorganisms can also be identified by growing them in a special nutrient in the laboratory; this technique is known as a *culture.* Some organisms can be cultured much more easily and accurately than others. Finding a microorganism in the blood does not always mean that this organism is causing disease. These tests are not part of standard panels of blood tests but must be ordered specially by your doctor.

▲ Urine Testing

Urine testing (*urinalysis*) measures the levels of protein, glucose (sugar), ketones, blood, and nitrites in your urine. Urine testing provides information about the functioning of the kidneys, the presence of diabetes, and possible infections of the urinary tract. Ask your physician to explain the specific laboratory test used.

You will be asked to provide a urine sample. Usually you will be given a specimen cup and pointed to the nearest toilet. If you have trouble urinating on demand, drink some water. Some people run the tap in the sink to provide psychological encouragement for urination.

▲ Stool Testing

Stool tests indicate the presence of bacteria and parasites in feces. Sometimes these tests need to be done following the administration of laxatives (*purged stool test*) in order to gather samples in which the parasites are still living and detectable. Stool can also be examined for the presence of blood, which suggests certain gastrointestinal diseases.

For a stool test, you go to a commercial parisitology laboratory and take a strong laxative. This is usually in the form of a small cup of neutral-tasting liquid. You will be told to return to the lab in half an hour—you may be encouraged to eat a meal while waiting. Within one hour the laxative will produce diarrhea that can then be examined for the organisms. The lab technician may ask you for more than one specimen, as the test needs stool of a particular consistency for best results.

The diarrhea caused by the laxative usually stops by itself after the initial flow—but you may want to bring an over-the-counter anti-diarrheal medication such as Imodium to take after the stool sample is successfully obtained.

IMAGING

Medical imaging techniques use various types of radiation in addition to visible light to obtain information about the interior of the body. These include X rays, radio waves, magnetic fields, and radioactivity.

▲ X Rays

Two medical imaging techniques use X rays: *conventional* X rays and *computerized tomography scans* (CT or CAT; the *A* in CAT stands for *axial*).

An X ray is a photograph that uses high-energy electromagnetic radiation (X rays) to penetrate the body and expose a piece of film. The actual X ray exposure is quick and painless. Radiation exposure is very small; the diagnostic benefit of X rays outweighs the tiny lifetime risk of their use. Radiation exposure accumulates over time, so lead cloth may be used to protect the parts of your body not being filmed from even this small amount of radiation. Since the technician performs many X rays each year, he or she must be completely protected from radiation to avoid the gradual accumulation of a dangerous dose.

X rays are done on many parts of the body (head, neck, chest, heart, lungs, organs in the abdomen or pelvis, and joints and bones throughout the body).

Some conventional X rays involve the use of a *contrast medium,* some kind of substance to enhance detail in the area being filmed. A dye or radioactive material may be injected into a blood vessel for X rays of the circulatory system and internal organs such as the liver or kidneys. A contrast medium such as barium may be swallowed in a "milkshake" or given in an enema for X rays of the pharynx, esophagus, stomach, or other parts of the gastrointestinal tract.

In either case, the use of the contrast medium may hurt or be uncomfortable. You may feel bloated from swallowing fluid or feel uncomfortable pressure from an enema. Some people have allergic reactions to the dye used, but this is unusual.

Electromagnetic radiation

Visible light is one type of electromagnetic radiation; X rays are another. If you have ever held your hand up to a bright light, you may have noticed that your hand is somewhat translucent: the light shines through. Flesh tends to block visible light, but is more transparent to higher-energy radiation such as X rays. The complete spectrum of *electromagnetic radiation* includes infrared radiation (such as that from heat lamps), visible light, ultraviolet radiation (black light, or the light from tanning lamps), radio waves, and X rays.

▲ Chest X Ray

A chest X ray is a conventional X ray done without using a contrast medium. It provides an image of the lungs and the inside of the chest cavity. Chest X rays may be done on an out-patient basis. They are performed by an X ray technician and interpreted by a radiologist.

You will get a chest X ray as part of many routine evaluations, especially if you have chest pain or respiratory problems such as coughing or shortness of breath. Lung infections and lung cancers (such as PCP, MAC, CMV pneumonia, KS, and lymphoma) may cause a chest X ray to look different from normal. Some infections have a tendency to appear in certain patterns. However, you cannot always distinguish between specific infections based on an X ray. Treatment decisions may require confirmation from other types of diagnostic tests.

You will stand up or lie down in front of an X ray machine. You will be asked to inflate your lungs and hold your breath for a few seconds while the X ray is taken. There is no pain and there are no aftereffects.

▲ Computerized Tomography Scans (CT)

A computerized tomography (CT) scan improves on conventional X rays by showing cross sections of the body instead of simple projections. CT scans are sometimes also known as computerized *axial* tomography (CAT) scans. CT scans take many X rays from different vantage points around the area being scanned. This information is then integrated by a computer to form an image of cross sections of the body that can be displayed on a video monitor. If done without a contrast medium, CT scans cause no pain or hazard. If dye is used for contrast, there may be mild discomfort or allergy. CT scans are most often used in HIV disease to examine the brain (to diagnose various neurological disorders) and the abdomen. CT scanning may be done on an out-patient basis. It is performed by a technologist or radiologist.

Head or brain CT scans are used to evaluate symptoms that suggest problems of the central nervous system (such as focal neurological deficits or dementia, see the neurology section in Chapter 10: Organ System Complications). A head CT scan is used primarily to obtain a preliminary diagnosis. Diagnosis is often confirmed by other methods. If a CT scan shows lesions characteristic of cerebral toxoplasmosis, your physician will want to begin immediate antitoxoplasmosis treatment without waiting for a confirmed diagnosis. A CT scan is also used before performing lumbar puncture to rule out cerebral mass lesions (displacements of brain tissue): lumbar puncture may change the pressure of cerebrospinal fluid and cause a dangerous collapse (*herniation*) of a mass lesion.

Be sure to tell the radiologist if you are allergic to iodine or to shrimp (some of the dyes used for CT scans may contain iodine). If you are going to have a CT scan, you may be asked to change into a hospital gown. You will lie on your back or stomach on a table that is then (partially) moved into a tunnel in the middle of a large machine. If you are having a head CT scan, then only your head will be in this space. The procedure takes about thirty minutes. There is no pain. Some people feel anxious about being in an enclosed space. You will be able to talk to the technologist via an intercom. There are no aftereffects.

▲ Magnetic Resonance Imaging (MRI)

Magnetic resonance imaging (MRI) obtains detailed three-dimensional images of the interior of the body without using X rays. MRI currently provides better images than the CT scan, but is more expensive. Consequently, many medical centers typically perform CT scans first, and use MRI only if necessary. MRI may be performed on an out-patient basis. The procedure is performed by a technologist and the resulting images are interpreted (or *read*) by a radiologist with special training in MRI.

It is possible that MRI scans may pose a hazard to a developing fetus. Because you will be exposed to an intense magnetic field, do not get an MRI if you have any metallic objects embedded inside your body such as bone pins or plates, or pacemakers. MRI will disrupt the functioning of a pacemaker.

The MRI device consists of a large structure with a tunnel-shaped space into which a movable table slides. The large structure contains the devices that produce the magnetic field and register the image. You will be asked to remove all metal from your person. You may be asked to change into a hospital gown. You will lie on your back on the movable table. A device that produces radio pulses will be attached to the part of your body that is to be examined. The table will move you into the tunnel and will continue to move slightly as the imaging progresses. When the magnets start you will hear a loud mechanical noise. The entire MRI requires forty to sixty minutes.

There is no pain. You may be uncomfortable because you have to lie very still for an extended period. Some people feel claustrophobic in the small enclosed space of the MRI instrument. You will be able to speak to the technologist via an intercom. If you tend to be claustrophobic, request antianxiety medication before the procedure. There are no after effects.

How an MRI works

An extremely intense magnetic field is used to align the molecules in the body. Pulses of radio waves of varying frequencies are then used to perturb the molecules, which selectively absorb the radio waves depending on the differing properties of each type of molecule. When a radio pulse ends, the molecules return to their resting state, causing a detectable change. The information is then integrated into a three-dimensional image that contains information about the distribution and composition of the area scanned.

▲ Gallium Scanning

A gallium scan is a *nuclear imaging* test that can give information about both the configuration of body parts and their functioning. Gallium scanning is performed on an out-patient basis by a technician. The resulting scan is then interpreted (or *read*) by a radiologist. In HIV disease, gallium scanning is used for evaluation of possible *Pneumocystis carinii* pneumonia (PCP) and for locating other infections or neoplasms in the abdomen.

There is no pain involved and you will be exposed to only a very small amount of radiation. The benefits of gallium scanning outweigh this small radiation exposure. Gallium scanning may pose some hazard to a developing fetus.

A solution of a radioactive isotope of the element gallium is injected in the body forty-eight to seventy-two hours before the scan takes place. This allows the gallium to be carried by the circulation to the area of interest. You will be asked to lie on your back on a table for about an hour. The gallium isotope undergoes *radioactive decay,* releasing particles that can be detected by a special instrument called a *gamma camera.* The gamma camera creates an image of the distribution and motion of isotope-carrying fluids as they move through the organ under examination. There are no aftereffects.

INVASIVE PROCEDURES

Invasive procedures generally involve the insertion of instruments into the body for inspection and possible removal of body tissue.

▲ Simple Biopsies

The examination of cells and tissues for abnormalities is called **cytology.** Samples of cells and tissues are obtained by procedures referred to as **biopsies.** Biopsies may be taken of skin (for instance to determine if a lesion is Kaposi's sarcoma), mucous membranes, or internal organs. Biopsies of skin or easily accessible mucous membranes are simple and straightforward. Tissue collection from internal organs is discussed later.

There are several different kinds of biopsies, including scraping, aspiration, and excision. With **scraping,** the cell sample is obtained by lightly scraping the area of concern with a wooden stick, much like a Q-Tip. It is rarely painful. A Pap smear is a type of scraping biopsy. With **aspiration,** a sample of cells (often with fluid) is obtained by inserting a needle and creating suction into a syringe. A local anesthesia is used first and pain is limited. With **excision,** the cells or tissue are cut out in a surgical procedure. The location and extent of the excision necessary determines whether the procedure is done under local or general anesthesia.

▲ Bronchoscopy

A bronchoscopy is a test to visually examine the airways (*bronchi*), collect secretions from the lung and bronchi for laboratory examination, and remove tissue samples (biopsies). The bronchi are the part of the respiratory tract that connects the lungs and the trachea (windpipe). In HIV disease, bronchoscopy may help to diagnose PCP, CMV pneumonitis, MAC, pulmonary KS, and other lung diseases. It is performed by a lung specialist called a *pulmonologist* and may be done on an out-patient or in-patient basis.

If you get this procedure on an out-patient basis, bring someone with you to keep you company and help you get home.

A local anesthetic will be sprayed into your mouth and throat. More local anesthesia will be put in your throat through a tube in your mouth. This will make you cough. The coughing is probably the worst part of the procedure.

The pulmonologist will insert a slender flexible fiber-optic tube (called a *bronchoscope*) in one nostril or in your throat. This tube will gradually be eased down your throat and into a bronchus (airway). The procedure is not very painful, but having something down your throat may make you anxious. You will be able to breathe, but the pressure of the tube may be uncomfortable.

The physician doing the procedure can examine the bronchi through the bronchoscope. In addition, the physician can withdraw secretions through the instrument. Fluid can also be introduced into the lungs to wash out cells for laboratory examination (*bronchoalveolar lavage,* BAL). Tiny devices on the end of the bronchoscope can remove tissue for cell biopsy.

The entire procedure takes about an hour. You may have a sore throat and a hoarse voice for a day or two.

▲ Endoscopy

Gastrointestinal endoscopies are procedures in which a slim flexible fiber-optic tube called an *endoscope* is inserted into the gut via the mouth or the anus. The inside of the gastrointestinal tract can be examined, photographed, and tissue samples removed through the endoscope.

Upper gastrointestinal endoscopy is used to examine the upper part of the gut. In HIV disease endoscopy (usually with removal of tissue for biopsy) can help diagnose esophageal candidiasis, or ulcers due to cytomegalovirus or herpes virus infection. Endoscopy is performed by a gastroenterologist and may be done either as an out-patient procedure or in the hospital.

Bring someone with you because you will be groggy after the procedure. You will be told to eat and drink nothing for the twelve hours preceding the endoscopy.

Immediately before an upper GI endoscopy you will gargle with a liquid local anesthetic. You will also receive intravenous medication (usually benzodiazepines) that will make you sleepy and reduce any pain. The gastroenterologist will insert the endoscope tube through your mouth and pharynx and gently move it down to the esophagus, stomach, or duodenum. The endoscope will be used to examine these areas visually. Tissue samples (biopsies) may also be taken. Intravenous medication ensures that the procedure is not painful. You will be able to breathe normally, but you may have some discomfort from the natural gagging reflex.

An endoscopy takes about fifteen minutes, although you will generally stay for rest and observation for one or two hours after the procedure. You will probably feel tired due to the medication. You may have a sore throat.

Colonoscopy is used to examine the lower part of the GI tract (the colon). In HIV disease colonoscopy (usually with biopsy) is used to diagnose CMV colitis and lymphoma. Colonoscopy is performed by a gastroenterologist and is done either as an out-patient or in hospital.

If you have the procedure done as an out-patient, bring someone with you to help you get home. To get a good view of the colon, it must be empty. This is accomplished with limited diet and laxatives the night before, and enemas on the day of the procedure.

Before the actual procedure you will be given intravenous medication that will make you feel very sleepy. The colonoscope will be inserted through your anus, into your rectum, and gently advanced up through your colon. The gastroenterologist will examine the walls of your colon for ulcers or other signs of disease. Samples of tissue can be removed with tiny instruments on the end of the colonoscope. With proper intravenous medication (usually benzodiazepines) you will feel no pain. The entire procedure takes about an hour. Because of the medication you may not remember anything about the procedure.

Because air is introduced to inflate the colon for better viewing, you may feel "gassy" for several hours. You may have mild rectal bleeding after the colonoscopy; if bleeding is heavy, report it to your doctor.

▲ Lumbar Puncture (Spinal Tap)

Tests of cerebrospinal fluid (CSF) help to diagnose infectious diseases that affect the central nervous system. A lumbar puncture (LP; commonly called a *spinal tap*) is used to obtain a small sample of fluid for testing. The LP is usually performed by a neurologist and may be done on an out-patient basis.

A CT scan should be done before performing lumbar puncture on an HIV-infected person to rule out cerebral mass lesions (displacements of brain tissue): lumbar puncture may change the pressure of cerebrospinal fluid and cause a dangerous collapse (*herniation*) of a mass lesion.

Bring someone with you to help you get home. To avoid headache you will want to lie down and stay still for several hours after the procedure. Your lower back will be locally anesthetized. The neurologist will insert a needle between two vertebrae and into your spinal canal. The neurologist will then remove a small amount of cerebrospinal fluid for testing.

The needle must pass through muscle tissue to reach the spinal canal. If the muscle is relaxed, the pain will be minimal. Deep breathing or taking relaxation medication before the LP may help. People usually feel that the actual procedure was not nearly as bad as its reputation.

Because the tap removes cerebrospinal fluid, it lowers the pressure of the fluid cushioning the brain. This may cause a long-lasting headache. To reduce headache after the procedure, lie down as much as possible and avoid moving your head suddenly.

▲ Bone Marrow Biopsy

Examination of bone marrow may help to diagnose lymphoma, certain types of thrombocytopenia (decrease in platelet count), and some fevers that are persistent and occur at the same time as anemias or other disorders of blood cells. The procedure is performed by a hematologist (blood specialist) and may be done on an out-patient basis. Bring someone with you to help you get home.

You will be given local anesthesia. The hematologist will insert a needle into your breastbone or one of the large bones at one side of the back of your pelvis. The needle is advanced into the cavity of the bone, where marrow is removed. You will feel pressure and a brief sharp pain. The whole procedure takes only a few minutes. You will stay for about thirty minutes after the procedure to make sure there is no bleeding. You may feel sore at the site for a few days.

▲ Brain Biopsy

The purpose of this procedure is to remove a tiny sample of brain tissue, primarily to help diagnose cerebral mass lesions that do not respond to antitoxoplasma medication. The procedure is necessary in order to choose the most effective therapy with the fewest side effects. Brain biopsies are performed by a neurosurgeon.

Brain biopsy sounds dramatic, but people who have had brain biopsies (of the *skinny-needle CT-guided* variety) report that it wasn't so bad. The main risk is infection: the procedure is therefore done only on an in-patient basis. The small amount of tissue removed does not damage the brain, nor will you experience any mental changes as a result of the procedure. Talk over the pros and cons of this procedure thoroughly with your physician.

"Skinny needle" CT-guided brain biopsy is now the method of choice. The CT scan eliminates the need to open the skull: open-brain biopsies present a greater risk of complications. A small area of your head will be shaved. Your head will be placed in a frame that provides a fixed reference point. A CT scan will be done to determine the exact location of the brain lesion relative to the frame. You will then be totally anesthetized and taken to an operating room (where the risk of infection is at a minimum). After you are unconscious a small hole will be made in your skull. A "skinny needle" will be inserted into the hole and guided to the lesion by information derived from the CT scan. A tiny sample of the tissue in the lesion will then be removed for examination.

You will be anesthetized during the procedure and therefore will feel no pain. A small area of the scalp and skull may be sore for a few days after the procedure. The brain itself cannot feel pain since there are no pain receptors in brain tissue.

▲ In-Dwelling Catheters

Certain medications are not absorbed properly by the body if they are taken orally or injected into a muscle. Such medications must be taken intravenously (IV). Small amounts of intravenous medication may be injected into a vein via a hypodermic needle. If the amount of medication necessary is greater than can be contained in a syringe, you can be given an *infusion* via a *temporary intravenous line.* For a temporary IV line a small needle is inserted into a vein and fixed in place with tape. A tube is attached to the needle so that liquid medication can drip slowly into the vein over a period of time. This is what people usually think of as "getting an IV."

In some circumstances you may need regular IV medication for an extended period, for instance to treat CMV retinitis or fluconazole-resistant cryptococcosis. Some people with serious weight loss or gastrointestinal problems also use a catheter in order to get intravenous feeding (partial or total *parenteral nutrition*—TPN).

Small veins near the skin are too fragile to provide long-term access to the bloodstream for ongoing IV medication. Such medication must be infused into a larger vein, one that is sturdier and farther from the surface of the body. For this purpose, long-term IV medication is given through a *central venous* catheter, also referred to as an *in-dwelling* catheter.

A catheter is a long narrow tube that is surgically inserted into the chest and through a large vein into a blood vessel near the heart called the *vena cava.* About six inches of the catheter remains outside the chest. A cap on the end prevents bleeding and infection. In order to take the required medication, you connect the catheter to tubing that leads to a bottle or plastic bag containing the liquid medication. For some medications a special pump ensures that the solution enters the body slowly and regularly. After the infusion is complete, the catheter and tube are disconnected. The catheter is then cleaned and taped against your chest.

Receiving an in-dwelling catheter requires a major psychological and practical adjustment. It requires (minor) surgery to install, it is visible when you are not dressed, it takes time to infuse the medication, and you must learn how to use the equipment properly to get the right amount of medication and avoid infection. However, if your physician suggests that an in-dwelling catheter is appropriate, it is likely that the catheter may help save your sight or keep you alive. Once you have a catheter, you can receive any medication through your catheter that needs to be taken intravenously. Blood can also be withdrawn through the catheter (no more needle-sticks).

As with many other aspects of dealing with AIDS, use of an in-dwelling catheter takes psychological adjustment and can be difficult and upsetting. Nonetheless, many patients have used catheters for extensive periods of time, dealt with the emotional issues, and continued to lead active and productive lives. You can swim, bathe, shower, participate in sports, and have sex with an in-dwelling catheter in place.

Types of in-dwelling venous catheters: Two major types of in-dwelling catheters have been used to administer medication to people with AIDS. The kind described above is known as a *Hickman catheter* and is the most frequently used device. A second kind of catheter is known as a *Port-a-cath.* It differs from the Hickman in that no tubing extends outside the body, and the infusion is started by injecting a needle into the catheter below the surface of the chest. This injection is not painful as the area at the insertion point has been permanently anesthetized during the installation surgery.

The advantage of a Port-a-cath is that it is less visible and therefore less intrusive. The disadvantage is that it is more likely to become infected than a Hickman catheter. Since infection is the main danger of catheter use, generally a Hickman catheter is preferred. People with vision problems should probably use a Hickman catheter since you have to be able to see the Port-a-cath to use it.

Installation: A catheter is installed in a brief surgical procedure. The procedure usually takes about a half an hour and is performed under local anesthesia. It is performed in an operating room by a surgeon; sterile conditions are crucial. An incision is made in the chest in the area where the tube will be inserted. A few sutures (stitches) will hold the catheter in place.

In about a week these sutures can be removed because fibrous tissue that grows around the tube will hold the catheter in place. A bandage (sterile dressing) is used to cover the site for a few weeks after the surgery. After that, the area is covered with a small dressing.

You may be hospitalized for a few days in order to have this procedure done. In some cases catheters may be installed in the out-patient surgical unit of a hospital. The pain during and after the surgery is minor; generally it is limited to the discomfort of the healing of a small incision.

Care: You may learn how to use the catheter to give yourself medication. This means learning how to set up the medication in the drip bag or pump, how to attach the catheter to the source of medication, how to make sure you are getting the correct dosage of medication at the correct rate, how to prevent clogging of the catheter, how to prevent air from getting into the catheter, how to disconnect the catheter, how to place a bandage (dressing) over the catheter, and how to change the catheter cap.

With practice, none of this is difficult. Home infusion is a simple repetitive procedure that anyone can be taught. On the other hand, using this equipment is a new skill and requires some time to learn. Get help using your catheter until you are confident that you can use it correctly. A home health-care service can send a professional to set up your home infusions until you feel comfortable doing it yourself. A visiting nurse and/or your physician will check periodically to make sure that your catheter is working properly.

If you intend to travel, plan carefully. You have to transport medication and equipment. Make certain that you will have access to a clean, orderly environment where you can care for your catheter properly.

Catheter sites can develop infection. Pay careful attention to correct sterile techniques when handling the catheter and setting up your infusions. Early signs of infection are redness, drainage of liquid from the site, swelling, fever, or pain. Contact your physician immediately if these signs occur. Contact your doctor if your catheter becomes dislodged or a hole develops (this is rare), or if the infusion does not flow through your catheter. If someone else is performing the catheter care, this person should wear gloves.

Psychological issues: There are several reasons why getting a Hickman catheter is emotionally difficult. A catheter is not visible to others under your clothes. However, it is visible when your chest is bare, and (more to the point) *you* always know it is there. It is a sign to others that you have a serious medical problem, and in communities where the disease is familiar, it is a sign that you have AIDS. You have to decide how to deal with a catheter if you have contact with a new sexual partner or if you are in any situation where your chest would normally be exposed (such as the beach or a gym locker room).

Taking medication by infusion takes time, sometimes several hours a day. This is an annoying intrusion in your daily routine and may be an unwelcome reminder of your illness. Caring for the catheter in order to prevent infection also takes time and is tedious. Planning for travel requires additional attention.

Some people feel more fragile after getting a Hickman catheter. The sense of an opening between the inside of your body and the outside world, as well as the realistic risk of infection, may make you feel vulnerable. Although catheters are rarely accidentally dislodged, this may at first feel like a danger, particularly if you are in a crowd or engaged in vigorous physical activity.

As time goes on you will become less aware of your catheter and less bothered by it. Infusions and catheter care will become routine. However, some people may alternate periods of ease and emotional discomfort about the catheter.

If you are about to get a catheter or have just had one installed, talk with someone who has used a catheter for a period of time. Firsthand information from a veteran may reduce your anxiety.

SUMMARY OF COMMON DIAGNOSTIC PROCEDURES

Procedure	Purpose	Staff or location	Precautions & premedication	Discomfort	Aftereffects
Blood test (Venipuncture)	Examine chemical & cellular components of blood, test for infections	Any health care provider	None	Small pain on insertion of needle	Possibly some bruising at site
Urine collection	Examine chemical & cellular components of urine	Any health care provider	None	None other than embarrassment	None
Purged stool collection	Microscopic exam and cultures for infection	Parasitology lab	Laxative 1 hr. prior	Requires 1 hr.; embarrassment	Diarrhea may continue briefly
Any scans using contrast media	Enhance detail of X ray, CT scan, or MRI	Technologist or radiologist	Benadryl if allergy known	Possible discomfort, flushing, allergy	None
X rays (radiography, "films")	Visualize inside of body (2D projection through body)	Technologist or radiologist	Lead cloths to protect areas not imaged	None	None
Computerized tomography (CT scan, CAT scan)	Visualize inside of body (3D image)	Technologist or radiologist	Use special dyes if allergic to iodine or shrimp	Possible claustrophobia	None
Magnetic resonance imaging (MRI)	Visualize inside of body (3D image plus composition info)	Technologist or radiologist	No metallic objects or pacemakers	Loud noise; possible claustrophobia	None

Procedure	Purpose	Staff or location	Precautions & premedication	Discomfort	Aftereffects
Gallium scan	Visualize inside of body, distinguish infectious processes	Technologist or radiologist	None	None	None
Simple biopsy	Collect skin or other tissue sample	Any health care provider	Local anesthetic	Minimal	Pain at site of biopsy
Bronchoscopy, bronchoalveolar lavage (BAL)	inspect airways; collect tissue, fluid, or microorganisms from lungs for diagnosis	Pulmon-ologist	Local anesthetic, relaxation medication (IV)	Possible gag reflex	Possible soreness
Upper GI endoscopy	Direct inspection of the esophagus, stomach, duodenum; tissue collection, medication	Gastro-enterologist	Relaxation medication (IV)	Possible gag reflex If out-patient, bring a care partner	Possible soreness
Colonoscopy (lower GI endoscopy)	Direct inspection of the bowel; tissue collection; medication	Gastro-enterologist	Relaxation medication (IV)	If done out-patient, bring a care partner	"Gassy" feeling; mild rectal bleeding
Lumbar puncture (LP)	Collect cerebrospinal fluid; administer medication	Neurologist	Local anesthetic; need head CT to rule out CML	Brief pain at site	Possible long-lasting headache
Bone marrow aspiration	Collect bone marrow to diagnose infection	Hematologist	Local anesthetic	Brief, sharp pain at site	None
Brain biopsy	Confirm diagnosis of lymphoma so that medication can begin	Neuro-surgeon	Total anesthesia (IV)	None	Possible soreness

IV = intravenous, CML = cerebral mass lesion, GI = gastrointestinal

QUESTIONS TO ASK ABOUT PROCEDURES

Here are some questions to ask your doctor before a procedure:

- Why is the procedure/test necessary?
- What information will the procedure/test provide?
- What actions will be based on the results?
- What are the risks associated with the procedure/test?
- How should I prepare for the procedure/test?
- Should I or can I bring a companion?
- When and where will the procedure/test be done?
- Who will perform the procedure/test?
- How long will it take?
- What happens during the procedure/test?
- What pain or discomfort should I expect?
- What pain medication will I receive?
- How will I feel immediately after the procedure/test?
- How will I feel later on?
- What symptoms are normal after such a procedure/test?
- What symptoms should prompt me to call my doctor?
- How quickly can I know the results of the procedure/test?

Chapter 14
The Experience of Hospitalization

It is likely that during the course of HIV disease you will have to spend some time in a hospital. Hospitalization is an experience that is necessary but one that most people find unpleasant. Hospitalization is required for serious acute illness and critical care, for surgery and recovery, and for complex diagnostic procedures. What follows is a description of some of the common facts of hospital life and some suggestions for making a hospital stay more bearable.

Sometimes it may be a relief to go to a hospital. The knowledge that you are in a situation in which you can get appropriate treatment for illness, close monitoring of your medical situation, and immediate high-tech care for emergencies may be quite reassuring when you are sick. Also, when you are feeling very bad, a hospital is a place where you will be relieved of many of the ordinary tasks of daily life.

What are the factors that make being a hospital patient difficult? First of all, you are likely to be feeling sick while you are in the hospital. You may be given medication that makes you feel sicker. You may have tests and treatments done that are anxiety-provoking, embarrassing, or painful. You have little privacy. Hospitals are run on routines that have little to do with your convenience or comfort and you have little control over many aspects of life while you are a patient in a hospital. You are sometimes separated from the people in your daily life. Finally, being confined to a hospital is often boring and the food is bad. None of these problems can be altogether avoided but some of them can be reduced.

CHOOSING A HOSPITAL

If you have a private doctor, you will routinely be admitted to the hospital with which your doctor is affiliated. If you are a patient at a clinic, you will be admitted to the hospital associated with the clinic. A doctor's right to admit someone to a particular hospital is known as *admitting privileges*. Hospital affiliation is one factor that you should take into account in choosing a physician.

It is generally desirable to receive treatment at a *teaching hospital*. These hospitals are affiliated with medical schools and generally provide

313

the best-quality care. Studies have indicated that patients treated in hospitals with extensive experience in treating HIV disease do better than patients at hospitals with little experience.

If your admission is not an emergency, a day will be arranged in advance for you to come into the hospital. If the admission is done on an emergency basis, you will often have to be admitted through the emergency room even if you have a private doctor. If you need to be in a hospital and no space (referred to in hospital lingo as a *bed*) is available at that hospital you may be transferred to another hospital or kept for a period of time on a bed or stretcher in the emergency room. This is a difficult experience. As much as is possible, plan ahead with your physician. Don't wait until the eleventh hour to report serious symptoms.

The most important factor in choosing a hospital is the quality of the medical care. Although it is desirable to be in a hospital that is physically pleasant and has good amenities, this is less crucial than the quality of the nursing and medical care you receive.

AIDS units: Hospitals are usually divided into units according to the kind of medical care or procedure you need (for example, obstetrics/gynecology, surgery, general medical, pediatrics).

Some hospitals in major urban areas have special AIDS units. Although it was initially feared that AIDS patients would be segregated in these units and receive inferior care, this has not turned out to be the case. In fact, you are often likely to get the best care for your HIV-related problem in an AIDS unit. The doctors there are knowledgeable in HIV care. The nurses have chosen to work in this unit; consequently they are unlikely to display homophobia or to act out of irrational fear of people with HIV infection. Sometimes AIDS units have special educational programs or support groups for people with HIV disease. In addition, you are most likely to meet fellow patients who share your interests and concerns.

EMERGENCY ROOMS

If you have a sudden serious medical problem and cannot reach your doctor, you can get help by going to a hospital emergency room (ER). It is best to go to the ER of the hospital with which your doctor is affiliated. However, if the problem is so severe that immediate attention is needed, you can go to the ER of the hospital nearest you.

Getting treatment through an ER is often a time-consuming and unpleasant experience. Therefore, you are going to want to use the ER only for real medical crises. Planning can sometimes help you avoid the ER. If a health problem is developing, contact your doctor during the week rather than waiting for the weekend.

You can also use the ER for psychiatric emergencies. It is appropriate to do so if you feel suicidal, unbearably anxious, or experience a sudden change in your thinking processes or level of consciousness.

Emergency rooms vary. If you live in a big city, the ER you go to is likely to be crowded with people with serious problems. Expect a long wait. Go with a friend if at all possible. The friend can keep you company and help you negotiate the system. Bring insurance information with you since hospitalization may be necessary. When asked, state your medical problems clearly and report any urgent problem; ERs treat the most urgent situations first. Bring with you medication that you take on a routine basis. Consider bringing a blanket or warm clothes, water, and something to eat. Emergency rooms are sometimes too frantic to provide even the basic amenities.

HOSPITAL PERSONNEL

Your hospital's staff will include doctors, nurses, social workers, and liaison psychiatrists.

Doctors and attending physicians. The doctor who is in charge of your medical care is referred to as the attending physician. If you are admitted to the hospital by a private doctor, he or she will be your attending physician. If you do not have a private doctor, one of the physicians on staff will be designated your attending physician.

The attending physician has the final decision-making power and responsibility for a case. This does not mean that the attending physician is the doctor you will see most often. Typically, your attending physician spends some time in the hospital and some time in an office setting. You will usually see your attending doctor once a day during the week. The chance to talk to your attending physician will be important to you. This is the person who makes most of the nonemergency decisions about such things as diagnostic procedures, diagnosis, medication and other treatment, and length of stay in the hospital.

For this reason, it is reassuring to most patients to know when they will next see their attending physician. Doctors often have unpredictable schedules, but you should ask your physician which days you can expect to see her or him and, if possible, at roughly what time of day. On weekends and holidays, if your doctor is not in the hospital, another physician will "cover"; you should know who this person is.

Because of this limited availability, you should also plan what you want to ask your doctor each day. Nurses and other doctors will be able to answer most general questions, but may refer you back to the attending physician for answers about treatment and discharge decisions.

Although we speak of the doctor as "making the decisions," you, the patient, can and should have a say in these decisions. You have a right to ask questions and to understand the costs and benefits of any treatment recommendation. Ultimately you have the right to refuse treatment, to consult or switch to another doctor, or to leave the hospital against medical advice. You do not, however, have the right to demand a particular treatment against the advice of your physician so, realistically, your say is limited.

House staff and medical students: House staff are physicians who have graduated from medical school and are receiving further advanced training. (The word house means "hospital" in medical lingo.) If you are a patient at a teaching hospital, you will deal with physicians who are *residents* or *fellows.*

After four years of medical school, doctors spend three or four years in further training primarily in a hospital setting before they are eligible to be licensed and practice on their own. At this stage doctors are called *residents.* First-year residents used to be referred to as *interns.* Residents specialize in one of several areas such as internal medicine, family practice, obstetrics and gynecology, surgery, or psychiatry. They do much of the day-to-day doctoring work with in-patients. After completing a residency, some doctors continue in further training and are referred to as *fellows.* Fellows sub-specialize in particular areas of medicine. Students in the last few years of medical school rotate through the various types of medical specialties, spending a few weeks or months observing, learning from, and assisting the house staff.

Various residents and fellows will be involved in your care during a hospital stay. Because they are involved in a period of intensive in-hospital training, they are often highly skilled and knowledgeable.

In general, attending physicians and fellows supervise residents. Advanced residents supervise beginning residents. Residents and fellows (and the medical students who work with them) often work very hard and are pressed for time. They take turns spending nights, weekends, and holidays in the hospital to do the medical work that is required. However, although they are busy, they sometimes have the opportunity and interest to spend time with you, explain things carefully, and get to know you.

The more you know the doctors who are treating you and the more they know you, the better. You will feel less powerless and less anonymous if you have some kind of relationship with the people who are treating you.

Specialists: Your doctor may consult with other physicians who have specialized in certain areas of medicine. These are doctors who have completed training in a particular area and are equipped to give your physician advice about a particular problem. Following is a list of the terms used to describe some of these specialists.

SOME SPECIALTIES

Name of specialist	Area of specialty
Cardiologist	Heart
Dermatologist	Skin
Gastroenterologist	Gut (including the esophagus, stomach, intestines, and colon)
Gynecologist/obstetrician	Women's reproductive system, childbirth
Hematologist	Blood
Infectious-disease specialist	Infectious diseases
Nephrologist	Kidneys
Oncologist	Cancer
Ophthalmologist	Eyes
Otolaryngologist (ENT)	Ears, nose, and throat
Pathologist	Interpretation of biopsies and other tests
Pulmonologist	Lungs
Radiologist	Interpretation of X rays and other tests
Urologist	Urinary system, male reproductive system

Nurses: Nurses are the heart of the hospital system. The nursing staff consists of RNs (registered nurses) and various kinds of nursing assistants. Nurses do most of the daily patient care in a hospital and perform or administer many basic procedures and treatments. The training and knowledge of RNs can vary widely; many of them are well trained and expert.

Nurse-practitioners, nurse-clinicians, and *nurse-midwives* are RNs with further advanced training. They perform functions traditionally done by physicians. These health care providers are highly trained, expert at performing certain procedures, and often have a sophisticated understanding of psychological issues. In some hospitals, *physicians' assistants* perform similar functions.

The **social work staff** consists of *social workers* (who have a master's degree in social work) and *social work assistants* (who usually have bachelor's degrees). Social workers in a hospital perform a variety of different functions. They are responsible for all the preparation necessary when a patient leaves the hospital. This *discharge planning* includes plans for follow-up care, nursing home and hospice placements, home care, applications for Medicare, Medicaid, welfare, Social Security Disability, food stamps, and other benefit programs. They are also responsible for providing psychological consultation and support for patients and their family members. Some hospital social workers perform both jobs. Their training and expertise, like that of doctors and nurses, is highly variable.

If you have particular arrangements to make for discharge, such as arranging for home health care, make plans as early as possible. Ask to speak to the social worker early on to find out what kind of paperwork needs to be done. Many of these things take time; waiting until the last minute can cause inconvenience and even delay discharge.

Liaison psychiatry: In addition to the psychological services provided by social workers, many hospitals have psychiatrists available to inpatients. They are referred to as *liaison psychiatrists* or *liaison/consultation psychiatrists.* They are expert in the psychiatric problems associated with medical illness and in the use of medications to treat these problems, including pain medication. They also help mediate between hospital staff and patients.

Usually your physician will request a consultation with a liaison psychiatrist if he or she feels it will be useful. If you are highly anxious, depressed, can't sleep, feel you are in too much pain, or are having ongoing problems in working with your doctor or other staff, you can request that your physician call in a liaison psychiatrist.

GETTING ALONG WITH HOSPITAL STAFF

Being on good terms with the hospital staff will make your stay in the hospital easier. How can you accomplish this? It is very difficult to think and act strategically when you are feeling sick, powerless, and worried. Nonetheless, a combination of self-control and assertiveness will be useful in your relations with hospital staff.

Many of the people in hospitals have too much to do. Residents are often fatigued and constantly busy. Nurses and social workers tend to be underpaid and overworked. When you are in the hospital you will often have to wait: wait for a nurse, wait for medication, wait to get a procedure started, wait for food. This waiting is generally not the fault of the staff but has to do with the complications of running a large understaffed system. Therefore, you have to decide about your attitude toward the typical delays and inconveniences you will face.

If you complain and get mad all the time, you are likely to alienate staff and feel disliked and more isolated. Since it is the system that is inefficient and clumsy, try not to direct your anger against the individuals who work in it. Try to remember that staff members on all levels are human and have problems and worries of their own. An effort to treat them like people rather than like machines will pay off in goodwill.

On the other hand, there are certain times when you may have to be assertive about making demands. For example, if you are in pain or feel that something is going wrong medically it is appropriate to demand immediate action. If you feel that you are being mistreated, you should certainly complain. Try to complain when you are feeling relatively calm and can present your complaints in a reasonable fashion. If the immediate staff you work with cannot address your complaint, you can ask to speak to a supervisor, for example the head nurse. In many hospitals you can ask to speak to an *ombuds officer* or *patient advocate,* who tries to resolve patient complaints.

HOSPITAL ROUTINE

Hospitals vary tremendously in terms of physical amenities. If you are a patient in a big hospital in a city like New York, the physical surroundings may be less than first class; the hospital may nevertheless provide excellent medical care.

You will probably be sharing a room with another patient. If you have problems with your roommate (noise, too many visitors, a medical problem that upsets you), speak to the nursing staff. At times, changes in room assignments can be made. However, the hospital staff has little flexibility and has to take nursing demands into account; you may have to tolerate problems with a roommate.

Daily routine: When you are an in-patient, certain procedures will be done over and over: measurements of temperature, pulse, blood pressure, and having blood drawn. These tests provide an ongoing source of information that is critical to evaluating your medical condition and your response to treatment.

Almost everyone who has been in a hospital complains about the odd schedule. You are often awakened early in the morning to have blood drawn, and your sleep may be disrupted to have your temperature checked or to be given medication. In an ideal system, it might be possible to avoid some of these inconveniences. In the complex real world of hospital life, the need to accomplish certain tasks takes precedence over patient comfort. For example, blood is drawn early in the morning so that test results arrive during the workday.

Staying in bed for protracted periods is bad for your body and leads to loss of strength quite rapidly. In addition, remaining in a lying-down position all the time can contribute to lung problems. Unless you are too ill, the nursing staff will probably urge you to get out of bed and walk around frequently. Try to cooperate because it is in the interests of your recovery.

Medication: Although nurses give you the medication, only physicians write the orders for medication. You can always refuse a medication but it is not possible for the nurse to give you a new medication without the written permission of the physician. Many medications are written as *standing orders* to be used on an "as necessary" basis (often indicated with the Latin abbreviation *PRN,* for *pro re nata*). In other words, the physician anticipates your need for a medication and writes an order for it on the chart so that the nurse can give it to you if necessary. For example, standing orders are often written for pain medication, sleep medication, antacids, or laxatives. If you anticipate concern with a particular problem, ask your doctor to arrange to have appropriate medication ordered in advance.

Many people with HIV disease enter the hospital already taking a variety of medications. Usually the hospital will provide all the medications while you are an in-patient but occasionally you may be told to bring a particular medication with you. You should bring a written list with you of all the medication that you are currently taking. Check with your doctor when you are admitted about *each* medication. Some medications may be discontinued or others started and you want to make sure that this is done by plan rather than oversight. For example, if you are taking an anti-depressant medication, you may have to remind the doctor that you need an order written for that medication.

Tolerating hospitalization: Being with people you are close to can make a hospital stay bearable. Many hospitals nowadays have extended visiting hours and some even allow someone to spend the night with you. If having people with you helps you feel better, let your friends and family know.

However, some people feel fatigued or stressed by too many visitors or visitors they do not particularly want to see. You also have a right to say no to visitors.

Being in the hospital is tough. Think of all the things you can do to make yourself more comfortable. For example, if you are going to be in the hospital for an extended period of time you may want to bring your own pillow or robe and pajamas.

One of the problems of being in the hospital is boredom and confinement. Anything you can think of to keep yourself entertained is a good idea. You may be able to rent television service. Consider bringing a tape machine or CD player with earphones so that you can listen to music. However, in some big-city hospitals you should be alert to the possibility of theft.

Feeling unwell and immobilized may reduce your appetite. Also, hospital food deserves its bland reputation. Sometimes it helps to have visitors bring you food that appeals to you. If you are not on a restricted diet, ask friends to bring you food from take-out restaurants or snacks that you can keep in your room.

Part Three
Understanding the Science

This part of the book contains short discussions of various technical topics for those who are curious. While learning more of the underlying scientific and technological material will enrich your understanding of HIV disease, you do not need to read these chapters in order to obtain good medical treatment. That's what you pay your doctor for.

Chapter 15: Details of Testing for HIV Infection covers technical aspects of various tests that help to detect HIV infection. Chapter 16: Immunology, Pathogenesis and Etiology combines a sketch of the functioning of the human immune system with a look at how HIV causes disease by disrupting immune function. Chapter 17: HIV—Virology and Therapeutic Strategies discusses the nature, structure, and operation of viruses, retroviruses, and HIV in particular. The chapter goes on to discuss how this information is used to design drugs and other therapies to control HIV. Chapter 18: Blood and Blood Cells provides in-depth information on this crucial body fluid. Chapter 19: Understanding Clinical Trials describes the medical experiments used to determine whether new drugs or other therapies are useful against HIV disease.

Chapter 15
Details of Testing for HIV Infection

LONG LATENCY STUDIES

The Centers for Disease Control (CDC) have long observed that virtually all HIV-infected people will develop detectable antibodies to the virus within three months of infection. In very rare cases people may take a little longer than three months following infection to test antibody positive. To leave a wide margin for error, the CDC recommends that a negative HIV antibody test should be considered fully meaningful only if six months has elapsed since the last possible risk for infection (episode of needle sharing or intercourse without a condom). This is sometimes called the *window period*. (Be careful to distinguish the relatively short window period for developing antibodies from the much longer eight- to twelve-year period that usually elapses between infection and serious illness from HIV.)

You may have read newspaper accounts that some people took longer than six months to test positive. The history of how this idea was proposed and then retracted is a good illustration of how scientists work.

In 1989, some researchers reported cases of HIV infection detectable by means other than the antibody test for long periods before the appearance of antibodies to HIV. They used the term *long latency* for the idea that HIV might have an unusually long period between infection and the generation of detectable antibodies. Reports of long latency greatly puzzled scientists and epidemiologists who had observed many thousands of actual cases: Why were these laboratory studies producing results that conflicted so dramatically with what epidemiologists observed in larger populations?

Most scientists do believe that long latency periods may occur in a tiny number of individuals. However, the overwhelming consensus is that these cases are likely to be very rare, particularly in people with low risk of exposure to HIV. The practical implications of this are that very few people will be infected, wait six months without risk, test negative, and then test positive at some later date.

At first glance the studies showing long latency raised many worries. But, after further examination of the experimental methodology used in these studies, scientists began to doubt that the results observed were necessarily correct or would necessarily carry over from small lab studies to the epidemiology of the general population. The methodological objections raised concerned chiefly the technique that was used to detect HIV in patients before the formation of antibodies. This technique—a DNA amplification technique called the *polymerase chain reaction,* or PCR—is based on a biochemical chain reaction that can be triggered by a single molecule of DNA. It is so sensitive that the tiniest contamination of test equipment with HIV genetic material from some source other than the sample being tested can cause a false positive. Contamination from previous tests (or even simply from samples of HIV stored nearby) is very hard to avoid.

Scientists observed that these results (based on quite a small number of subjects) contradicted the large body of experience acquired by observing many tens of thousands of cases of HIV infection over the past decade. In 1991 the authors of the long-latency studies confirmed that they could not reproduce their own results. At this point, it is safe to assume that long latency is very rare. Six months allows plenty of time for HIV antibodies to develop—in most cases they will be detectable within three months.

TECHNICAL DETAILS OF THE ELISA TEST

HIV from a laboratory source is grown in human white blood cells in the test tube. The resultant virus is chemically disrupted and then used to coat a small container or well. *Serum* (the cell-free portion of blood) from the person being tested is added to the coated well. If antibody to HIV is present, it will bind with the viral fragments lining the well. The serum is then washed away, leaving only the attached antibody behind. Another preparation is then added to the well. This preparation contains antibodies to human antibodies. These antiantibodies have been chemically attached to an enzyme, and the whole complex binds to the HIV antibody left in the well from the subject's serum. The well is then washed again to remove any material that has not bound to HIV antibody. Finally a substance is added that reacts with the enzyme linked to the antiantibody, producing a visible color change. This color change is then measured with a photometer (a device that measures the color of light reflected from the well). If the color change is over a preset threshold, the result is positive.

TECHNICAL DETAILS OF THE WESTERN BLOT TEST

The Western blot is performed by exposing a specially prepared paper test strip to the blood sample. This strip is made in the following way. A quantity of HIV is grown in test tube cultures of human cells. The virus is isolated from the growth medium and disrupted into its component pieces. Each of these components is a molecule with a characteristic *molecular weight.* These components are then sorted by weight through a process called *gel electrophoresis.* In this process the solution of disrupted virus with the different component molecules mixed together is applied to one end of a sheet of polyacrylimide gel, a special porous material. An electric field is applied across the sheet, and this field accelerates molecules of different weights at different rates. At the end of a period of time, the mix of different components will separate into *bands* across the gel, with the lighter molecules at one end and the heavier molecules at the other. Each band contains molecules of a certain molecular weight—that is, each band contains only one kind of antigen. The gel is then blotted onto a sheet of paper, and this sheet is then cut into strips, each of which contains the full set of bands (complement of antigens).

As with the ELISA, the strip is exposed to the blood sample to allow any antibodies in the blood to react with the antigens in the strip. The strip is then washed so that any free unbound antibody is removed. Then the strip is exposed to a special anti-human globulin that binds to any human antibody. This anti-human globulin will combine with HIV antibodies that may have bound to bands in the test strip. The anti-human globulin is tagged with a normally colorless enzyme that reacts with a substrate to produce visibly colored bands wherever HIV antibody binds to the test strip. The intensity and location of these visible bands indicates the presence and relative proportion of the different antibodies that were present in the blood sample.

The formal interpretation of the Western blot depends on which combinations of two or more bands are present in a particular sample.

TECHNICAL DETAILS OF DNA AMPLIFICATION

DNA amplification is a method of detecting the presence of very small amounts of a known DNA sequence. One DNA amplification test uses a technique known as the *polymerase chain reaction,* or PCR, to increase the number of copies of the target DNA sequence to the point where the DNA can be detected by conventional chemical assays. DNA amplification is enormously useful for a variety of purposes, including testing for HIV infection in those situations where HIV antibody testing may not provide information, such as soon after infection or in newborns who passively carry maternal antibodies to HIV. However, this test is difficult to perform correctly—false positives may occur if the sample is contaminated with even a single copy of the target DNA.

DNA replicates if four conditions are met: the ordinarily double-stranded DNA is separated into single strands at a certain point; the single strand is chemically primed for replication; the enzyme *polymerase* is available to catalyze the replication reaction at this site; and sufficient quantities of raw materials for replication (called *nucleotide triphosphates*) are available near the replication site.

In PCR, the sample DNA is heated (*denatured*) to separate the double strands into single strands. DNA polymerase and raw nucleotides can be synthesized in quantity and added to the denatured sample DNA. That leaves the problem of priming the single strands. In order to use PCR to detect a target region of DNA, two short sequences of bases at either end of the region are synthesized to provide a large quantity of *primer molecules* that attach to the single-stranded samples on either side of the target region.

If you start with a sample that contains at least two complementary strands of known target DNA sequence, the steps involved in DNA amplification are as follows:

- Add appropriate synthetic primers to the sample
- Heat the mixture to separate the DNA into single strands
- Lower the temperature to allow the primers to bind onto the DNA strands
- Now you have two single strands with short double-strand primers
- Add polymerase and nucleotide triphosphates (raw materials for DNA replication)
- The polymerase makes new DNA in between the primed segments
- When finished, the process has doubled the number of copies of the target sequence

Repeat this cycle until a detectable amount of the target DNA has been made.

These primer sequences must be conserved across genetic variants of the organism if the test is to be sufficiently sensitive. If genetic variability among different strains of HIV allows mutants that have different sequences than those used as primers, then PCR will not amplify the mutant HIV DNA, and the test will have a falsely negative result. This problem can be reduced if multiple pairs of primers are used so as to increase the chance that at least one pair will work with any strain of HIV that might be present in the sample.

Chapter 16
Immunology, Pathogenesis, and Etiology

IMMUNOLOGY: A SKETCH OF THE IMMUNE SYSTEM

Consider the task facing the human immune system. The human organism is a huge collection of billions of cells, substances, and structures, adapted to protect and propagate each individual's genes. The human body exists in an environment populated by other organisms, some of which are cooperative, some neutral, and some harmfully competitive.

Just as thousands of years of evolution have produced instincts and capabilities that help humans survive when threatened by large complex organisms (e.g., tigers), evolution has also guided the development of a complex set of strategies for coping with threats on a microscopic scale. Such tiny threats include both infections by microorganisms and the misbehavior of the body's own cells (such as cells transformed by cancer or viruses).

It is hard to understand what is currently known about the immune system. Partly this is due to the fact that we simply do not know enough about the immune system to have formed good coherent models. But part of the untidiness of the immune system is inherent in the nature of evolutionary development. Evolution is ingenious but unscrupulously opportunistic. It operates incrementally, is fabulously crafty, and loves to use its creations for multiple purposes and in overlapping ways. It cares little for tying up loose ends or for making systems that we might find compact and simple to understand.

We have presented here a simplified model of the immune system, focusing on those aspects most relevant to HIV. With these caveats, let's begin with a description of the actual composition of the immune system.

▲ Parts of the Immune System

The immune system is composed of the lymphatic circulatory system, the white blood cells, and the lymphoid organs.

Lymphatic circulatory system: When we think of the circulatory system, we generally think of blood vessels such as veins, arteries, and capillaries. There is, however, an entire parallel circulatory system called the *lymphatic system,* set aside for the use of the immune system. This system circulates *lymph,* a yellow watery fluid that surrounds the body's tissues—*lymph* is Greek for "water." Lymph transports white cells and dissolved material around the body. The system consists of a network of lymph vessels that drain lymph from around all the body's tissues. These vessels deliver lymph to *lymph nodes,* numerous pea-sized structures scattered through the body that store white cells and allow them to communicate with each other. Smaller lymph vessels drain into larger lymph vessels until finally the entire lymphatic system discharges into the bloodstream through a vessel in the chest called the *thoracic duct.*

White cells in blood, lymph, and tissue: White blood cells (or *leukocytes*) are the major active component of the immune system. Although they are commonly called white *blood* cells, they also appear in fluids other than blood and throughout body tissue as well.

White cells come in a great variety of types. We will briefly describe the major categories here and leave detailed description of the function of various types for later.

White blood cells are divided into *phagocytes* and *lymphocytes.* Phagocytes (or "eater cells") are large cells that engulf and digest all sorts of debris and unwanted material in the body, both foreign microorganisms and worn-out body cells.

Phagocytes are divided into *macrophages/monocytes* and *granulocytes* (granule-containing cells). Macrophage/monocytes begin activity in the bloodstream: at this point they are called *monocytes* (the "mono-" prefix refers to the monocyte's single-lobed nucleus). When monocytes enter tissue they change and develop into *macrophages* of various types. Macrophages ("big eaters") have many regulatory and transport functions that they carry out in addition to their general search-and-destroy mission throughout the body. Some examples of macrophages are microglial cells in the brain, Langerhans cells in the skin (a type of *dendritic* or "treelike" cell), and Kupffer cells in the liver.

Granulocytes share the property that they contain special sacs (or granules) that store certain useful chemicals for quick release. Often these sacs of chemicals are used to destroy microorganisms. The nuclei of granulocytes have multiple lobes, hence the distinction from monocytes. Granulocytes in circulation include *basophils, neutrophils,* and *eosinophils* (named as to whether they take up basic, neutral, or acidic stains used for microscopy). Granulocytes in tissue are called *mast cells.*

Lymphocytes will be the cells we discuss in most detail. They are so called because they are often found in lymph fluid. They are smaller than phagocytes and come in three basic types: T lymphocytes, B lymphocytes, and "natural killer" or NK lymphocytes.

There are also noncirculating parts of the immune system located all over the body. **Primary lymphoid organs and tissues** include the bone marrow, the thymus gland (located under the breastbone), and the spleen (in the abdomen). There are also smaller clumps of lymphoid tissue in the tonsils, adenoids, appendix, in areas of the gastrointestinal tract called Peyer's patches, and in miscellaneous places throughout the body.

▲ Distributed Rather Than Centralized Activity

Immune cells interact as populations of individuals: It is easier to understand organs such as the heart than to understand the immune system. The heart is a discrete organ with a definite size and location. We can use our everyday ideas about electricity and fluids to imagine how the heart's signals and pumping action might work. The immune system is quite different in two ways. First, it is made largely of many different populations of physically separate, widely distributed individual cells. Second, these cells are not controlled from some central source or signal, but instead act like a hive of bees, or like a city of people. Each cell is on its own, but information from other cells nearby guides its behavior and development. The overall behavior of the immune system is actually the statistical aggregate of the individual actions of its component cells.

Immune cells communicate in two ways: either by directly touching another cell or via the release and detection of messenger chemicals called *cytokines* (literally, "cell-movers").

Cells interact directly via receptors: Cells protect their contents from the environment with a *membrane,* a flexible envelope composed of a double layer of fat molecules. Embedded in every cell's membrane are thousands of copies of various gateway molecules called *receptors.* Receptors give the cell information about its chemical environment and help control the passage of substances into and out of the cell.

Two immune cells can communicate if they are in close proximity and each has the appropriate receptor for the other. If the receptors bind chemically this information is communicated to the contents of the cell, and various events may occur in response.

There is a great variety of receptor types. Immune cells spend a lot of time bumping up against one another, looking for the correct fit. One of the functions of lymph nodes is to provide a good place for immune cells to contact one another. This increases the chance that a cell can give its message to the correct type of recipient.

Cells use cytokines to talk to cells both nearby and far away: Different types of cells manufacture different types of cytokines—the messenger chemicals. Lymphocytes make *lymphokines,* and macrophage/monocytes make *monokines.*

Some cytokines operate on one cell at close range. For instance, by binding directly to receptors on certain cells and then releasing lymphokines, one type of T cell gives permission for other cells to develop and complete their function.

Some cytokines operate at a distance and may affect the behavior of many other cells. For example, the activation of an immune cell may result in the release of cytokines that diffuse away from the site and attract other immune cells to the site of an infection.

Movement of foreign material through system: Material from outside the body generally enters through the gastrointestinal tract, lungs, or through other mucous membranes. Before being passed into the bloodstream, useful material such as food is broken down into simple molecules that do not attract the attention of the immune system. Anything more complex may get eaten by part of the nonspecific defenses of the body, such as phagocytes. Phagocytes and other cells transport the things they eat to the lymph nodes to show to lymphocytes. Lymphocytes look at these pieces and selectively generate further immune responses. Some lymphocytes then record having seen this type of foreign material, ready to respond quickly if they see it again in the future. Remaining foreign material processed by the immune system is ultimately digested by macrophages in the liver called Kupffer cells or by macrophages in the spleen.

▲ Nonspecific ("Native") Immunity

The immune system has evolved many separate (but interrelated) defense mechanisms. Some threats are common in the environment and easily chemically identified as a general class. For instance, bacteria are ubiquitous and most have cell walls that can be identified and easily distinguished from human cells. Evolution has consequently favored organisms with substantial fixed resources constantly devoted to defending in a nonspecific fashion against common ubiquitous problems. These defenses are always in place and do not require previous exposure to the threat. This is sometimes called the "native" immune system.

Some threats are less common, or may appear only in certain subpopulations. It is desirable to be able to defend against rarer threats, but it is costly (given finite resources) to maintain such defenses continuously. Evolution has favored organisms that, rather than devoting a large fixed set of resources to defending against relatively rare problems, instead developed a flexible system of *specific* and *adaptive* defenses that can be mobilized as needed. The *adaptive* branch of the immune system requires a small amount of time to become effective after initial exposure to a specific threat. Once a specific threat has been successfully countered, the adaptive immune system is thereafter vigilant for and able to respond quickly to that threat.

The native immune system includes phagocytes, natural killer cells, and a collection of chemicals called *complement*.

Phagocytes are programmed to destroy a variety of predictable threats. Phagocytes have distinct appetites—for instance, neutrophils nonspecifically eat many types of bacteria. A decline in neutrophils (such as occurs as a side effect of some drugs) thus may disastrously hurt the body's ability to control bacterial infections.

Natural killer cells are a type of lymphocyte that resemble phagocytes in their ability to bind nonspecifically to undesirable cells and release destructive chemicals.

The term **complement** describes a large group of circulating proteins that act in a coordinated *cascade.* These proteins coat foreign material to make it appetizing to phagocytes, stimulate other immune cells to respond, and form themselves into an amazing molecular "can opener" that punctures the membranes of undesirable cells.

▲ Immune Globulins Allow Specific ("Adaptive") Immunity

The adaptive immune system depends on proteins called *immune globulins* to recognize and respond to less common threats. Each immune globulin is able to recognize only one specific molecule, called an *antigen.* Examples of immune globulins are *antibodies,* and the antigen-specific *receptors* on lymphocytes.

The variety of human immune globulins evolved (like the variety of animal or insect species) via mutation and natural selection. Two pressures have affected the evolution of the body's repertoire of immune globulins. It is clearly desirable to protect against as many different threats as possible, so there is a strong pressure toward diversity and variation of immune globulins. The body is in fact able to recognize hundreds of millions of different antigens.

The second pressure is for a compact genetic encoding of these globulins. Humans have a lot of DNA, but not enough to code straightforwardly for hundreds of millions of immune globulins. The DNA instructions required to manufacture a large number of different immune globulins would simply be impossibly long if the instructions were placed end to end. Human DNA therefore contains instructions for only a few thousands of different *pieces* that are then mixed together (*recombined*) in many different ways to produce the ultimate immune globulins.

The immune system has thus evolved to recognize a bigger repertoire of antigens than it might otherwise. But this brings problems of its own. The recombination process means that there is less control over which immune globulins get made. As a result, some immune globulins are useful, some are useless, and some are actually harmful. In our discussion of T4 helper/inducer cells, which follows, we will describe how the body prevents the expression of harmful immune globulins.

Antibodies typically are Y-shaped complex proteins. The tips of the two branches of the Y bind to the antigen and differ for each type of antibody. When antibody binds to antigen the result is called *immune complex.* The stem of the Y is similar for all antibodies, and provides an easily recognizable "handle" so that the native immune system can continue the processing and disposal of immune complexes.

There are nine types of antibody, which fall into five classes. Immune globulin type G, or IgG, comes in four types and is present throughout the circulation and in tissue. IgM is found in circulation and is good at killing bacteria. IgA comes in two types and is secreted from cells in mucous membranes—it provides an immediate barrier against antigen that might enter through the mucosa. IgE is found only in small amounts—it is responsible for allergic reactions, although its useful function is not well understood. IgD is found in the membranes of B lymphocytes, and its function is not well understood either.

Antibodies and immune complex have a number of functions. Some antibodies attach directly to toxins and chemically neutralize them. Some antibodies coat cells, forming immune complexes that mark the cells for disposal by scavengers or destruction by natural killer cells (a process known as *antibody-dependent cellular cytotoxicity,* or ADCC). Antibodies and immune complex can activate the complement cascade. Some antibodies block the access of viruses to cells by occupying the surface receptors used for entry.

Normally, immune complex is removed from circulation and digested by Kupffer cells (a type of macrophage) in the liver and macrophages in the spleen. If too much immune complex accumulates in the body, it can clog up circulation and lymph nodes. The presence of large persistent immune complexes plays a role in many autoimmune diseases.

Lymphocytes have antigen-specific receptors: In addition to floating freely as antibodies, immune globulins appear in the form of antigen-specific receptors that occur in the membranes of lymphocytes. Lymphocytes are divided into three main groups: B lymphocytes, T lymphocytes, and natural killer cells (NK cells, described above). All lymphocytes are derived from precursor cells in the bone marrow. Some lymphocytes then migrate to the thymus gland to develop further and are therefore called T cells (T = thymus), while those that develop further in the bone marrow before entering general circulation are called B cells (B = bone marrow).

B (bone marrow) and T (thymus) lymphocytes both have the ability to recognize specific antigens by virtue of the receptors embedded in their surfaces. B cells have the additional ability to secrete a soluble immune globulin that is a variation of these receptors. This protein product of B cells is what we call antibodies. As described above, genetic recombination provides a large variety of basic templates for B cells to use in making receptors and antibodies. B cells also mutate, potentially producing totally new immune globulins. Each B cell can make exactly one type of immune globulin matching exactly one antigen. While there are hundreds of millions of different possible globulins that can be made, each globulin is initially represented by only a small number of B cells. Some B cells are programmed to make useful immune globulins, some can make useless globulins, and some can make potentially harmful globulins.

B cells are distinguished by their ability to recognize raw, free antigen.

Receptors on a B cell's surface bind to such antigen. The immune complex thus formed is brought into the B cell and broken apart. This *processed* antigen is then displayed on the surface of the B cell for inspection by T helper cells. B cells present processed antigen to T helper cells to determine whether the antigen is native to the body (*self*) or foreign (*nonself*). If a T helper cell recognizes the processed antigen, it gives its permission to proceed. Once it has obtained permission from a T helper cell, the B cell divides repeatedly (*clonal expansion*). The resulting daughter cells then develop into large antibody factories called *plasma cells*. Some activated B cells become *memory cells* instead of plasma cells. Memory cells do not produce antibody but instead wait, ready to respond quickly in the future to the same antigen.

T (thymus) cells differ from B cells in a number of respects. Although they share a common origin in the bone marrow, T cells migrate to a gland under the breastbone called the thymus to continue their development and differentiation. Before arriving at the thymus gland, T cells (like B cells) recombine for variety. The thymus gland somehow eliminates those T cells that might allow a harmful immune response against the body's own cells. In this way, the thymus works by manipulating the original population of T cells. In order to preserve the work of the thymus, T cells (unlike B cells) do not mutate.

T cells evolve into three different forms, named after characteristic receptors on their membranes and characteristic behavior. *Helper/inducer* T4 cells that implement the self/nonself distinction are marked with a receptor molecule named CD4; *killer* T8 cells carry the receptor named CD8 and destroy cells bearing a specific matching antigen; *suppressor* T8 cells also carry the CD8 receptor and act to damp down specific immune responses. Nomenclature is often used interchangeably: you will often hear the same set of cells called helper cells, inducer cells, T4 cells, CD4+ cells, or even called OKT4 cells, after the substance used to detect them in the laboratory (the OKT4 *monoclonal antibody*).

▲ Self/Nonself Distinction and MHC Restriction

The body needs to be able to recognize and protect its own cells and recognize and attack foreign cells. The body also needs to be able to identify cells belonging to the immune system.

Every cell in an individual human is labeled with copies of a special "password" molecule called the *class I major histocompatibility complex* (Class I MHC). These molecules are all the same within one individual, but differ from person to person. In addition to Class I MHC, immune system cells also carry molecules of Class II MHC, which (like the badge of a police officer) confer extra rights and duties. The presence and recognition of these two types of password molecules is called *MHC restriction*.

One of the functions of mature T4 cells is to implement the lesson learned in the thymus: the distinction between *self* and *nonself*. All types of T cells require some interaction with antigen-presenting cells or with mature T4 cells to complete their maturation and become fully active.

The surface membrane of a T4 helper lymphocyte is studded with receptor molecules called CD4. T4 cells recognize processed antigens presented with Class II MHC marker (found only on macrophages and B cells). As described above, mature T4 cells stimulate the correct clonal expansion of B cells. Mature T4 cells also act with macrophages to stimulate the maturation of killer T8 cells.

T8 suppressor and T8 killer cells have CD8 receptors: T8 lymphocytes carry CD8 receptor molecules in their membranes. T8 cells fall into two classes: *cytotoxic* or *killer* T8 cells, and *suppressor* T8 cells.

Cytotoxic T8 cells recognize processed antigen with Class I MHC marker (found on most body cells). Incompatible Class I MHC marker may be made by cells transformed by cancer or viral infection—such cells will be attacked by killer T8 cells.

T8 suppressor cells have a different function: they balance the activation of T4 help cells to help to turn off the immune reaction to a specific antigen.

Antigen presentation: Lymph nodes and other lymphoid tissue provide good opportunity and environment for presentation of antigens to lymphocytes. Antigen-presenting cells include macrophage/monocytes, B cells, and dendritic cells.

▲ Normal Immune Processes Cause Tissue Damage

The operation of the immune system normally involves some damage to tissue at the area of the infection or cancer under attack. The heat, swelling, and redness associated with inflammation are characteristic signs of the immune system at work, as lymphokines and complement cause blood vessels to dilate and cause membranes to allow fluid and cells to enter the area.

Inflammation works well as a weapon against relatively localized problems: if only a small amount of tissue is sacrificed the body can usually recover and heal. If the inflammation is more generalized and more intense, much healthy tissue may be destroyed, resulting in a loss of function or even death. Inflammation may in and of itself be dangerous: pneumonia may be deadly not because the causative organism is directly toxic but because the immune response inflames the lungs so much that breathing becomes impossible.

Evolution has favored this type of aggressive immune response to protect relatively healthy individuals of child-bearing age who suffer from minor infections and microscopic cancers. However, this aggressive immune response may sometimes be more dangerous than the disease itself. Evolution plays the percentages: the immune response protects those sick individuals who have a better chance of recovery (and hence reproduction) and sacrifices other sick individuals in the process.

Physicians will sometimes use steroid medications to suppress such harmful immune responses. For instance, acute *Pneumocystis carinii* pneumonia is now often treated with a combination of antibiotics and steroids.

▲ Immune System Problems

In addition to immune deficiencies such as AIDS, there are a number of serious problems that can affect the immune system: autoimmune diseases, allergies, and cancers.

In **autoimmune disease** the body's mechanisms for distinguishing self from nonself break down. The immune system attacks healthy tissue in the body. Harmful antibodies may begin to be produced against antigens that appear in normal tissue, causing the immune system to destroy cells bearing that antigen. The immune system may attack any of a number of cell types, causing different problems: blood cells, causing anemia; insulin-producing cells in the pancreas, causing diabetes; the fatty myelin lining of nerve fibers in the central or peripheral nervous system, causing multiple sclerosis or myasthenia gravis; or connective tissues, causing systemic lupus erythematosus.

Allergy/sensitivity: Allergies are inappropriate immune reactions to harmless elements in the environment such as dust, pollen, or animal fur. Familiar symptoms of allergy include runny nose, congestion, and teary or itchy eyes. Less common symptoms may include fever or rash as is seen with many allergies to medications.

Allergies appear to be caused by a specialized immune mechanism of unclear purpose. Anything that causes an allergy is called an *allergen.* When the immune system is initially exposed to an allergen, B cells manufacture immune globulin type E (IgE) in response. This IgE then migrates to granulocytes (mast cells in tissue or basophils in circulation), where it becomes embedded in the cell membrane. The next presentation of the allergen is quickly detected by the IgE in the membrane of these mast cells or basophils, which cause allergic symptoms when they release chemicals stored in their granules such as *histamines* and *prostaglandins.*

Allergic reactions vary in severity from very mild to potentially fatal. Very dangerous allergic reactions may be controllable with steroids that suppress the immune system.

Cancers: Since the cells of the immune system are widely distributed and often in circulation, cancers of the immune system may not necessarily appear as discrete localized tumors. Examples of such distributed cancers are *leukemia,* or cancer of white blood cells, and *multiple myeloma,* or cancer of the antibody-producing plasma cells that derive from activated B cells. Immune system cancers also include *lymphomas,* cancers of clusters of lymphoid tissue such as lymph nodes.

PATHOGENESIS: A SKETCH OF HOW HIV CAUSES DISEASE

▲ HIV Causes Immune Deficiency

CD4 receptor: Each particle of HIV carries many copies of a protein called gp120 attached to its membrane. This protein has a strong affinity for (or ability to bind to) the CD4 molecule that characteristically appears on the surface of T4 lymphocytes.

T4 lymphocytes are therefore subject to infection by HIV. This subset of immune cells seems to bear the brunt of HIV infection. **But many other body cells are also capable of being infected with the virus.** Cells that present processed antigen to T cells for recognition (including many varieties of macrophages/monocytes) may also carry the CD4 molecule and therefore may be infected with HIV. The virus has a variety of effects on different cells.

▲ T Cell Defects

The most noticeable consequence of HIV infection is *leukopenia,* or a decrease in the number of white blood cells. This decrease is largely attributable to a decline in the number of T4 lymphocytes. HIV is hypothesized to destroy T4 cells in a number of ways.

In T4 cells in which HIV is replicating quickly, so many particles of virus may accumulate that the cell simply breaks open, an event called **lysis.**

Syncytia formation: HIV-infected T4 cells make and display the viral product gp120 on their surfaces. This gp120 may then bind to the CD4 molecules on the surfaces of uninfected T4 cells. Once bound at multiple points the two cell membranes may fuse, creating a large cell with more than one nucleus. The process of fusion may then continue with more and more uninfected T4 cells. These *giant multinucleated cells,* or *syncytia* ("cells together"), are not able to function properly, clog up the works, and eventually die or are destroyed by the immune system.

Natural killer cells or killer T8 cells may be alerted by the display of viral proteins and attack infected T4 cells directly.

In addition to the fact that HIV infection reduces the number of T4 cells available, it also seems to **reduce the effectiveness of the T4 cells that remain.** HIV-infected T4 cells react sluggishly to antigen-presenting cells and provide decreased stimulation to the immune cells that depend on T4 signals.

Killer T8 cells require permission from T4 cells before they can mature and begin their cytotoxic function. **HIV-infected T4 cells are less able to provide the signals that killer T8 cells need to mature.**

Normally, activated T4 cells stimulate other T cells to divide repeatedly, forming large genetically identical groups of cells *(clones).* This **decreased clonal expansion of T cells** limits the intensity of specific immune responses.

Failure to mount immune response to new antigens: HIV-infected T4 cells do not respond normally to antigen-presenting cells. If an antigen was seen before T4 cell dysfunction began, then part of the immune response is already in place. For instance, memory B cells are ready to become antibody-producing plasma cells, and may do so to some degree independently of T4 cells. However, the cell-killing branch of the immune system requires permission from T4 cells even to operate against an antigen seen once before.

HIV-infected T4 cells often do not respond correctly to new antigens. This means that a new antigen may provoke neither cell-killing nor even an antibody response (neither *cellular* nor *humoral* immunity). As an example, HIV-infected people may not respond at all to standard doses of common vaccines.

▲ Macrophage Dysfunction

Macrophages are a major reservoir of HIV in the body. HIV does not destroy macrophages as it does T4 lymphocytes. Because macrophages move about the body and communicate with many other immune cells, they have great potential to transmit HIV to all the cells they touch. In addition to being vectors of infection, the function of macrophages is affected for the worse.

HIV-infected macrophages seem to lose much of their appetite for consuming bacteria and immune complexes. This *decreased phagocytosis* is the first in a number of ways in which HIV interferes with the normal steps in the processing of antigen.

Even if antigen has successfully been eaten, HIV-infected macrophages are less efficient at presenting it to T4 cells. This only adds to the problem that T4 cells have in responding.

▲ B Cell Defects

B cells are also affected by HIV infection. B cells, like macrophages, become less able to present antigen to T4 cells. Many different genetic types (or clones) of B cells also become inappropriately activated simultaneously (*polyclonal B cell activation*) in the absence of the correct antigenic stimulus. This results in the purposeless manufacture of large quantities of antibodies, called *hypergammaglobulinemia.* These useless antibodies may form immune complexes that are difficult to clear from the body.

In the setting of HIV infection, B cells may make antibodies against a variety of healthy body components, including lymphocytes, platelets (clotting elements in the blood), myelin (the fatty covering of nerve fibers), and components of cell nuclei. This autoimmune response may occur because T4 cells fail to maintain the distinction between self and nonself. HIV-induced autoimmunity is not well understood but may be responsible for many mysterious symptoms of the disease, including various anemias and neuropathies.

337

▲ NK Cell Dysfunction

As has been described above, natural killer (NK) cells are a vital part of the natural or nonspecific immune system. NK cells, phagocytes, and killer T8 cells together provide the only protection against infected or cancerous body cells. NK cell activity is markedly decreased in an HIV-infected individual.

▲ Other Lymphoid Tissue Damage

In addition to destroying or interfering with white blood cells, HIV infection also seems to cause damage to lymphoid tissue. Part of the thymus gland (the *epithelium*)—critical for T4 cell function—is damaged in what appears to be an autoimmune reaction. Also, the internal structure of lymph nodes changes and degenerates in a manner visible under the microscope. The exact cause and meaning of this damage is not known, but it seems significant.

▲ Clinical Consequences

Opportunistic infections: HIV-related immune deficiency causes resurgence of a certain limited group of latent pathogens that are usually controlled by reliance on cell-killing mechanisms:

- Viruses reside inside body cells, where they cannot be neutralized by antibodies.
- Intracellular parasites hide from the immune system inside body cells. Other parasites may have stages of their life cycle in which they hide in cysts or other enclosures.
- Mycobacteria and encapsulated bacteria may also escape antibodies.

Some disease in HIV-infected people is due to new infection, not to the reactivation of latent infection. Because HIV-infected T4 cells are less responsive to new antigens, the immune response to a new infection is sluggish. The new infection has more opportunity to establish itself before the mobilization of the body's defenses.

General immune deficiency may also increase disease caused by common pathogens. On the other hand, overactivation of the immune system in some phases of disease may actually reduce the incidence of some common illnesses. Some people in the early stages of HIV disease "haven't had a cold in years."

Neoplasms (cancers): There are three main theories about why certain cancers appear in HIV disease. It may be that opportunistic cancer-causing viruses take advantage of the immune deficiency to flourish. Failure of cellular immune surveillance secondary to HIV infection may allow microscopic cancers to grow that would otherwise have been detected and destroyed. Immune dysregulation may cause overproduction of selected growth factors. Thus, a vascularization growth factor may be responsible for the abnormal growth of the lining of blood vessels seen in Kaposi's sarcoma.

Direct HIV or HIV-product damage: The viral product gp120 or the direct action of the virus itself may kill cells in the brain or the lining of the intestines. This may explain the dementia and wasting associated with the disease.

ETIOLOGY: CAN WE BE SURE THAT HIV CAUSES AIDS?

During the course of the AIDS epidemic, there has been some controversy about whether HIV is the cause of AIDS. Although this debate continues in some areas, it is no longer considered a question among almost all scientists who are expert in HIV disease; scientific consensus is that infection with HIV is necessary to cause AIDS. This does not

CRITICISMS OF HIV AS THE CAUSE OF AIDS, WITH RESPONSES

Duesberg's Argument	Response
Not everyone with HIV develops the symptoms of AIDS	Development of AIDS in HIV infected people increases over time. At least 30% of HIV-infected people get AIDS within five years. Over time, increasing percentages of HIV-infected people develop AIDS. The best mathematical models project that over 90% of HIV-infected people will develop serious symptoms within 14 years of infection.
Circulating particles of HIV cannot be found in all AIDS patients	Earlier in the epidemic, laboratory techniques for culturing HIV were not well developed, and consequently the virus was often hard to detect in the blood of patients. Now that better laboratory tests exist for establishing the presence of the virus, 90% to 100% of people with AIDS can be shown to have circulating virus.
HIV does not infect enough of the white blood cells called T4 lymphocytes to be fatal	Although HIV may infect only a minority of the white blood cells called T4 lymphocytes, it does damage to many more by indirect mechanisms, including suppression of T4 cell growth factor, agglomeration of infected and uninfected T4 cells into dysfunctional giant multinucleated cells (*syncytia*), and binding of free gp 120 to uninfected T4 cells, marking them for elimination. The principal reservoir of HIV in the body is not T4 cells but other white blood cells called monocytes/macrophages and lymphoid tissue.
Since the body develops a relatively high level of antibodies to HIV, HIV cannot cause serious disease	A number of viruses provoke production of antibodies that do not neutralize virus inside cells. These include herpes simplex, varicella zoster, hepatitis B, and a number of slow-activating animal viruses. In fact, a number of diseases caused by slow-activating animal viruses resemble HIV disease in their form: long latency, slow damage to the immune system, and killing of white blood cells in culture.

address the question of whether some other factor(s) may play a role in determining the course of the disease.

Peter Duesberg, a molecular biologist, is the most respected critic of HIV's causative role in AIDS. A few of his arguments and the scientific refutations follow, drawn from reports of a scientific forum on the topic sponsored by the American Foundation for AIDS Research (AmFAR) in Washington, D.C., on April 9, 1988.

Chapter 17
HIV: Virology and Therapeutic Strategies

VIROLOGY OF HIV

VIRUSES AND RETROVIRUSES

Viruses are protein-shelled particles containing genetic material (composed of *nucleic acids*). Viruses also sometimes contain *enzymes*, which are complex proteins that enable very specific chemical reactions, in effect acting as tiny machines that assemble and disassemble other molecules. Viruses sometimes have an enclosing fatty (*lipid*) membrane. Viruses have no ability to reproduce on their own and are completely reliant upon the host cell to make the proteins the virus needs for reproduction.

HIV is an unusual type of virus called a *retrovirus,* or "reverse virus." The name stems from the fact that retroviruses reverse part of the usual path by which genes make proteins.

▲ Protein Synthesis
The normal course of human protein synthesis follows a strict sequence of events. The instructions that define and operate the human cell are encoded onto a few dozen very long, double-stranded molecules of *deoxyribonucleic acid* (DNA, the famous double helix). Each of these molecules of DNA contains tens of thousands of individual genes. Each gene describes a protein.

Based on complex chemical cues that reach the nucleus, a gene may become *activated.* An activated gene is *transcribed* by enzymes into ribonucleic acid (RNA), a single-stranded copy of that gene's DNA. The new RNA molecule then leaves the nucleus. Outside the nucleus, cellular machines called *ribosomes* use this RNA to make proteins from chemical building blocks called *amino acids* or *peptides.*

Just as we combine the letters of the alphabet into sequences that form words, DNA strings together a small repertoire of codes to "spell" or encode instructions for each amino acid. There are only four letters in the genetic alphabet, each one a single molecule called a *base* or *nucleotide.* There are only sixty-four words in the genetic vocabulary, and each one is exactly three letters long. Each genetic word (or *codon*) stands for just one of twenty amino acids (the code overlaps, so that some words stand for the same amino acid). Just as we string words together to form sentences, ribosomes join a long string of amino acids together, forming a protein. Every protein folds itself into a characteristic shape by virtue of chemical bonds that form between its parts. The varied properties of the many thousands of proteins and enzymes used by the human body derive from this shape.

In the ordinary course of events, DNA is always transcribed into RNA, which is then used by ribosomes to make protein.

▲ Normal Viral Behavior

Classic viruses use either DNA or RNA as their genetic material. If the virus uses RNA, the host cell uses the viral RNA to make proteins in the usual way. The resulting viral proteins are then assembled into new virus particles (*virions*). If the virus uses DNA, then its first step is to force the host cell to transcribe the DNA into RNA. After this, protein synthesis proceeds as usual. The usual flow of information from DNA to RNA to protein is respected.

▲ Retroviral Behavior

Retroviruses use RNA as their genetic material, but use an enzyme called *reverse transcriptase* to reverse the usual DNA-to-RNA transcription process. Reverse transcriptase forces the cell to copy the virus's RNA into DNA, the opposite of the usual flow of information in the cell.

Newly made viral DNA migrates to the nucleus, where it is incorporated into the cell's own native DNA. The part of an infected host's DNA that encodes the retrovirus is called the *provirus*. If the host cell divides, the provirus divides right along with rest of the host DNA, and the latent retroviral infection is passed along to the daughter cells. Some nonretroviral DNA viruses such as the herpes viruses may also integrate their genetic material into the host cell's DNA. In consequence, infections such as herpes and HIV are lifelong: once part of cellular DNA, the provirus cannot be eradicated with current medical technology.

HIV'S PHYSICAL STRUCTURE

A particle of HIV is encapsulated with a lipid (fatty) membrane studded with protein spikes. The viral membrane is derived from the membrane of the host cell. Inside the virus's membrane is a spherical protein shell. Inside this shell is a tapered cylinder of protein that with its contents forms the *core complex* of the virus. The core complex contains both the genetic material of the virus (RNA sheathed in a protein coat) and the virus's enzymes (*reverse transcriptase/ribonuclease H, HIV integrase,* and *HIV protease*).

Many of HIV's component molecules are named on the basis of their chemical type and their molecular weight. For instance, the viral core protein is named *p24* while the viral spike protein is named *gp120*. The prefix *p* stands for protein and the prefix *gp* stands for *glycoprotein,* a molecule made of a complex sugar (*carbohydrate*) and a protein. The numbers that follow these prefixes are an abbreviation of the molecular weight (roughly, the size) of the molecule, expressed in the unit *kilodaltons.* Thus, gp120 is a 120-kilodalton glycoprotein.

The accompanying diagram shows the name and location of the components of the virus. Of particular importance for our purposes are gp120 (which is responsible for the virus's preference for the CD4 receptor that appears on many immune system cells) and p24 (which provides a useful measure of viral activity).

DRUG STRATEGIES TO DISRUPT HIV'S REPRODUCTIVE CYCLE

There are six major steps in the course of the reproductive cycle of the virus that may provide opportunities for anti-HIV drug therapy: attachment, uncoating, reverse transcription, protein synthesis, particle assembly, and budding. A description of each of these steps follows, together with a brief sketch of possibilities for intervention with drugs.

Of the drugs mentioned, the vast majority are experimental, not

Physical Structure of HIV

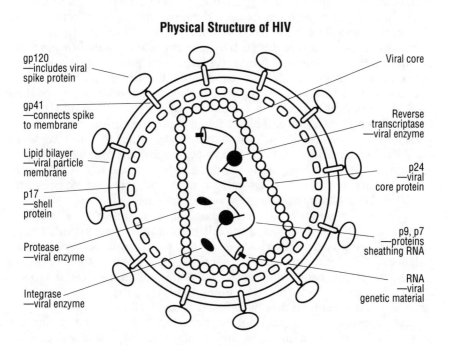

gp120
—includes viral spike protein

gp41
—connects spike to membrane

Lipid bilayer
—viral particle membrane

p17
—shell protein

Protease
—viral enzyme

Integrase
—viral enzyme

Viral core

Reverse transcriptase
—viral enzyme

p24
—viral core protein

p9, p7
—proteins sheathing RNA

RNA
—viral genetic material

widely available, and lack sufficient evidence of safety and efficacy to be approved or recommended by physicians. With exceptions noted below, the only antiretroviral drugs in common use as of late 1991 are AZT, ddC, and ddI. Sources of detailed and up-to-date information about experimental drugs are listed in Chapter 9: Learning About Experimental Treatments and in the appendices.

▲ Attachment, Cell-Cell Transmission

Free virus attaches to an uninfected cell when gp120 on the surface of the virus binds with a compatible receptor molecule on the cell's surface. This is usually the CD4 receptor that appears on T4 lymphocytes, macrophage/monocytes, and neural tissue, but other receptor molecules may also allow gp120 to bind. After binding, the core complex of the virus enters the cell, either by being engulfed or when the membranes of the cell and the virus particle fuse.

In addition, gp120 displayed on the surface of an infected cell may bind to receptors on an uninfected cell, causing the two cell membranes to fuse. This process may continue until many cells are joined in one membrane, forming nonfunctional giant multinucleated cells called *syncytia*. In this way many healthy cells may be destroyed even if relatively few free virions are in circulation.

A number of approaches to interfere with the binding of gp120 to cell surface receptors have been suggested to prevent attachment and membrane fusion, but none have yet been demonstrated to be effective.

Recombinant soluble CD4 (rsCD4): One idea is to "use up" the binding sites on the gp120 molecules so that they are not available to bind to cellular receptors. Proposed substances for this purpose include made-to-order antibodies and a soluble version of the CD4 molecule itself.

Recombinant soluble CD4, or rsCD4, is a human-made copy of the CD4 receptors that appear on the surface of T4 cells. CD4 and gp120 have a high mutual affinity. If high enough concentrations of rsCD4 were present in the body, HIV might bind to the drug rather than to receptors on T4 cells. Variations of rsCD4 have been considered in which other substances would be attached to the drug: either a toxin to kill the virus or something to make the CD4 remain in the body longer. At present, rsCD4 is available only through experimental trials.

Lipid-active agents: Viral infections have been shown to affect the composition of fats that make up cell membranes. One hypothesized treatment uses certain lipid-active agents to attempt to restore the balance of cell membranes' fats so that the virus is less able to enter cells. One such agent is made from egg lecithin and is commonly referred to as *AL721*. Since it is made from a common food AL721 is almost certainly harmless, but several studies have failed to show efficacy.

Other substances suggested but not proven to affect viral attachment include a short chain of eight amino acids called **peptide T** and a substance called **dextran sulfate.** No data are yet available on peptide T.

Dextran sulfate is a long chain-like molecule of sugars with sulfur groups attached—a *sulfated polymer*. Small preliminary trials of dextran sulfate showed acceptable toxicity but no efficacy, whether taken by mouth or intravenously. Other sulfated polymers under study are more effective than dextran sulfate in test tube studies.

Both peptide T and dextran sulfate are available from underground sources.

▲ Uncoating

Once the core complex is inside the cell an incompletely understood process causes the dissociation of the core's protein shell and the uncoating of the viral genetic material. This releases the viral RNA and enzymes to do their work. It is hypothesized that certain of the naturally occurring human cytokines (cellular messenger chemicals) called *interferons* may be able to interfere with this stage of the viral reproductive cycle.

▲ Reverse Transcription and Integration

Reverse transcription is the step against which most drug development has been targeted.

As described on p. 342, retroviruses are characterized by the activity of the enzyme reverse transcriptase (RT). This enzyme is able to act after the core complex and viral RNA have been uncoated. The enzyme uses raw materials available inside the host cell to copy viral RNA back into a piece of DNA. *Ribonuclease H,* a viral enzyme packaged with reverse transcriptase, removes the RNA from the newly synthesized DNA strand. Completed viral DNA is referred to as *provirus.* Provirus migrates into the nucleus of the cell, where the cell's own DNA resides. The viral enzyme *integrase* also enters the nucleus, where it snips open the cellular DNA and inserts (or integrates) the provirus.

Reverse transcriptase is not a native human enzyme. If a drug could selectively inhibit the activity of reverse transcriptase only, then such a drug would prevent the replication of HIV without interfering with any normal human cellular functions. Because of this reasoning there has been an intense focus on the development of drugs that interfere with reverse transcription. Some RT inhibitors are available by prescription and some are available from underground sources.

(No *integrase inhibitor* drugs are available; none has been shown effective in preventing the integration of free circular viral DNA once reverse transcription is complete.)

Most research on reverse transcriptase inhibitors has concerned a specific family of drugs called *nucleoside analogs.*

The nucleoside analogs approved so far against HIV attack this stage of the viral reproductive cycle. AZT is effective against HIV, but it is unfortunately not ideally selective for reverse transcriptase. Because it also inhibits normal human enzymes necessary for cell division (*DNA polymerase),* AZT has significant adverse side effects. Drugs that inhibit cell division will particularly affect rapidly dividing cells such as the bone marrow cells which generate red and white blood cells. Thus, anemia and leukopenia (decrease of red and white blood cells) may be side effects of any insufficiently specific RT inhibitor. The drugs ddI and ddC do not appear to cause the anemia and leukopenia associated with AZT.

Nucleoside analog reverse transcriptase inhibitors: Reverse transcriptase takes a piece of RNA and makes a DNA copy. Each of the two strands of whole DNA is a chain of bases or *nucleosides* "holding hands" along a common backbone of sugar. Each nucleoside uses its "left hand"—actually a chemical bond—to hold the "right hand" of its neighbor.

RT starts at one end of the RNA, reads the first base, and grabs the matching type of nucleoside out of the supply floating freely in the cell. RT then moves one base down the RNA and starts over. It reads the next base, grabs another nucleoside, and attaches the new nucleoside's left hand to the previous nucleoside's right hand. The process normally continues until all bases on the RNA have been processed, creating a matching DNA chain of nucleosides. (The viral enzyme *ribonuclease H* then degrades the RNA strand. The single-stranded DNA remaining is then completed by cellular enzymes to form conventional double-stranded DNA.)

Nucleoside *analogs* such as AZT look very similar to nucleosides, but they have no "right hand"—they lack one of the two necessary chemical bonds. If RT can be fooled into attaching a nucleoside analog onto the end of the chain it is building, then the following nucleosides have nothing to hold on to and the chain will remain only a fragment. Nucleoside analogs are sometimes called *chain terminators* for this reason.

SUMMARY OF NUCLEOSIDE-ANALOG REVERSE-TRANSCRIPTASE INHIBITORS

Common Name	Brand Name	Chemical Name	Structural Name	Manufacturer & Status
AZT (azido-thymidine)	Retrovir	Zidovudine (ZDV)	3'-azido-3'-deoxythymidine	Burroughs-Wellcome FDA approved in 1987
ddI	Videx	Didanosine	2',3'-dideoxyinosine	Bristol-Myers FDA approved in 1991
ddC	Hivid	Zalcitabine	2',3'-dideoxycytidine	Hoffman-LaRoche FDA conditionally approved in 1992

Researchers are working on **new nonnucleoside reverse transcriptase inhibitors** that work in different ways from the nucleoside analogs AZT, ddI, and ddC. Some of these drugs are listed in the chart below. So far, the development of nonnucleoside reverse transcriptase inhibitors has been difficult and discouraging. Trials have generally shown limited antiviral effect, high toxicity, and inability for the drug to be sufficiently absorbed when taken by mouth *(limited oral bioavailability)*. Since these drugs are very specific for HIV's reverse transcriptase, viral resistance is expected to develop rapidly. Therefore these drugs are likely to be used in combination with other antivirals to reduce resistance.

EXPERIMENTAL NONNUCLEOSIDE REVERSE TRANSCRIPTASE INHIBITORS

Drug & Mfr.	Trials	Comment
BI-RG-587 Boehringer-Ingelheim	Phase I/II	BI-RG-587 is related to a class of drugs known as benzodiazepines (Valium is a benzodiazepine). The drug has greater test tube activity against HIV than AZT, and may be synergistic with AZT.
L compounds Merck, Sharp, & Dohme	Phase I/II	Side effects appear to be limited in the short term. No efficacy data are yet available. Development of L-697,661, the first Merck L compound, has been halted. Other L drugs continue in development.
TIBO compounds or derivatives (R82913) Janssen	Pilot studies	Unlikely to be available in any form in the United States in the near term. TIBO compounds resemble the class of drugs called benzodiazepines (e.g., Valium). R82913 is the first TIBO compound to be used in clinical trials. A European pilot study showed few side effects and some decrease in p24 antigen levels but no conclusions could be made as to efficacy.

▲ Expression and Manufacture of Viral Proteins

Two HIV proviral genes (called *env* and *gag*) code for structural proteins like gp120 and p24. Another gene (called *pol*) codes for enzymes like reverse transcriptase and HIV integrase.

Regulatory genes: Three viral genes have been identified that regulate other HIV genes. One regulatory gene (called *tat*) encourages expression of HIV genes; another may suppress it (*nef*); and the last provides feedback to the other two (*rev*).

The virus's sophisticated regulatory apparatus gives it a complex potential pattern of activity. The level of expression of viral genes (and hence the generation of new virus particles) can vary considerably. Once integrated, proviral DNA may remain latent at a low level of activity for years. Then, in response to unknown cues, the provirus may radically increase its activity. This variable pattern may help HIV elude the immune system's defenses. It may also explain why HIV-infected people remain healthy for so long before an episode of serious illness.

Hoffman-LaRoche developed a drug, RO-24-7429, that operates against the gene called *tat*. This gene encourages the activity of other HIV genes. If RO-24-7429 works in humans, it might permanently force the virus to remain latent and inactive. RO-24-7429 is also reported to have activity against *pol*, the enzyme gene. Unfortunately, this *tat* inhibitor may be toxic and difficult to study.

It would be tremendously useful to understand and control *nef*, the gene that may suppress HIV, but such efforts are still very much in the research stage. If a suppressing gene could be turned on permanently, HIV infection might never cause illness at all.

Viral protein synthesis: Once the provirus does become active, the normal cellular processes transcribe proviral DNA to RNA using the human enzyme *RNA polymerase*. This RNA then leaves the nucleus. Some of the RNA becomes the genetic material of new virus particles. Ribosomes (cellular protein factories) outside the nucleus use other pieces of the RNA to string together amino acids to make a precursor protein that is destined to become new viral structural proteins and enzymes. HIV's *protease* enzyme cuts and shapes the precursor protein to make the required viral components.

The level of activity of the virus in the body is often measured by the relative quantity of viral proteins that are being manufactured. One protein, p24, has come to be a standard measure used to evaluate the efficacy of new anti-HIV drugs.

The manufacture of viral proteins closely resembles the manufacture of proteins that the cell needs to survive and function. A drug that nonspecifically suppresses the cell's ability to make proteins from RNA will cause unacceptable side effects.

Interferons may be able to selectively suppress the synthesis of viral proteins. In the ordinary immune response to viral infection interferons are produced well in advance of any antibody response. In this context interferons seem to suppress the synthesis of viral proteins only, via some specific but unknown mechanism.

Alpha-interferon is currently approved as a therapy against Kaposi's sarcoma and is available by prescription. However, its efficacy as an anti-HIV drug has not yet been demonstrated. Studies are proceeding but preliminary data show significant side effects (severe flu-like symptoms, possible anemia and neutropenia) and mixed efficacy. Combinations of alpha-interferon with AZT are also being studied.

Other proposed drugs are **antisense oligomers,** short pieces of nucleic acid constructed to be complementary (hence antisense) to a specific segment of HIV's genetic material. A molecule so designed could bind to proviral DNA and block its transcription into RNA. Antisense oligomers might also bind to viral RNA and block protein manufacture from this RNA.

Protease inhibitors: Some novel compounds inhibit the activity of HIV protease in the test tube, preventing the enzyme from splicing together viral proteins out of the precursor proteins. A successful protease inhibitor drug would block infected cells from making necessary viral enzymes and structural proteins. RO-31-8959 is a protease inhibitor manufactured by Hoffman-LaRoche. The drug is poorly absorbed and so difficult to synthesize that only very small studies will be possible in the near future. Other protease inhibitors are in development by other firms (e.g., Upjohn). No reliable data are yet available. Protease inhibitors are not available to the public from any source.

Ribavirin is a drug that is hypothesized to prevent the processing of a type of RNA called *messenger RNA*. Messenger RNA is the RNA that travels out from the nucleus to be used by ribosomes to make protein. It is distinguished from another type of RNA called *transfer RNA* that ribosomes use to decode triplets of messenger RNA bases into the various amino acids, the constituents of proteins.

Early reports of ribavirin's efficacy have been questioned. Ribavirin antagonizes (interferes with) the anti-HIV activity of AZT in the test tube. Ribavirin has at times been available from underground sources.

GLQ223 (tricosanthin, Compound Q): Compound Q is a drug derived from the Chinese cucumber root, *Tricosanthes kirilowii*. It has been used for years in humans to cause abortion. Compound Q has the remarkable test tube effect of selectively killing HIV-infected cells while leaving healthy cells alone. It is thought to operate by inactivating the ribosomes that synthesize viral proteins. Trials are being conducted both by the drug's manufacturer (Genelabs) and by Project Inform, a community-based HIV treatment research and information organization in San Francisco.

Small early studies are inconclusive for efficacy. In contrast to most other drugs, side effects seem to diminish with use. This implies that higher doses can be used over time, possibly leading to increased efficacy. Compound Q can have dangerous or even fatal side effects, especially in those with prior neurological problems. Compound Q is often administered in combination with a steroid (such as Decadron) to reduce these side effects.

Compound Q is available from underground sources, but be very cautious. Use compound Q only as part of an established research protocol or, after thorough investigation and discussion, under the supervision of a well-qualified physician experienced in the use of this drug.

▲ Viral Assembly and Glycosylation

New viral particles assemble themselves from viral RNA and the newly synthesized viral enzymes and structural proteins. Many copies of the viral proteins p7 and p9 stick to viral RNA, forming a protective sheath and preparing the genetic material for encapsulation.

Enzymes (reverse transcriptase, integrase, protease) and sheathed RNA gather together and are then enclosed in many copies of the viral core protein (p24) to form the core complex. The completed core complex is enclosed in shell protein (p17).

The viral spikes (gp41 and gp120) are glycoproteins (made of proteins and carbohydrates). The process of attaching the necessary carbohydrate molecules to the proteins is called *glycosylation.* After glycosylation many copies of gp41 and gp120 become embedded in the cell membrane, with gp120 sticking outside of the host cell membrane, anchored by gp41. This is in preparation for the final stage of the virus particle's development, in which it will wrap itself in part of the host cell's membrane.

Glycosylation is also necessary for the normal processing of some cellular proteins. However, HIV glycoproteins require significantly more glycosylation than do cellular proteins. Glycosylation-inhibiting drugs therefore preferentially but not specifically affect the processing of viral products over normal cellular products.

(In an attempt to defend itself, the host cell also displays viral proteins other than gp120 on its surface. This is done to give the immune system an opportunity to recognize the foreign proteins, i.e., via lymphocytes or antibodies to p24.)

It may also be possible to interfere with the addition of the sugars *(glycosylation)* necessary to make gp41 and gp120. One possible **glycosylation inhibitor** under investigation is a drug called castanospermine, a substance found in the seeds of the Australian chestnut tree. This drug inhibits glycosylation of HIV proteins in the test tube. Small human studies have shown limited toxicity but no data on efficacy are yet available. Another proposed glycosylation inhibitor is N-butyl-DNJ (deoxynojirimycin), but even less data are available than for castanospermine.

▲ Budding, Free Virions

The final step in the reproductive cycle of the virus occurs when the assembled protein component wraps itself in a portion of the host cell's lipid membrane studded with viral spike proteins, and then buds free as a completed particle of HIV, called a *free virion.* Spike proteins on free virions may then attach to CD4 on uninfected cells, starting the cycle over again.

Alpha-interferon may suppress the budding process. Neutralizing antibodies would remove free virions from circulation and might inactivate gp120 displayed on host cells. Unfortunately, the antibodies produced in the natural immune response do not neutralize HIV. Neutralizing antibodies could possibly be produced in response to specially designed vaccines

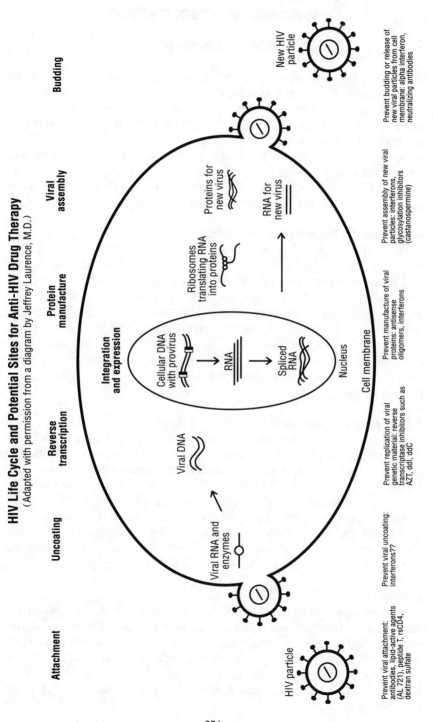

HIV Life Cycle and Potential Sites for Anti-HIV Drug Therapy

(Adapted with permission from a diagram by Jeffrey Laurence, M.D.)

HIV: Virology and Therapeutic Strategies

Attachment

Prevent viral attachment: antibodies, lipid-active agents (AL 721), peptide T, rsCD4, dextran sulfate

HIV particle

Uncoating

Prevent viral uncoating: interferons??

Viral RNA and enzymes

Reverse transcription

Prevent replication of viral genetic material: reverse transcriptase inhibitors such as AZT, ddI, ddC

Viral DNA

Integration and expression

Cellular DNA with provirus → RNA → Spliced RNA

Nucleus

Cell membrane

Protein manufacture

Prevent manufacture of viral proteins: antisense oligomers, interferons

Ribosomes translating RNA into proteins

Viral assembly

Prevent assembly of new viral particles: interferons, glycosylation inhibitors (castanospermine)

Proteins for new virus

RNA for new virus

Budding

Prevent budding or release of new viral particles from cell membrane: alpha interferon, neutralizing antibodies

New HIV particle

IMMUNOLOGIC THERAPEUTIC STRATEGIES

VACCINES AGAINST HIV

We are all familiar with vaccines that protect uninfected individuals from certain diseases such as polio or measles. These vaccines operate by stimulating the immune system to produce immunity to a specific infection. When a harmless form of a specific antigen is introduced into the body, the immune system generates *memory B lymphocytes.* These memory cells then patrol the body, ready to multiply and transform themselves into antibody factories at the next sign of infection with the antigen. Vaccination primes the body to respond very quickly to infection—so quickly that infection can never result in disease.

▲ Rationale for Postinfection Vaccination

The body does develop an immune response against HIV, in the form of antibodies. Antibodies to HIV remove viral particles from circulation, and probably suppress viral activity to a considerable degree. Yet, the antibodies produced naturally in response to HIV infection do not provide complete protection against HIV disease. It may be that the immune system could be artificially encouraged to respond more effectively to HIV infection long after the initial infection, an idea called *postexposure vaccination.* This is an unfamiliar type of vaccination, since we do not usually vaccinate people who have already been infected with a specific disease.

▲ Safety and Efficacy Issues

Postexposure HIV vaccines necessarily work by increasing the activity of the immune system. Increased immune system activity might also make the virus more active. This makes some researchers worry that HIV vaccination might in itself be dangerous to those already infected.

For those who are not HIV infected, a different issue arises. How could researchers ever test the efficacy of an HIV vaccine in preventing initial infection with HIV? Who would volunteer for such a test? It will be very difficult to guarantee the safety and efficacy of a vaccine to protect the uninfected.

▲ Strategies

A number of post-exposure vaccination strategies are under investigation. These strategies are designed to provoke an effective response without aggravating existing disease. An ideal vaccine would both improve the neutralizing power of antibodies produced against HIV and—crucially—improve the immune system's ability to destroy HIV resident inside host cells, where it is largely protected from the influence of antibodies.

Subunit vaccines are created by synthesizing certain components of the virus in quantity. The immune system may mount a more effective response against certain parts of the virus. One difficulty is that the parts of the virus accessible to the immune system undergo rapid variation, presenting a moving target that complicates the efforts of vaccine designers. Another is that some parts of the virus may be harmful in and of themselves.

A **whole-virus vaccine** uses actual particles of HIV that have been tampered with so as to destroy their ability to cause infection. The advantage of whole-virus vaccines is that the immune system responds better to viral antigens presented on the surface of particles than to "naked" subunit antigens. However, the antigens that naturally appear on the surface of HIV particles may not be able to provoke a completely effective immune response. The safety of whole-virus vaccines may also be hard to guarantee.

Vaccinia-vector recombinant vaccines combine the favorable aspects of subunit vaccines and whole-virus vaccines. Vaccines get their name from the cowpox virus, *Vaccinia*, which was first used by Pasteur to immunize humans against smallpox. (The two viruses share an antigen, so that infection with the benign cowpox virus confers immunity against the dangerous smallpox virus.) Through genetic engineering, genes for specific HIV antigens may be inserted into the genetic material of a strain of *Vaccinia*. The altered *Vaccinia* then expresses HIV antigen on the surface of its particles. When injected, the altered virus displays HIV antigen in a way that is more likely to provoke an effective immune response and should not cause disease.

Another problem of vaccine development is that the desired immune response may occur but be too weak, perhaps due to the enfeebled state of the HIV-infected immune system. The **prime-boost strategy** is designed to overcome this problem. The priming step is done by vaccination with antigen presented either as whole virus or via a *Vaccinia* vector. Subsequently, boosters are given that flood the immune system with subunit copies of the antigen in an attempt to rouse a vigorous response.

▲ Status of Vaccine Development

All these strategies are under study. Some subunit vaccines began clinical trials as of early 1992. Other human trials are planned, and many researchers are optimistic that the 1990s will be the decade of the vaccine. Yet, we must note that this type of immunotherapy research takes place at the extreme boundaries of human knowledge and technological sophistication. An effective postexposure vaccine against HIV is at least years away, and a vaccine to prevent initial infection may take decades to develop and test. Keep up-to-date about the status of vaccine development by following the suggestions given in Chapter 9: Learning About Experimental Treatments.

"IMMUNE MODULATORS"

Immune modulators is a term used to describe a hoped-for class of drugs that might improve the functioning of the immune system. At this point no proposed immune modulators have been shown to work.

The only immune modulator tested in large trials—Imuthiol (ditocarb sodium, sodium diethyldithiocarbamate, DTC), has been withdrawn from development by the manufacturer after preliminary data showed no benefit and possible harm in terms of progression of disease.

Recombinant gp160 (rgp160) is a genetically engineered molecule under consideration as an immune modulator. The drug may provoke a heightened immune response against this component of HIV. It is controversial, but is being pursued in a number of clinical trials and by several biotechnology companies.

A compound called *n-acetylcysteine* (NAC) has shown some anti-HIV activity in vitro and is currently in clinical trials.

Other compounds proposed as immune modulators include ampligen; DHEA; hypericin; tacrine; thymotrinin (TP3); methionine enkephalin (MEK); and pentoxyfiline.

Earlier in the book we described granulocyte colony stimulating factor (G-CSF) and granulocyte-monocyte colony-stimulating factor (GM-CSF). These are synthetic versions of two of the messenger chemicals of the immune system that are used to boost production of certain white blood cells. These drugs are used to repair hematologic toxicities caused by other drugs (such as ganciclovir). While these drugs might fairly be called immune modulators, and while they certainly are useful in the context of HIV disease, they are not generally thought of as immune modulators in the sense implied in this section.

Chapter 18
Blood and Blood Cells

Blood is a liquid suspension of specialized cells and other elements. It contains diverse structures and performs multiple functions. Blood extends to every tissue in the body and maintains the balance of the entire body. Many diseases cause blood disorders; blood disorders can produce malfunctioning of many parts of the body. Blood is a prime indicator of problems in the body and it is easily accessible. In the course of medical care you will have samples of blood taken and examined many times with many different tests.

Blood is composed of almost equal volumes of *formed elements* and *plasma* that can be separated by spinning a test tube of blood at high speed in a centrifuge ("spinning down" blood). Formed elements are red cells, white cells, and platelets. Plasma is nine-tenths water. The remaining tenth of plasma is various dissolved substances: proteins, electrolytes (charged particles or *ions*), sugars, vitamins, minerals, hormones, and drugs.

The *hematopoietic system* (the "blood-growth" system) is composed of blood cells, the organs that produce these cells (bone marrow, lymph nodes, thymus, spleen), the organs that help blood cells mature and grow (such as the liver), and the channels that carry blood cells to every part of the body (veins, arteries, and lymph vessels).

Bone marrow is the soft material filling the cavities of bones. Red blood cells and some white blood cells are produced in the bone marrow.

The lymphatic system drains excess fluid from the tissue of the body and returns it to the blood. Lymphocytes are produced in the lymph nodes, spleen, and thymus. (Lymphoid tissue is the major reservoir of HIV in the body).

DEVELOPMENT OF BLOOD CELLS

Blood cells have a developmental history in the body. They start in one form and then go through multiple stages during which they change their form and function. All blood cells are produced by one small population of *stem cells* that differentiate as they develop. These cells exist throughout the hematopoietic system, including circulating blood, spleen, and bone marrow. Other organs are involved in the complex biochemical process of maturation of blood cells. The stomach and kidney produce factors that are involved in maturation of red blood cells.

Other elements in the blood that influence cell growth and differentiation include *granulocyte colony-stimulating factor* (G-CSF), and *granulocyte-monocyte colony-stimulating factor* (GM-CSF).

If some factor (genetic, infective, drug-related) interferes with the development of elements in the blood, the earlier in the developmental process it causes the defect, the more broadly it will affect the whole system.

TYPES AND FUNCTIONS OF BLOOD CELLS

There are a number of different kinds of mature cells in blood. The three major types of mature cells are red blood cells (*erythrocytes*), white blood cells (*leukocytes*), and platelets. There are many different types of white blood cells.

▲ Red Blood Cells (Erythrocytes)

Red blood cells are smaller than average cells and lack a nucleus (for which reason they are properly called *corpuscles*). They transport oxygen from the lungs to body tissues using an iron-containing substance called *hemoglobin*. Attaching oxygen to hemoglobin in red corpuscles allows the blood to carry enough oxygen for a five-minute supply, much more than if oxygen were simply dissolved in blood.

The number of red corpuscles in a healthy individual tends to remain constant. Men have more red corpuscles than women, and adults have more than children. Levels of red blood cells are lower in African-Americans than in whites; this does not seem to be dependent on socioeconomic variables.

Red blood cells are formed in the marrow of the skull, ribs, and vertebrae and in children at the ends of bones in the arms and legs. This formation process is referred to as *erythropoiesis*. This process is regulated by the hormone *erythropoietin* and dependent on an adequate supply of nutrients: most especially, iron, folic acid, and vitamin B_{12}.

Once a mature red blood cell is formed, it can no longer grow and divide. A red blood cell has a 120-day life span. About 1 percent of the circulating red blood cells must be replenished each day.

Anemia occurs if the blood cannot carry enough oxygen to nourish tissues. Common symptoms of anemia are fatigue, headache, and shortness of breath. Anemia may be caused by too few red blood cells or too little hemoglobin or both. Anemia may develop if the demand for red blood cells increases or the production capacity of bone marrow decreases. Demand may go up if blood is lost through bleeding or if red blood cells die too quickly. Production may go down because of infection or lack of raw materials such as iron for hemoglobin. Since anemia is always a symptom of some underlying problem, it is usually not sufficient to treat the anemia alone.

Blood and Blood Cells

▲ Reticulocytes

As a red corpuscle precursor cell develops, it gains hemoglobin, divides and redivides, shrinks, and finally loses the nucleus to become an actual erythrocyte. The cell has different names at different stages of development. *Reticulocytes* are new red blood corpuscles that have just entered the bloodstream. One red blood cell in every 200 is a reticulocyte. The success of treatments for anemia can be judged by measuring the increase in reticulocytes in blood (the *reticulocyte count*).

▲ White Blood Cells (Leukocytes)

White blood cells, also known as *leukocytes,* are a part of the immune system. There are many fewer white blood cells than red blood cells. White blood cells contain nuclei.

A *white blood count* (WBC) is the number of white blood cells per cubic millimeter of blood. White blood cell count rises when infection is present. It can also rise very high in leukemia, in which cancerous white blood cells proliferate to a degree that they interfere with the functioning of organs.

A total white blood cell count is the sum of several types of white blood cells—neutrophils, eosinophils, basophils, lymphocytes, and macrophage/monocytes. A rise in the number of white blood cells (leukocytes) is called *leukocytosis.* A decrease in the number of white blood cells is called *leukopenia.*

Neutrophils make up the largest percentage of white blood cells and work to prevent bacterial infections. Consequently, the level of neutrophils rises in response to bacterial infections and some other infections. Neutrophil counts drop in response to certain diseases and medications. Neutrophils are produced in bone marrow.

Neutrophils can travel in tissue by squeezing between other cells. This is important in their role in fighting infection. Neutrophils travel to the area where bacteria or other microorganisms have invaded, enter the tissue, and devour the invader. Bacteria contain toxins that eventually kill white blood cells.

A rise in the number of neutrophils (*neutrophilia*) can be caused by infection (with bacteria, mycobacteria, fungi, parasites), local or metabolic disorders, some cancers (including lymphoma), and some drugs that affect the kidneys and liver.

A drop in the number of neutrophils (*neutropenia*) can be caused by viral infection (rubeola, hepatitis), certain bacterial infections (typhoid, brucella), and all very serious systemic bacterial infections (bacteremia). It can also be caused by drugs (including AZT, ganciclovir, Bactrim), lack of folic acid or vitamin B_{12}, enlargement of the spleen, and other disorders (e.g., systemic lupus, immunodeficiencies, anaphylaxis).

Lymphocytes are white blood cells that play an important role in the immune system. They are chiefly produced in the lymph nodes, spleen, and thymus. There are two types of lymphocytes, T cells and B cells. T4 cells are one type of T lymphocyte (the number 4 in T4 is an arbitrary label—the various types of T lymphocyte were numbered in the order in which they were characterized).

A rise in the number of lymphocytes (*lymphocytosis*) may be caused by some acute infections (mononeucleosis, pertussis, mumps, measles, infectious hepatitis), the convalescent stage of many acute infections, and some chronic infections (tuberculosis, syphilis, brucellosis). Also, some metabolic disorders and some cancers including lymphomas cause lymphocytosis. A drop in the number of lymphocytes is called *lymphopenia* or *lymphocytopenia.* Lymphopenia may be caused by HIV itself over the long term or as a side effect of medication.

Macrophage/monocytes: Monocytes are white blood cells that form in the spleen and lymph nodes, are transported in the bloodstream, and settle in various tissues of the body, where they develop into macrophages. Macrophages are an important reservoir of HIV and the vehicle by which HIV enters the central nervous system.

Eosinophils are a type of white blood cell that becomes elevated in certain illnesses: allergies (hay fever, asthma, dermatitis, drug reactions); parasitic infections (of intestines or tissues); skin disorders (dermatitis); some cancers including non-Hodgkin's lymphoma; and some other disorders (such as scarlet fever and pernicious anemia). They are produced in bone marrow.

Basophils: These white blood cells are infrequently elevated. Several diseases including leukemia, Hodgkin's disease, varicella, and contact dermatitis can result in an elevation. They are produced in bone marrow.

▲ Platelets (Thrombocytes)

Platelets are central in the process of blood clotting. They arise from *megakaryocytes,* cells formed in bone marrow that are twenty-five times the size of platelets. Megakaryocytes fall apart into thrombocytes. A low platelet count is called *thrombocytopenia.* HIV infection can cause lowering of platelets. This does not necessarily cause symptoms and does not necessarily indicate a general decline in the immune system. AZT can both lower and raise platelet count in various circumstances.

Chapter 19
Understanding Clinical Trials

AZT's value has been proved by repeated clinical trials of the drug performed over the last seven years. Clinical trials are the scientific experiments that judge the safety and efficacy of drugs used on humans. To understand why certain drugs are recommended, it helps to understand how the evidence was gathered that shows the drug's benefit.

HIV disease has focused close attention on the conduct of clinical trials over the past ten years. Articulate and politically mobilized HIV-infected people have raised many questions about the drug development process. This process is slow and full of ethical and scientific pitfalls, yet we must have some way of determining the relative value of different treatments. Clinical trials using the scientific method provide reliable and useful information when carefully performed and carefully interpreted. However, many factors affect *which* drugs are tried. Some of these factors—such as patentability or profitability—do not necessarily operate to the benefit of HIV-infected people.

Clinical trials have also provided the only access to some experimental treatments. However, trials have not historically been a significant source of drugs or other care, since only a small percentage of HIV-infected people have ever participated in a formal clinical trial. The introduction of *expanded access programs* has recently allowed more people access to experimental medications.

This section describes the drug development process in the United States as of early 1992. Read this section: if you want to understand why AZT or other drugs are recommended; if you want to know more about how drugs are tested; or if you are thinking of becoming a subject in a clinical trial.

DRUG DEVELOPMENT, THE FDA, AND PHARMACEUTICAL COMPANIES

The Food and Drug Administration (FDA) is the government agency responsible for regulating the manufacture and sale of medical drugs. In the past, this agency's mandate has been to protect the public from harmful or useless drugs. This has been done chiefly by requiring elaborate documentation of safety and efficacy from pharmaceutical companies before licensing a new drug for sale. The FDA is not in the business of developing new drugs: the agency simply approves or rejects the drugs presented by the pharmaceutical industry.

The history of the drug thalidomide provides insight into the FDA's behavior. Thalidomide was used in other countries as a tranquilizer and subsequently was discovered to cause fetal deformities. The FDA had refused to approve thalidomide in this country, and consequently the public here was spared the thalidomide-induced deformities observed elsewhere in the world. This incident confirmed the FDA's conservatism in granting approval to new drugs. Thalidomide was a graphic illustration of the danger of approving any drug.

AIDS activists took issue with this conservatism, arguing that this philosophy arbitrarily denied consenting, informed adults access to potentially beneficial treatments. Activists also turned the spotlight on the extraordinary difficulties and delays that FDA-drug-approval procedures imposed on the release of new drugs. To the credit of all involved, both the FDA and the biomedical research establishment have shown some flexibility in responding to the activist critique.

STEPS IN DRUG DEVELOPMENT

There are many steps that must be taken before a drug can be marketed. First, it must be discovered or invented. A drug may be discovered as one of the huge number of compounds that are randomly screened in the test tube each year for efficacy against disease; or a drug may be chemically synthesized based on a theorized mechanism of action. Drugs are therefore found either through *random screening* or *targeted discovery.*

Once a drug has been identified to have potential benefit against a disease, researchers perform intensive test tube studies (often called *in vitro* studies, Latin for "in glass"). In vitro studies provide preliminary information on the concentration of drug needed to have a desired effect. An important goal in drug development is to achieve this effective concentration of the drug in the diseased tissue without causing intolerable damage or toxicity.

The next step is to find the best form in which to administer the drug. The *formulation* of the drug is designed to minimize toxicity and maximize *bioavailability*—the amount of the drug that actually is available for therapeutic use in the affected tissue rather than simply being metabolized or directly excreted.

Before testing an untried drug in humans, researchers perform animal studies to see how the drug is absorbed and tolerated by a living system. Information about a drug's physical distribution and concentration over time is called *pharmacokinetics* (Greek for "drug movement"). There are two important pharmacokinetic issues in humans.

- How quickly is the drug removed from the body? This rate is often measured in terms of *half-life,* the length of time required for the concentration of drug to drop by half. A drug's half-life affects the dosage used and the chance of toxicities.

- Does the drug get into brain tissue? The brain is protected from diseases and toxins with a special mechanism called the *blood-brain barrier*. Some drugs cannot penetrate this barrier and so cannot be effective against brain disease. Since HIV disease involves not only direct infection of microglial cells in the brain (a type of macrophage) but secondary complications involving the central nervous system, it is important that drugs against HIV cross the blood-brain barrier.

A problem in the study of HIV disease has been the lack of good *animal models*. This virus causes disease in only a few animals: humans and a few other primates (principally chimpanzees). The number of chimpanzees available for drug research is extremely limited. Researchers recently genetically engineered a new type of laboratory mouse that may provide a useful animal model for HIV disease. This new animal is called the SCID-HU mouse. SCID refers to the fact that these mice have a genetically determined *severe combined immune deficiency*—that is, they are born without major components of an immune system. The HU refers to the fact that these mice are then artificially provided with components of the human immune system, including the white blood cells that HIV affects. The use of the SCID-HU mouse may speed development of drugs against HIV. Another promising animal model is the pig-tailed macaque. This macaque develops symptoms relatively soon after infection and easily breeds in captivity, in contrast to the chimpanzee.

If in vitro and animal studies show promise, a pharmaceutical company may then file an *investigational new drug* application (IND) with the FDA. This signals the company's intention to test the drug in human beings, tests known as *clinical trials*. The ethics of clinical trials are very complicated. Ethical drug testing in humans is based on the notion of *informed consent,* which means that the cooperation of human subjects is not coerced in any way and that the subjects are aware of all the risks involved, known and potential. Before clinical trials recruit subjects, a committee called an *institutional review board* (IRB) is formed to oversee the trial and ensure that subjects are protected.

Clinical trials have traditionally been divided into three *phases,* ranging from quick studies of a small number of subjects to huge multiyear studies of tens of thousands of subjects.

Phase I clinical trials are done on a small number of subjects (usually tens of people). Phase I trials are done primarily to determine any obvious adverse side effects of the drug and the dosage needed to achieve the blood levels deemed therapeutic in test tube studies. These *toxicity* and *dose ranging* trials may last only a few weeks. Phase I trials may provide some suggestion of the efficacy of the drug, but the small number of subjects precludes conclusive evidence.

Phase II clinical trials provide the first reliable evidence of safety and efficacy. These trials involve more subjects, typically in the hundreds. They may last a few months or more.

If Phase II trials promise some efficacy with reasonably tolerable side effects, the drug company may decide to proceed with phase III trials — large-scale studies of safety and efficacy in thousands of subjects over several years.

The process traditionally took many years to go from test tube studies to animal studies to phase I through phase III clinical trials. AIDS activists complained bitterly about the delay and suggested a number of ways to streamline the process. Time is now saved in some cases by performing phase II and phase III trials simultaneously. Activists and others suggested that trials use laboratory values such as T4 count or p24 antigen level to substitute for clinical endpoints such as death or the development of opportunistic infections. The use of such *surrogate markers* is attractive to activists for reasons of both efficiency and ethics.

Armed with masses of data from clinical trials, a drug company may then file a *new drug application* (NDA) asking for FDA approval and licensing of the drug. The FDA reviews all the data and makes its decision.

Experimental drugs have in the past been made available to patients who had no other options for treatment through so-called *compassionate-use* protocols. These protocols required that patients be very sick. Relatively few patients have obtained drugs through compassionate-use protocols.

Access to experimental drugs was recently improved by a remarkable collaboration between drug companies, AIDS activists, and the government. Some drugs are now available to patients through *parallel track* or *expanded access* programs. These programs allow people who cannot participate in formal clinical trials to have supervised access to new drugs before formal approval.

CONTROL AND BLINDING

The central issue in the design of clinical drug trials is how to distinguish the effect of the drug itself from random chance and the confounding effects of all the other factors that affect the subjects. If the effect of chance is eliminated, the experiment is described as a *controlled trial.* Observed changes in an uncontrolled experiment cannot reliably be attributed to any one variable.

In clinical drug trials, no reliable conclusion can be drawn if all subjects receive exactly the same regimen. Controlled drug trials randomly assign each subject into one of two groups: the *treatment group* receives the drug being tested; the *control group* does not receive the drug.

The attitude of the subjects can affect the clinical outcome. It has been shown that the treatment group may do better than the control group even if instead of an active drug they are secretly treated with a neutral inert compound (termed a *placebo*). This is called the *placebo effect.* Researchers counter the placebo effect by treating both groups of subjects: the treatment group is given active drug while the control group is given an inactive substitute. This is called *placebo control.*

Subjects in a controlled trial must not know whether they are in the treatment group or the control group. This is called *blinding.* If subjects did know which group they were assigned to, the trial would be distorted by the differing impact of the placebo effect on the two groups.

It has been shown that unconscious biases on the part of the researchers can also distort clinical trials. Researchers who know which subjects are on drug and which are on control may subtly and unconsciously alter the way they treat subjects, or they may unconsciously reveal to the subject his or her group assignment. In a *double-blind* controlled clinical trial, neither the subjects nor the researchers who treat them know which subjects are in the treatment group and which subjects are in the control group.

The classic standard of proof for new drugs has been the double-blind placebo-controlled clinical trial. There are ethical problems in the use of placebo control in subjects with life-threatening disease. If an existing treatment has been proved safe and effective in a clinical trial, then it is unethical to deny treatment to the control group. For example, Bactrim for PCP prevention was proved effective in leukemic children in the 1970s. Was it ethical to conduct placebo-controlled trials of Bactrim for PCP prevention in people with AIDS?

One possible solution to this problem is to treat the control group with a different drug from the one being tested. This is referred to as a *positive control.* Researchers have resisted the use of positive controls because it complicates the interpretation of trial data and possibly limits the significance of the results. Increasingly trials do compare an unknown drug against a known drug rather than an unknown drug against a placebo.

There are also ethical problems in use of blinding. If the treatment group is obviously doing much better than the control group, the blinding should be broken so that the controls may get the benefit of the treatment. This has in fact become standard for large clinical trials of drugs against HIV disease. Blinding was broken in several large trials of AZT because the treatment group was doing so much better than the control group. Breaking blinding gains better short-term health for the control group by sacrificing information that might have been gathered by letting the trial continue longer.

ISSUES IN TRIAL DESIGN

A number of complicated factors affect the design of clinical trials.

Understanding the Science

▲ Inclusion-Exclusion Criteria

Researchers pick a particular population of subjects for the experiment by designing *inclusion-exclusion criteria.* Criteria commonly involve sex, age, route by which HIV was transmitted, T4 count, the history of opportunistic infections, what drugs are being taken currently or were taken in the past. Many of the early trials required a formal diagnosis of AIDS for subjects to be included. Many trials explicitly excluded people who had been infected by needle sharing (to eliminate what were seen as potentially uncooperative subjects) and women of childbearing age (which was intended to protect any potential fetus from possibly harmful drugs, but which also denied women access to these drugs).

▲ Number of Subjects

The number of subjects in a trial greatly affects the significance of any results. In general, the more subjects the better. However, a large trial means a more complicated trial: large expenses, possible difficulties in recruiting subjects, and problems with providing services to subjects.

▲ Population Bias

Characteristics of the subject population have to be examined carefully if trial results are to be meaningful. For instance, one trial found that women with AIDS have in general died much more quickly than men with AIDS. Some people took this to mean that there was a biological difference between the sexes that influenced the course of disease. However, women with AIDS are a very different population from men with AIDS. Half of women with AIDS were infected by sharing needles. Another quarter were sexual partners of men who shared needles. Both these groups tended to be poor and in bad health to begin with. Also, needle sharers and poor people are less likely to have access to the health care they need: for complex reasons, they tend not to be diagnosed with AIDS until they are very ill. Thus, the time from diagnosis to death is likely to be shorter on average for women, not because they are female, but for reasons of health history and socioeconomics.

Subject characteristics that affect interpretation of results are called *population biases.* Factors that may cause population bias include general health and specific medical history, age, socioeconomic factors, and transmission route. Population bias can be minimized through *matching,* in which subjects are chosen so that demographic characteristics are the same for both treatment and control groups.

▲ Recruitment and Compliance

Some clinical trials for HIV drugs have had difficulty recruiting the planned number of subjects. Some subjects may not cooperate with the study in various ways: subjects may drop out of the study, may miss appointments, may not take the drugs on schedule, or may take other drugs that compromise the interpretation of trial results. Some drugs

364

under study are also available underground or through expanded access: this is one reason why expanded access programs attempt to limit availability to those who cannot participate in formal trials. HIV-infected people may need special services such as daycare for children or incentives such as comprehensive medical care to persuade them to enroll as subjects. Recruitment and compliance remain significant problems that delay trials and reduce the reliability of results.

▲ Duration and Dosage

Trials are also characterized by the length of time that they run. Clearly, a trial provides most information if you let it run a long time. However, there is tremendous pressure to identify promising results as early as possible, given the serious nature of HIV disease. So the reliability of results from clinical trials (and information about long-term consequences of drugs) is balanced against the ethical need to protect subjects from harm or neglect and to get information to other infected people at the earliest opportunity.

▲ Clinical Endpoints and Surrogate Markers

The efficacy of experimental drugs has traditionally been determined by reference to *clinical endpoints* such as the death or acute illness of subjects. Since prophylaxis now exists, it is unethical to use the development of PCP as a clinical endpoint in the evaluation of antiviral drugs. Many consider it unethical to use any placebo in antiviral trials, since several effective antiviral drugs are now known.

Various laboratory values such as T4 count or p24 antigen level have been proposed as substitutes for clinical endpoints. These proposed substitutes are often called *surrogate markers.* While clinical endpoints are unambiguous indicators of clinical efficacy, the significance of surrogate markers is necessarily indirect. A drug trial using death as a clinical endpoint provides clear information on survival, whereas results based on p24 antigen as a surrogate marker may be hard to translate into increased months of survival. Clearly, surrogate markers are desirable, but we need to understand the relation between these markers and clinical benefit.

▲ Analysis

Statistical arguments can be subtle. The interpretation of results may depend not only on mathematical gymnastics but on commonsense definitions. As an example, a recent study observed that the time from formal diagnosis with AIDS to death had actually *decreased* in a certain population. Thus, one could argue that improvements in treatment had *decreased* survival. However, a closer look revealed that this population was benefiting from treatment so much that their diagnosis with AIDS was delayed until a much later stage of immune deficiency: that is, people were kept healthy for a longer time, and then got sick and were formally diagnosed. Survival from the initiation of treatment was actually greatly *increased.* The lesson here is that, for the purposes of evaluating treatment, survival should not be measured from diagnosis but from the start of the treatment.

SHOULD YOU BE IN A CLINICAL TRIAL?

You may be interested in participating in a clinical trial of an experimental treatment for some aspect of HIV disease. If so, consult with your physician carefully. If possible, learn as much as you can about the drug, the researchers, and the details of the trial. To get information about clinical trials in your area that are open for enrollment, call the Centers for Disease Control (CDC) AIDS drug trial information service at 800-TRIALS-A (800-874-2572, Monday to Friday, 9:00 A.M. to 7:00 P.M. EST). Information is available in both Spanish and English. You will get to speak to someone in person who will give you information about government-approved clinical trials and also about specific drugs, both antivirals and for opportunistic infections. They will also do computer searches for you. Services are free. Refer to Chapter 9: Learning About Experimental Treatments for other sources of information about experimental drugs and clinical trials.

Part Four
Practical Matters

This part of the book discusses some practical matters that are not, strictly speaking, medical in nature but which have a great impact on people with HIV disease: medical insurance, money to live on, and legal matters such as discrimination, power of attorney, and wills.

Chapter 20
Medical Insurance

NEED FOR MEDICAL INSURANCE

If you are infected with HIV, it is crucial for you to have adequate medical insurance. Medical care without insurance is almost always prohibitively expensive. Try to arrange medical insurance that will help you pay for care for all stages of HIV disease including early intervention. If you are forced to rely on government-funded medical insurance (such as Medicaid), your likely choices about medical care are limited. Plan your medical insurance carefully: do not let your medical insurance lapse at any time.

The insurance industry is regulated on a state-by-state basis, and regulations and laws relevant to AIDS and HIV infection are changing. Familiarize yourself with the regulations in your home state. Learn any new regulations or industry practices before buying or changing insurance policies. Ask your local AIDS service organization for advice. It is sometimes difficult to get accurate information from insurance companies—you may want to check the information they provide against that available through your state insurance agency. Some AIDS organizations provide written material, seminars, and individual consultation on insurance matters.

▲ Plan Ahead

Medical insurance is so crucial for you if you are HIV infected that you must often give it priority in making plans. For example, you may need to make decisions about taking, leaving, or changing jobs partially on the basis of the medical insurance benefits offered. This is a bitter pill to swallow. Especially if you are young it is difficult to have to make decisions based on insurance. It may make you more acutely aware of your HIV disease. It emphasizes the feeling of unfairness that comes with being HIV infected.

In addition, it is difficult to do the practical work necessary for evaluating the adequacy of your insurance and making changes. Concentrating on details of medical insurance means having to consider issues such as medication, hospitalization, disability; this is likely to be upsetting. Insurance policies make dull reading. Trying to get information from an insurance company can be infuriating.

Nonetheless, getting your insurance in order must be a priority for anyone who is HIV infected. If you are having trouble doing this, try to get support from a friend in taking the practical steps.

▲ The Changing State of Insurance

Payment for health care is undergoing a crisis in the United States. In 1989, about 33 million United States citizens had no medical insurance. More and more U.S. citizens are ending up with either no health care insurance or inadequate insurance. The opportunity to buy medical insurance privately is shrinking and employer-based insurance is also less available and more restricted than in the past. In 1965, 76 percent of the poor were covered by Medicaid (government sponsored medical insurance); in 1991, fewer than 38 percent of the poor were covered.

▲ Figures on Uninsured

What will happen in the future? The gloomy prediction is that this problem will grow and millions more will be left with inadequate access to medical care. The optimistic prediction is that the government will adopt some kind of more just and rational system of payment for health care. Since you as an individual cannot count on things changing for the better—though you can work toward this—you should be as careful and cautious as possible in making your personal arrangements for medical insurance. Unfortunately, because of the changing nature of this system, it is impossible to predict all the potential changes and difficulties.

INSURANCE YOU PAY FOR (NON-GOVERNMENT INSURANCE)

▲ Employer-Based Insurance

One of the easiest and best ways for you to obtain insurance is through your place of employment. At many jobs you get group medical insurance, often partially financed as a component of your job's compensation. Group medical insurance is often fairly comprehensive and affordable. At companies with at least twenty-five employees, insurance policies usually do not refuse to cover you because you have a medical problem; no "proof of insurability" is required. However, there may be a six- to twelve-month waiting period before you are eligible to get benefits for pre-existing conditions—such as any HIV-related disorder you had at or before the effective date of the policy.

▲ Changing Jobs and Continuing Insurance (COBRA)

If you leave your job, you can maintain your medical insurance at least temporarily. Under the federal Consolidated Omnibus Budget Reconciliation Act of 1985 (COBRA), if you work for an employer that has at least twenty employees, you are entitled to continue your group insurance for eighteen months after you leave your job, at your own expense. If you are disabled at the time you leave your job you are entitled to continue for twenty-nine months. If you change jobs, you may use COBRA to maintain your old group coverage during the waiting period before pre-existing conditions are covered under the group insurance at your new job. Similar laws exist in some states to cover people who work for institutions with fewer than twenty employees.

Converting your insurance: Check the terms of your policy and state insurance regulations to see if you can convert your group policy permanently to individual insurance after you leave your job. These individual policies usually cost more and cover much less than does the group insurance. Your employer does not have to notify you specially that such an option is available; the listing in the employees benefits handbook or contract is considered adequate. *To take advantage of continuation or conversion options, you must take action to change your policy immediately (often within twenty days) after leaving your job, so act promptly.*

▲ Other Group Insurance

If you are not employed, or if your employment does not offer medical insurance benefits, then you should investigate joining a social group or professional organization that offers a group insurance plan. Such plans are often more expensive than employment-based group insurance.

▲ Individual Insurance

Individual medical insurance (also referred to as direct pay or nongroup insurance) is usually expensive. Commercial insurance companies are not required to write policies for people who have an increased chance of falling ill. Consequently, they will refuse you insurance coverage if they think you are at high risk for developing AIDS. For this purpose, insurance companies have the legal right to require HIV antibody testing so your choice of buying such a policy will be very limited. However, if you already have a good individual policy, hold on to it if possible. This insurance cannot be changed or canceled and gives you the most control.

▲ Blue Cross/Blue Shield Open Enrollment

In a few states you can obtain individual insurance through a Blue Cross/Blue Shield open enrollment program. These policies are available without medical evidence of insurability; you may purchase such a policy even if you have AIDS. However, these policies have a number of disadvantages: some coverage may be limited, you may have to pay a certain amount of the medical bills before your insurance begins, there may be a waiting period between buying the insurance and being able to use it, and in some locations only basic hospitalization coverage is available. These policies are available for purchase year round in some states and only during specified periods in other states. You can check about the availability of an open enrollment policy by calling the Blue Cross/Blue Shield office in your area and, if necessary, double-check by calling your state insurance regulatory agency.

▲ Risk Pools

As of December 1990, twenty-six states had created risk pools through which citizens who are otherwise uninsurable can obtain health coverage, although at an increased premium (typically about 150 percent of the median insurance rates). The cost of risk pool insurance is quite high for the level of coverage provided. Contact your state insurance commission for information.

▲ What Your Policy Should Include

If you have medical insurance, whether group or individual, you should read the provisions of your policy carefully. If you do not have a detailed description of the provisions of your medical insurance policy, get one by contacting your personnel office or insurance company.

There are two basic types of medical insurance: hospitalization, which pays for hospital expenses other than doctors' bills; and basic medical/major medical, which pays for some or all of doctors' fees both in and out of the hospital and out-patient laboratory and procedure bills.

Check the following provisions of your policy. If the answers are not satisfactory, consider what options you have for improving your coverage. You may have the option of choosing different levels of coverage. If you are HIV infected and have an increased likelihood of becoming ill, you should choose the highest level of coverage you can afford—that is, the policy that pays for the most extensive health care costs.

- Is there a limit on reimbursement for hospitalization on either a yearly or lifetime basis? If you have HIV disease this limit should be very high because of the possibility of prolonged and expensive hospitalization.
- What percentage of your medical costs does your policy pay for? Policies typically cover 80 percent to 100 percent of your medical bills. Can you afford to pay for the uncovered portion if your bills are extensive?
- Does your policy have a pre-existing-condition clause? What are the details of this provision? A pre-existing condition is a medical condition that existed prior to the effective date of an insurance policy. Coverage may or may not be provided for pre-existing conditions under the terms of a particular policy. Some policies cover all illnesses, whether or not they are pre-existing conditions. Other policies will never pay for any pre-existing condition. Still other policies pay claims relating to pre-existing conditions after a specified waiting time, often eleven months from the effective date of the policy. Definitions of pre-existing conditions vary widely.

372

- Are you free to choose your doctors both for regular medical care and for specialists' visits? Some policies allow you to choose any licensed doctor. Others, known as Health Maintenance Organizations (HMOs) limit your choice to a panel of physicians who are enrolled with them. HMOs provide comprehensive services for a fixed, prepaid amount that is independent of the number of services actually used. The advantage of HMOs is that they pay for 100 percent of medical expenses and are often a good bargain financially. The (very significant) disadvantages are that there may be no doctors expert in treatment of HIV-related illnesses affiliated with your HMO, you will have a limited choice of hospitals to which you can be admitted, and there may be long waits for appointments. Another type of program is referred to as a Preferred Program Organization (PPO). This type of plan functions like an HMO but also allows you to choose a physician outside the approved panel, paying for a higher percentage of the fee than for that of a panel doctor.
- Does your policy pay for prescriptions? Medications for HIV disease can be very expensive. It is highly desirable to have a policy that pays for drugs. If your policy does cover prescription drugs, then in some states (including New York) it has to pay for any drug that has been FDA approved, such as AZT and ddI. It does not have to pay for experimental drugs but often will.
- Does your policy pay for home care and non-hospital institutional care? If you become seriously ill, you may need housekeeping or nursing services at home. This becomes crucial for some people who can remain out of the hospital if they have the appropriate support at home. Some insurance policies pay for such home care. The number of visits allowed per year varies from policy to policy. It is best if your policy covers at least two hundred visits per year. In addition, some policies pay for hospice or nursing home care which gives you increased options if you do become very ill.

▲ The Issue of Disclosure

What you put down on an insurance form is not really confidential. HIV-infected people face a dilemma of when to start using their health care insurance to pay for HIV-related medical care. On the one hand, it does involve a potential loss of confidentiality. On the other hand, most people cannot pay for medical care without insurance; that's the point of obtaining such insurance.

It is important to think about the consequences of loss of confidentiality in your particular situation. If you get your insurance through your job, your claims may be seen by someone in your firm who processes such forms. This is much more likely to happen in a small company where claims may be handled in the office than in a large company where forms are processed by the insurance company. If your claims will be seen by someone in the office, it is usually best to disclose your situation to someone who is in a position of authority. Pursue your right to have the information treated in a careful and confidential manner, and not spread to many people throughout the company.

If you file an insurance form that indicates either directly or indirectly your HIV status, you do lose some control of the information. Clearly, this could affect your ability to get individual medical insurance in the future. However, at this point virtually all such insurance requires HIV antibody testing for acceptance. Consequently, you won't be able to get such insurance if you are HIV infected.

Generally speaking, you might as well use your insurance. An exception to this may be if you are in a situation where you are about to change jobs and have to take into account the pre-existing-condition clause of your next insurance policy. Insurance companies at this point share information only about applications, not about claims.

GOVERNMENT MEDICAL INSURANCE

Either Medicaid or Medicare is a possibility if you cannot get employer-based insurance or individual insurance. There are many problems with using Medicare or Medicaid, but with persistence and energy it may be possible for you to get adequate or even good medical care with this type of insurance. For more information about applying for Medicare or Medicaid, contact an entitlement worker from an AIDS service organization. Application is made at a local welfare office.

▲ Medicare

Medicare is a federally funded program that pays for partial medical costs for anyone who is over 65, has permanent kidney failure, or has been entitled to Social Security Disability Insurance (SSDI) benefits for two years. This two-year delay often makes the Medicare program useless to those with AIDS.

Medicare pays for hospitalization (with some deductible and some limit), a limited amount of skilled nursing-facility care, some hospice care, a very limited amount of home care, and for eighty percent of out-patient doctors' visits.

Application is made at the local Social Security office. Those receiving SSDI (see pp. 378–79) will automatically receive the benefits after two years.

▲ Medicaid

Medicaid (known as MediCal in California) is a federally, state, and locally funded program that covers health care expenses for some people who do not have medical insurance and whose income falls below the poverty level. If you receive Social Security Disability Insurance (SSDI) or Aid to Families with Dependent Children (AFDC), you are automatically entitled to Medicaid in some states. In other states you will have to make a separate application.

If you are uninsured but have some savings, you will have to spend most of your savings ("divesting assets," or "spending down") before you are eligible for Medicaid. Sometimes Medicaid will pay the premium of a pre-existing individual insurance policy that you can no longer afford to pay. For example, it will pay the premium on a Blue Cross/Blue Shield open enrollment policy in New York. If you are on Medicaid, you will probably not be able to find a private doctor who will see you as a patient. However, if you have been seeing a private doctor in the past through insurance and then become dependent on Medicaid, your physician will probably continue to treat you, although sometimes through the hospital clinic with which she or he is affiliated.

If you are on Medicaid the best place to find treatment is through a clinic connected to a teaching hospital that has experience with HIV disease. Although there is a gross shortage of such services, there are such clinics in New York, San Francisco, Los Angeles, and a number of other cities. Call your local AIDS organizations and find out which clinic they suggest. Some of these clinics may have waiting lists; sign up as soon as possible and be sure to keep your first appointment.

Chapter 21
Money to Live On

If you are ill with HIV disease you may be unable to work. This means that you will have to find an alternate source of income. This source of money may come either through the job you held (benefits) or through government programs (entitlements). Explore this topic in depth and be sure you are getting all the funding for which you are eligible.

GET HELP AND INFORMATION

The information provided below is only a brief outline of a complex and frequently changing topic. Get help. See what lectures, pamphlets, and individual assistance is available from local AIDS organizations. A book called *The AIDS Benefits Handbook* by T.P. McCormack (Yale University Press, 1990) contains excellent and detailed information about a large variety of private and government programs. Another excellent resource that is constantly updated is *Personal Finances and HIV Disease* by David Petersen. It is available from Multi-Tasking Systems, 636 Avenue of the Americas, Rm. 3D, New York, NY 10011.

BENEFITS

▲ Life Insurance
Life insurance is an issue for HIV-infected people for two reasons. First, like anyone else you may wish by means of a life insurance policy to provide for someone financially if you die. In addition, at this point it is possible for people who are gravely ill to collect on their life insurance policies while they are alive or to sell them for a significant amount of money. If you have limited resources financially, this money might make a crucial difference if you become seriously ill and need greater resources to lead a more comfortable life.

If you are HIV infected, you will not be able to buy life insurance privately. Life insurance companies do HIV-antibody testing and reject anyone who tests positive.

However, your job may provide life insurance, generally in institutions with greater than twenty-five employees. If this is the case, no medical underwriting is required and you are not HIV tested.

If you leave your job, you are entitled to take over payment of your life insurance policy. You must take action within thirty days of leaving your job. This provision is not nearly as well known as the COBRA rule for medical insurance (see pp. 370–71). If your job denies that this option is available or does not know about it, check immediately with your state insurance agency.

It is possible to get payment on your life insurance policy while you are still alive. Many insurance companies have provisions known as "accelerated benefits." This plan allows seriously ill people to collect a portion of their life insurance. The amount that you can collect on the policy is less than face value but can be as much as 96 percent of this value. Some policies allow you to collect some of the funds, with the remainder to go to your beneficiary.

It is also possible to sell your life insurance policy. Policies are being bought by private companies that use the name "viatical settlement companies." These companies pay you a sum of money (usually 50 percent to 70 percent of the face value of the policy) in return for naming them as the beneficiary of your life insurance. You have to provide information to them about your medical status. You can get information about these programs by calling an AIDS organization.

▲ Disability Insurance

If you become ill and are unable to work, you will need another source of income. Short-term disability insurance (generally six months) is commonly provided through employers. Some jobs (usually in large institutions) also provide long-term disability insurance, which will pay a significant portion of your former earnings, usually 60 percent to 70 percent. These policies can also be purchased privately, but are not sold to people who are HIV infected.

ENTITLEMENTS (GOVERNMENT PROVIDED)

If you have HIV disease and have limited means financially, some government entitlements are available. Medicaid, described above, is relevant to anyone with HIV disease who does not have medical insurance. A number of other programs provide financial assistance if you do not have a job, generally when you are too ill to work.

Following are some guidelines to help you with entitlements:

- Entitlement regulations vary from state to state and city to city and are often confusing. Entitlements tend to be higher in northern industrial states and California and lower in the sunbelt. It is best if you can get information and help from an entitlement worker who is expert in the laws and regulations in your local area. Sometimes you can get such assistance through a local AIDS organization. Some hospital social workers are expert in benefits programs, others are not.
- Time is always an issue in applying for benefits. The bureaucracy

can be—and usually is—slow, confusing, and inefficient. Although you may need extensive documentation to get various entitlements, you should start the application process as soon as you have reason to feel you might be eligible. You can assemble documents at a later date. Sometimes AIDS service organizations have special arrangements or informal relationships with government offices that can reduce waiting time and cut through red tape.

- Documents are important. Your case will move faster if you can provide clear written evidence of any medical statements or financial claims. Always make a photocopy of anything you give to a government office; things get lost.
- Be thorough and assertive. If you do not hear from an entitlements office in the expected period of time, follow through with a phone call, preferably followed by a personal visit. However, try to remember that the workers in these offices are frequently under great stress and that it is in your interest to establish a positive relationship, if possible, with the entitlement worker.
- It may become clear to you that you will need to apply to some kind of entitlement program while you are hospitalized. If you suspect this is the case, begin the process while you are in the hospital and as soon as possible. Ask to speak to the social worker or other staff member who deals with benefits. Some entitlements can be arranged faster while you are an in-patient in the hospital.

Following are the major programs that can provide you with assistance.

▲ Social Security: Social Security Disability Insurance (SSDI)

SSDI is a federally funded program that provides money to aged, blind, and disabled people who have worked and paid funds into Social Security. It is not means tested; that is, you are eligible for SSDI regardless of your financial status if you meet other requirements. Benefits start five full calendar months after the onset of disability. The definition of disability is complex and changing. A diagnosis of AIDS has qualified people for SSDI, while other forms of HIV disease have received varying responses. However, as the new definition (1992) of AIDS becomes effective, not all people with an AIDS diagnosis will qualify for SSDI although the total number of people with HIV disease who can get SSDI will increase.

Benefits vary depending on your lifetime average earnings. You can continue to work and receive a very limited amount of income while receiving SSDI or return to work on a trial basis.

▲ Supplemental Security Income (SSI)

SSI is another source of income provided by Social Security and is similar to SSDI in many of its eligibility requirements. However, it is intended to provide money for poor, aged, blind, or otherwise disabled persons who have not worked enough to get the full amount of SSDI. It is means-tested. It can become effective immediately at the onset of a disability and can be a bridge until you are eligible for SSDI.

Apply for SSDI and SSI at your local Social Security office. Someone else can apply for you if you are hospitalized or sick and generally you can begin the application procedure while in the hospital with the help of an entitlement worker.

▲ Help Paying for AIDS Drugs

The AIDS Drugs Reimbursement Program provides funding for drugs for eligible HIV-infected people. It is jointly run by federal and state government, and provisions and entitlements vary widely from state to state. Some states pay only for AZT. Other states, such as California and New York, pay for a variety of drugs used to treat HIV disease. In both New York State and California, these programs have performed exceptionally well. The red tape is limited, response time is fast, and the programs pay for many drugs needed in treating HIV disease.

Eligibility consists of proof of medical need (a form filled out by your doctor) and certain financial requirements. The financial requirements are that you do not have an insurance policy that covers prescriptions, are not on Medicaid, and earn below a certain amount of money per year, varying by the particular state. In New York State, the limit is $44,000 per year. In California, the limit for full reimbursement is $27,000 per year; Californians with income between $27,000 and $50,000 per year are responsible for a copayment that depends on your taxable income. In some states the income cap is as low as $6,000 per year. In some states the program has run out of funds. Information about the AIDS Drug Reimbursement Program is generally available by calling the Department of Health in your county. Some direct sources of information are:

US Health Resources and Services Agency   (301) 443-9086
    AIDS Drug Reimbursement Program

NY State AIDS Drug Assistance Program   (800) 542-2437
    (ADAP)

CA State Office of AIDS   (916)-324-8429

▲ Aid to Families with Dependent Children (AFDC)

AFDC is one of the programs usually referred to as welfare. It is jointly run by the federal and state government. It provides assistance to certain low-income families with at least one child below the age of 18. AFDC is means-tested. Both these standards and benefits vary from state to state. You are automatically eligible for Medicaid if you qualify for AFDC. Application is made at your local welfare office. Someone else may apply for you if you are hospitalized or sick.

▲ General Assistance

General assistance is another term for what people call welfare. It is also referred to as *public assistance* and *income maintenance.* It is available in most but not all localities in the United States. The programs are state and locally run and provide money to people who are not eligible for AFDC or SSI. Because these programs are locally run, the requirements, benefits, and red tape vary from location to location. Waits and confusion are common and you should attempt to file all applications as promptly as possible and follow through aggressively.

Application is made at your local welfare office. You can also apply at these offices for Emergency Assistance, which in some states will pay for one-time emergency expenses for eligible people. They may pay for such things as overdue rent and utility bills, food, and shelters, or hotel bills for the homeless. Requirements and benefits vary state by state.

▲ Food Stamps

The Food Stamps program is federally funded and state run. It provides money for food for disabled individuals on SSDI and SSI and others who meet the income requirement. Application is made at your local welfare office.

▲ New York State AIDS Health Insurance Program (AHIP)

This New York State program will pay insurance premiums for those with income below $1,049 per month and any amount of assets. It is particularly useful for people who are on SSDI and not Medicaid-eligible.

Check what other benefits might be provided to people with AIDS by local government in your area. For example, reduced fare on public transportation is available in many areas and rent subsidies are paid in some locations. Student loans are canceled with the onset of disability.

FREE PRIVATE SERVICES

Many voluntary, private, and religious organizations provide a number of important services to people with AIDS. For example, in several cities qualified applicants can receive free meals delivered to the home.

Transportation to medical appointments is another option in some areas. Volunteer services from a "buddy" who will do tasks and provide company and support are available through some AIDS organizations. A variety of other services are available. You should check with your local or state AIDS organizations to find out what services may be available and useful to you.

Chapter 22
Some Legal Matters

DISCRIMINATION

▲ General

You face the possibility of harassment and discrimination because of your HIV infection. People with AIDS have suffered discrimination in employment, health care, insurance, education, housing, and the use of public accommodations. Discrimination against people with AIDS or HIV infection is illegal in most situations. Almost all the court cases have been decided against discrimination and in the favor of the person with HIV disease.

However, this does not resolve the issue of discrimination for people with HIV disease. If you face discrimination you will have to take action to get relief from your grievance. This requires effort, time, energy, and, sometimes, money, and all these resources may be in short supply if you are a person with AIDS. Furthermore, fighting discrimination can be enormously taxing psychologically.

If you face discrimination, you will have to make a decision about what to do about it. In principle, it would be helpful for people with HIV disease if every person who faced discrimination fought back in various ways, including through the use of the legal system. However, it may not be the right decision for you as an individual to do so. This will depend on how you have been discriminated against, what you have lost by the discrimination, and what you stand to gain by taking action. It will also depend on your physical state of health, your psychological state, what kind of practical and emotional resources are available to you and what kind of support you can get from people and institutions around you.

If you are facing any situation that you think is discriminatory—even if you are not sure—you should at least take the step of getting expert advice. Many AIDS organizations can arrange for you to speak without charge to someone who can advise you about your situation. Such advice has been available directly through staff members at some AIDS organizations, through gay and lesbian legal-rights groups, and, in some areas, from local Human Rights Commissions.

Even if you decide not to take legal action, this consultation can be useful. People who are dealing with HIV discrimination can give you an accurate idea about how much work would be necessary for you to take legal action. It may not be as difficult as you fear. They may also be able to give you advice on other methods of lessening discrimination. Some people feel empowered if they know about possible action and therefore feel less vulnerable and better able to protect themselves.

So—the first thing to do if you face possible discrimination is to call your local or state AIDS organization and get a referral to talk with someone. If you live in a small town or isolated area, you can call an AIDS organization in the nearest major metropolitan area.

It is important to investigate your rights quickly, because time may be a factor in what options are available to you. Laws may invalidate complaints filed too long after the offending action—this means you may have to act within a few weeks of the date of any incident.

Lawyers are expensive. The majority of people with HIV disease cannot afford private legal services to fight discrimination. Free legal services are available in many communities; check with your local or state AIDS organization. If you can afford to get help privately, get a referral to a lawyer who is experienced in HIV-related discrimination law.

It is a good idea to keep careful notes and documents about any discrimination you face. Such documentation could be vital in taking action. If it is possible, record names, dates, and descriptions of discriminatory occurrences. If you are facing possible employment discrimination, it is in your interest to establish a "paper trail" in the form of a written record of positive job evaluations.

The laws surrounding discrimination are complicated, changing, and vary depending on whether federal, state, or local law is invoked. Only a brief summary of some important points can be given here.

Until recently, a primary source of protection against discrimination in employment and education for people with AIDS has been Section 504 of the United States Federal Rehabilitation Act of 1973. This act prohibits discrimination against the handicapped and courts have ruled this to include HIV disease. The limitation of Section 504 of the United States Federal Rehabilitation Act is that only institutions receiving federal funds are protected.

In 1990 the United States Congress passed the Americans with Disabilities Act (ADA), to take effect in 1992. ADA extends the provisions of Section 504 of the Rehabilitation Act to a much broader group of people and covers public accommodations, transportation, and public services. As of 1992, employers with twenty-five or more employees must comply. In 1994, employers with fifteen or more employees also have to comply. ADA specifically covers people with HIV disease.

HIV antibody testing is not permitted in an employment setting, since the use of tests to screen out disabled persons is explicitly prohibited by Section 504 of the Rehabilitation Act. Employers have tried to justify termination of HIV-infected employees on the grounds that medical costs associated with the illnesses of some HIV-infected employees impose an economic burden on businesses by increasing the cost of employee benefit programs. The courts have rejected this argument in several instances.

Until the federal ADA is enforced, some who suffer discrimination may be protected only under state and municipal laws. About forty states have laws prohibiting discrimination against the disabled in employment, and many states have recently strengthened these laws. Laws are different in each state: some cover only public employees or employees of organizations with more than sixteen workers; some exclude those with communicable diseases.

If you are a union member, your collective-bargaining agreement may provide additional protection because it places limits on the arbitrary dismissal of an employee.

People have also faced discrimination in housing, education, and access to services, particularly medical and dental care and nursing homes. Again, the vast majority of cases that have been litigated have been decided in favor of the person with HIV disease. Get advice.

▲ Federal Employment

The federal government requires all applicants for employment or service in certain programs to take the HIV antibody test. These include the Peace Corps, the Foreign Service of the State Department; the Armed Forces; the state National Guard; and residential training programs of the Job Corps. Those testing positive are excluded.

▲ Military Personnel

All military and National Guard personnel and all recruits are subjected to HIV antibody testing. Relevant to the United States military's policies regarding AIDS, note that "homosexual conduct" and intravenous (IV) drug use are charges for which any member of the military may face court-martial. If you are diagnosed with HIV disease while you are in the military, get legal help *immediately*. Some sources of help:

Military Law Task Force (National Military Project on AIDS)	(619) 233-1701
Citizen Soldier	(212) 777-3470
Midwest Committee for Military Counseling	(312) 939-3349
CCCO	(415) 474-3002, (215) 545-4626

Some Legal Matters

▲ Prisoners

A large number of HIV-infected Americans are incarcerated in federal, state, or local prisons. Medical care in prison systems is very poor: it is difficult for an HIV-infected prisoner to get the sophisticated medical care that HIV-related illness requires. The United States Supreme Court has ruled that prisoners have a constitutional right to adequate health care. In some cases, prisoners have been able to obtain legal assistance to improve the quality of health care they receive. Prisoners may also be able to obtain help from local AIDS service organizations.

▲ Immigration

Since December 1987, all applicants for citizenship and resident alien status ("green card") have been obliged to be HIV antibody tested, and if positive are (with rare exceptions) excluded. All applicants for amnesty under the 1986 Simpson-Rodino Immigration Act are also required to be tested. If you have already gained citizenship or resident alien status, you are not required to be tested. Get expert help with immigration problems: the laws are highly specialized and complex.

▲ Travel to Foreign Countries

Over fifty countries now place some travel restrictions on HIV-infected people. These restrictions apply primarily to those visitors who are planning long-term stays, such as students or migrant workers. Permanent immigration of HIV-infected people is barred by many countries.

The regulations vary widely. Check with the embassy of foreign countries you plan to visit to get up-to-the-minute information about their visa requirements. Ironically, the United States has one of the most restrictive travel policies in the world.

▲ Information Sources for Help Against Discrimination

For information and help regarding discrimination, contact your state and local Human Rights Commissions. A good collection of legal information available in bookstores is *AIDS and the Law,* edited by H. Dalton, S. Burris, and the Yale AIDS Law Project, Yale University Press, 1987. Contact Lambda Legal Defense to get their pamphlet *Living With AIDS* and their *AIDS Legal Guide,* a more detailed technical work. The National Lawyers' Guild AIDS Network publishes an *AIDS Practice Manual* for lawyers as well as *The Exchange,* a newsletter on legal and political issues around AIDS. The Intergovernmental Health Policy Project has published *AIDS: A Public Health Challenge* which contains information on state and federal legislation, plus broad discussions of AIDS policy issues. You may also wish to contact the following national organizations:

American Civil Liberties   (212) 944-9800, ext. 545
Union—AIDS Project

National Lawyers' Guild AIDS
Network

(415) 285-5066

Intergovernmental Health Policy
Project—AIDS Policy Center
(George Washington University)

(202) 872-1445

WILLS, LIVING WILLS, AND DURABLE POWER OF ATTORNEY

▲ Wills

It is difficult to think about the topic of wills because it means thinking about your death. Nonetheless, wills are generally easy to do and give you control over what happens to your property. It is particularly important if you are unmarried (gay or straight) and you want your property to go to a life partner or to a charity. If you do not have a will, any property you leave will go automatically to your spouse or nearest living relative.

If you cannot afford the help of a private lawyer, most AIDS organizations will provide free assistance in making a will.

▲ Living Wills

A living will is a document that gives you some say about the kind of medical care you will get if you are very seriously ill and are unconscious or incompetent to make decisions. Provisions for living wills vary from state to state.

It is not complicated to make a living will. You can obtain a sample copy of the type suitable to your location from your local AIDS organization and then make specifications after speaking to your doctor. Two witnesses sign the document, and you give a copy to your physician and one to someone close to you. You can always rescind or change the living will.

Living wills cover topics such as when resuscitation should occur, pain medication, artificial feeding, surgery, dialysis, transplantation, use of a respirator, and use of medical "heroic measures."

You can often get free help with making a living will through your local AIDS organization. If you wish to make out a living will while you are in the hospital, speak to the social worker.

▲ Durable Power of Attorney

As part of the living will, or separately, you can get a "durable power of attorney" that will specify someone close to you to help make medical decisions if you are unable to do so. This is also referred to as a "health care proxy."

This person can then make decisions that are not covered by the living will. This person can be a friend or family member; it cannot be your physician. Obviously, you need have the agreement of the person you are designating and should have a discussion with this person about the type of care you wish. Your health care proxy cannot be held legally or financially responsible.

You may wish to give someone you trust power of attorney so that they can handle financial and practical matters should you be unable to do so.

Sources

ABBREVIATIONS USED

ACC	*AIDS Clinical Care*
AIDS	Acquired Immune Deficiency Syndrome
AIM	*Annals of Internal Medicine*
CDC	Centers for Disease Control
J	Journal
J of AIDS	*Journal of the Acquired Immune Deficiency Syndromes*
JAMA	*Journal of the American Medical Association*
J Inf Dis	*Journal of Infectious Diseases*
Med	Medical *or* Medicine
MMWR	*Morbidity and Mortality Weekly Report*
NEJM	*New England Journal of Medicine*
Rev Inf Dis	*Reviews of Infectious Diseases*

We would like to acknowledge our indebtedness throughout the text to the following excellent medical textbooks, abbreviated as indicated below:

COHEN	Cohen, P., Sande, M., Volberding, P., eds. *The AIDS Knowledge Base.* Massachusetts Medical Society, Waltham, MA, 1990.
HARVEY	Harvey, A., ed. *The Principles and Practice of Medicine.* Appleton & Lange, East Norwalk, CT, 1988.
SANDE	Sande, M., and Volberding, P., eds. *The Medical Management of AIDS.* W. B. Saunders, Philadelphia, PA, 1990.
WORMSER	Wormser, G., ed. *AIDS and Other Manifestations of HIV Infection,* Noyes Publications, Park Ridge, NJ, 1987.

CHAPTER 1—HIV ANTIBODY TESTING

Burke, D., et al. Measurement of the false positive rate in a screening program for human immunodeficiency virus infections. *NEJM,* 1988; 319:961–64.

CDC. Interpretation and use of the Western blot assay for serodiagnosis of human immunodeficiency virus type 1 infections. *MMWR,* July 28, 1989; 38:S-7:1–7.

_____. Update—Serologic testing for antibody to human immunodeficiency virus. *MMWR,* 1988; 36:833–40, 845.

_____. Update—HIV-2 infection—United States. *MMWR,* Aug. 25, 1989; 38:33:572–80.

Cleary, P., et al. Compulsory premarital screening for the human immunodeficiency virus: technical and public health considerations. *JAMA,* 1987; 258:1757–62.

Demkovich, L., ed. HIV reporting in the states. Intergovernmental AIDS Reports, AIDS Policy Center, George Washington University, Washington, D.C., Nov.–Dec. 1989; 2:5:3.

Genesca, J., et al. What do Western blot indeterminate patterns for human immunodeficiency virus mean in EIA-negative blood donors? *Lancet,* Oct. 28, 1989.

Groopman, J., et al. Antibody seronegative human T-lymphotropic virus type III (HTLV-III)-infected patients with acquired immunodeficiency syndrome or related disorders. *Blood,* 1985; 66:742–44.

_____. Lack of evidence of prolonged human immunodeficiency virus infection before antibody seroconversion. *Blood,* 1988; 71:1752–54.

Horsburgh, R., et al; Pan, L. Z., et al. Correspondence on "Imagawa, D., et al.: Human immunodeficiency virus type 1 infection in homosexual men who remain seronegative for prolonged periods." *NEJM,* Dec. 14, 1989; 321:24:1678–81.

Imagawa, D., et al. "HIV-1 in seronegative homosexual men." Letter, *NEJM,* Oct. 24, 1991; 325:17:1250–51.

_____. Human immunodeficiency virus type 1 infection in homosexual men who remain seronegative for prolonged periods. *NEJM,* June 1, 1989; 320:22:1458. *Later retracted in the following letter to the editor.*

Pan, L., et al. Lack of detection of human immunodeficiency virus in persistently seronegative homosexual men with high or medium risks for infection. *J Inf Dis,* Nov. 1991; 164:5:962–64.

Phair, J., et al. Diagnosis of infection with the human immunodeficiency virus. *J Inf Dis,* Feb. 1989; 159:2:320–23.

Ranki, A. Long latency precedes overt seroconversion in sexually transmitted human-immunodeficiency-virus infection. *Lancet,* Sept. 12, 1987, vol. 2 for 1987, 8559:589–93.

Rutherford, G., et al. Course of HIV-1 infection in a cohort of homosexual and bisexual men: an 11-year follow-up study. *British Med J,* Nov. 24, 1990; 301:1183–88.

Ward, J., et al. Risk of human immunodeficiency virus infection from blood donors who later developed the acquired immune deficiency syndrome. *AIM,* 1987; 106:61–62.

Wolinsky, S., et al. Human immunodeficiency virus type 1 (HIV-1) infection of a median of 18 months before a diagnostic Western blot. *AIM,* Dec. 15, 1989; 111:12:961–72.

CHAPTER 2—YOU AND YOUR DOCTOR

No sources.

Sources

CHAPTER 3—MONITORING THE IMMUNE SYSTEM

Crowe, S., et al. Predictive value of CD4 lymphocyte numbers for the development of opportunistic infections and malignancies in HIV-infected persons. *J of AIDS,* 1991; 4:770–76.

Davey, R., and Lane, H. Laboratory methods in the diagnosis and prognostic staging of infection with human immunodeficiency virus type 1. *Rev Inf Dis,* Sept.–Oct. 1990; 12:5:912–30.

Hecht, F. Prognostic Markers I: T-lymphocytes. *ACC,* March 1991; 3:3:20.

————. Prognostic Markers II. *ACC,* Apr. 1991; 3:4:28–29.

Krämer, A., et al. Neopterin: a predictive marker of acquired immune deficiency syndrome in human immunodeficiency virus infection. *J of AIDS,* 1989; 2:291–96.

Machado, S., et al. On the use of laboratory markers as surrogates for clinical endpoints in the evaluation of treatment for HIV infection. *J of AIDS,* 1990; 3:1065–73.

Moss, A., and Bacchetti, P. Natural history of HIV infection. AIDS, 1989; 3:55–61.

Polis, M., and Masur, H. Predicting the progression to AIDS. *American J Med,* Dec. 1990; 89:701–05.

Reddy, M., and Grieco, M. Neopterin and alpha and beta interleukin-1 levels in sera of patients with human immunodeficiency virus infection. *J of Clinical Microbiology,* 1989; 27:1919–23.

Taylor, J., et al. CD4 percentage, CD4 number, and CD4:CD8 ratio in HIV infection: which to choose and how to use. *J of AIDS,* 1989; 2:114–24.

Yarchoan, R., et al. CD4 count and the risk of death in patients with HIV receiving antiretroviral therapy. *AIM,* Aug. 1991; 115:3:184–89.

CHAPTER 4—AZT, DDI, AND DDC

Bach, M., et al. Long-term follow-up of patients with HIV isolates resistant to zidovudine (AZT) treated with dideoxyinosine, abstract TUB91, Seventh International AIDS Conference, Florence, 1991.

Beswick, T. DDC. Fact sheet, Project Inform, San Francisco, May 1, 1991.

Broder, S., et al. Antiretroviral therapy in AIDS. *AIM,* Oct. 15, 1990; 113:8:604–18.

Collier, A., et al. Effect of combination therapy with zidovudine (ZDV) and didanosine (ddI) on surrogate markers, abstract TUB2, Seventh International AIDS Conference, Florence, 1991.

Cooley, T., et al. Once-daily administration of 2'3'-dideoxyinosine (ddI) in patients with the acquired immune deficiency syndrome or the

AIDS-related complex: a phase I trial. *NEJM,* May 10, 1990; 322:19:1340–45.

Crowe, S., et al. Predictive value of CD4 lymphocyte numbers for the development of opportunistic infections and malignancies in HIV-infected persons. *J of AIDS,* 1991; 4:770–76.

Dalakas, M., et al. Mitochondrial myopathy caused by long-term zidovudine therapy midochondrial myopathy. *NEJM,* Apr. 19, 1990; 322:16:1098–1105.

Don, P., et al. Nail dyschromia associated with zidovudine. *AIM,* Jan. 15, 1990, 112:2:145–46.

Edwards, P., et al. Esophogeal ulceration induced by zidovudine. *AIM,* Jan. 1, 1990; 112:1:65–66.

Eron, J., et al. Synergistic inhibition of HIV-1 by the combination of zidovudine (AZT) and 2'3'-dideoxycytidine (ddC) in vitro, abstract WB 2110, Seventh International AIDS Conference, Florence, 1991.

Fischl, M., et al. Prolonged zidovudine therapy in patients with AIDS and advanced AIDS-related complex. *JAMA,* Nov. 3, 1989; 262:17:2405–10.

———. Response to T. Odell letter to the editor "Prolonged zidovudine therapy: confounded by *Pneumocystis carinii* prophylaxis?" *JAMA,* March 23, 1990; 263:12:1635.

———. The efficacy of azidothymidine (AZT) in the treatment of patients with AIDS and AIDS-related complex. A double-blind, placebo-controlled trial. *NEJM,* July 23, 1987; 317:185–91.

———. The safety and efficacy of zidovudine (AZT) in the treatment of subjects with mildly symptomatic human immunodeficiency virus type 1 (HIV) infection. *AIM,* May 15, 1990; 112:10:727.

———. Dideoxynucleoside antiretroviral therapy. In Volberding, P., ed. *AIDS Clinical Review,* 1991, Marcel Dekker, 1991.

———. Randomized controlled trial of a reduced daily dose of zidovudine in patients with the acquired immunodeficiency syndrome. *NEJM,* Oct. 11, 1991, 323:15:1009–14.

———. Recombinant erythropoietin for patients with AIDS treated with zidovudine. *NEJM,* May 24, 1990; 322:21:1488–93.

Friedland, G. Editorial: Early treatment for HIV. *NEJM,* Apr. 5, 1990; 322:14:1000–02.

Gottlieb, M., et al. 2'3'-Dideoxycytidine (ddC) in the treatment of patients with AIDS and ARC, abstract ThBO3, Fifth International AIDS Conference, Montreal, 1989.

Graham, N., et al. The effects on survival of early treatment of human immunodeficiency virus infection. *NEJM,* Apr. 16, 1992; 326:16:1037–42.

———. Zidovudine use in AIDS-free HIV-I seropositive homosexual men in the multicenter AIDS cohort study (MACS), 1987–1989. *J of AIDS,* 1991; 4:3:267–76.

Sources

Hamilton, J. A controlled trial of early versus late treatment with zidovudine in symptomatic HIV infection. *NEJM,* Feb. 13, 1992; 326:7:437–43.

Hirsch, M. Azidothymidine. *J Inf Dis,* March, 1988; 157:3:427–30.

Jackson, G., et al. Human immunodeficiency virus (HIV) antigenemia (p24) in the acquired immunodeficiency syndrome (AIDS) and the effect of treatment with zidovudine (AZT). *AIM,* Feb. 1988; 108:2:175–80.

Joseph, E., et al. Synergistic inhibition of HIV-1 by the combination of zidovudine (AZT) and 2'3'-dideoxycytidine (ddC) in vitro, abstract WB 2110, Seventh International AIDS Conference, Florence, 1991.

Kahn, J. Clinical issues in using Didanosine (ddI), *ACC,* Dec. 1991; 3:12:90–91, 95.

Lambert, J., et al. 2'3'-dideoxyinosine (ddI) in patients phase I trials: reduction of serum p24 and sustained increases of T4 cells in patients with the acquired immune deficiency syndrome or the AIDS-related complex. *NEJM,* May 10, 1990; 322:19:254–61.

Lane, C., et al. Zidovudine in patients with human immunodeficiency virus (HIV) and Kaposi's sarcoma. *AIM,* July 1, 1989; 111:1:41–50.

Larder, B., et al. HIV with reduced sensitivity to zidovudine (AZT) isolated during prolonged therapy, *Science,* March 31, 1989; 243:1731–34.

Lemp, G., et al. Improved survival for persons with AIDS in San Francisco, abstract TUC 41, 1991, Seventh International AIDS Conference, Florence, 1991.

Meng, T. Combination therapy with zidovudine and dideoxycytidine in patients with advanced human immunodeficiency virus infection, *AIM,* Jan. 1, 1992, 116:85–86.

Merigan, T., et al. Circulating P24 antigen levels and response of dideoxycytidine in human immunodeficiency virus (HIV) infections. *AIM,* Feb. 1, 1989; 110:3:189–94.

Metroka, C. Failure of prophylaxis with dapsone in patients taking dideoxyinosine (letter). *NEJM,* 325:10:737.

Montaner, J. The effect of zidovudine on platelet count in HIV-infected individuals. *J of AIDS,* 1990, 3:6:565–70.

Moore, R., et al. Zidovudine and the natural history of the acquired immunodeficiency syndrome, *NEJM,* May 16, 1991; 324:20:1412–16.

Oskenhendler, E. Zidovudine for thrombocytopenic purpura related to human immunodeficiency virus (HIV) infection, *AIM,* March 1, 1989; 110:5:365–68.

Project Inform (San Francisco) fact sheet on AZT, March 27, 1990.

Rachlis, A. Zidovudine (Retrovir) update. *Canadian Med Assoc J,* 1990, 143: 1177–85.

Sources

Reudy, J., et al. Editorial: Zidovudine for early human immunodeficiency virus infection: who, when, and how? *AIM*, May 15, 1990, 112:10:721–23.

Richman, D., et al. The toxicity of azidothymidine (AZT) in the treatment of patients with AIDS and AIDS-related complex. A double-blind, placebo-controlled trial. *NEJM*, July 23, 1987; 317:185–91.

Richman, D. Effect of stage of disease and drug dose on zidovudine susceptibilities of isolates of human immunodeficiency virus. *J of AIDS*, 1990; 3:8:743–46.

Rosenberg, P. National AIDS incidence trends and the extent of zidovudine therapy in selected demographic and transmission groups. *J of AIDS*, 1991; 4:4:392–401.

Rozencweig, M. Overview of phase I trials of 2'3'-dideoxyinosine (ddI) conducted on adult patients. *Rev Inf Dis*, July–Aug. 1990; 12:Supplement:S570–S574.

Sattler, F., et al. Acetominophen does not impair clearance of zidovudine. *AIM*, June 1, 1991; 114:11:937–40.

Schecter, M., et al. Effect of zidovudine on progression to AIDS in cohort study, (letter), *Lancet*, May 6, 1989; 1026.

Shaunak, S. Zidovudine-induced neutropenia: are we too cautious? *Lancet*, July 8, 1989; 91–92.

Shirasaka, T., et al. HIV may develop resistance preferentially to azidothymidine (AZT) as compared to dideoxycytidine (ddC) or dideoxyinosine (ddI) in patients receiving antiviral therapy, abstract WA9, Seventh International AIDS Conference, Florence, 1991.

Singer, J., et al. Clinical significance of in-vitro HIV resistance to zidovudine in early HIV-infected individuals after four years of therapy, abstract WB2414, Seventh International AIDS Conference, Florence, 1991.

Skowron, G. Phase II trials of alternating and intermittent regimens of zidovudine (ZDV) and 2'3'-dideoxycytidine (ddC) in AIDS and ARC, abstract ThB23, Sixth International AIDS Conference, San Francisco, 1990.

Steffe, E. The effect of acetominophen on zidovudine metabolism in HIV-infected patients. *J of AIDS*, 1990; 3:7:691–94.

Torres, G. Highlights from the VII International AIDS Conference, June 16–21, 1991, Florence. Treatment Issues, Gay Men's Health Crisis, New York, 1991.

Unadkat, J., et al. Pharmacokinetics of oral zidovudine (azidothymidine) in patients with AIDS when administered with and without a high-fat meal. AIDS, 1990; 4:3:229–32.

Volberding, P., et al. Zidovudine in asymptomatic human immunodeficiency virus infection. *NEJM*, Apr. 5, 1990; 322:14:941–49.

Yarchoan, R., et al. Administration of 3'-azido-3'-deoxythymidine, an inhibitor of HTL VIII/LAV replication, to patients with AIDS or AIDS-related complex, *Lancet*, 1986; 1:575–80.

————. Clinical pharmacology of 3'-azido-2'3' dideoxythymidine (zidovudine) and related dideoxynucleosides. *NEJM*, Sept. 14, 1989; 321:11:726–38.

————. In vivo activity against HIV and favorable toxicity profile of 2'3'-dideoxyinosine. *Science*, 1989; 245:412–15.

————. Long-term toxicity/activity profile of 2'3'-dideoxyinosine in AIDS or AIDS-related complex. *Lancet*, Sept. 1, 1990; 336:526–29.

————. Phase I studies of ddC in HIV infection as a single agent and alternating with zidovudine. *Lancet*, Jan. 16, 1988; 1:8576–81.

CHAPTER 5—PREVENTING PCP AND OTHER COMPLICATIONS

Beecham, H., et al. Decreasing incidence of *Pneumocystis carinii* pneumonia in a human immunodeficiency virus positive population [abstract], In Programs and Abstracts of the 30th Interscience Conference on Antimicrobial Agents and Chemotherapy, Atlanta, 1990.

CDC, Public Health Service Task Force Report. Antipneumocystis prophylaxis in human imunodeficiency virus-infected individuals. *MMWR*, 1989; 38:1–9.

————. Guidelines for prophylaxis against *Pneumocystis carinii* pneumonia for persons infected with the human immunodeficiency virus. *MMWR*, 1989; 38:S5.

Clotet, B., et al. Twice-weekly dapsone-pyremethamine as pneumocystis prophylaxis, abstract ThB414, Sixth International AIDS Conference, San Francisco, 1990.

Crowe, S., et al. Predictive values of CD4 lymphocyte numbers for the development of opportunistic infections and malignancies in HIV-infected persons, *J of AIDS*, 1991; 4:8:776.

DeGans, J. Pyrimethamine alone as maintenance therapy for central nervous system toxoplasmosis in 38 patients with AIDS toxoplasmosis. *J of AIDS*, Feb. 1992; 5:2:137–43.

Fischl, M., et al. Safety and efficacy of sulfamethoxazole and trimethoprim chemoprophylaxis for *Pneumocystis carinii* pneumonia in AIDS. *JAMA*, 1988; 259:1185–89.

Girard, P. Prévention des rechutes de pneumocystose par les aerosols de pentamidine: Étude prospective randomisée chez les patients SIDA traités par AZT, abstract TBP 49, Fifth International AIDS Conference, Montreal, 1989.

Hardy, D. Prophylaxis of AIDS-related opportunistic infections (OIs): current status and future strategies. In Volberding, P., ed. *AIDS Clinical Review*, 1991, Marcel Dekker, 1991.

Sources

HHS News, U.S. Department of Health and Human Services, Bulletin, for release Sept. 6, 1991.

Hirschel, B., et al. A controlled study of inhaled pentamidine for the primary prevention of *Pneumocystis carinii* pneumonia, *NEJM,* Apr. 18, 1991; 321:16:1079–83.

Hughes, W., et al. Successful chemoprophylaxis for *Pneumocystis carinii* pneumonia, *NEJM,* 1977; 297:1419–26.

Jenkins, R., et al. Prophylaxis for opportunistic infections, PI Perspective, Project Inform, Apr., 1991; 10:8–11.

Kovacs, J., et al. Prophylaxis of *Pneumocystis carinii* pneumonia: an update. *J Inf Dis,* Nov. 1989; 160:5:882–86.

Leoung, G., et al. Aerosolized pentamidine for prophylaxis against *Pneumocystis carinii* pneumonia, *NEJM,* Sept. 20, 1990; 232:12:769–75.

Masur, H. Prevention of *Pneumocystis carinii* pneumonia. *Rev Inf Dis,* Nov.–Dec. 1989: II:S7:S1664–S1668.

Metroka, C., et al. Desensitization to dapsone in HIV-positive patients. *JAMA,* Jan. 22/29, 1992; 267:4:512.

———. et al. Successful chemoprophylaxis for Pneumocystis with dapsone or Bactrim, abstract TBO4 Fifth International AIDS Conference, Montreal, 1989.

———. Failure of prophylaxis with dapsone in patients taking dideoxyinosine (letter). *NEJM;* 325:10:737.

Montaner, J., et al. Aerosolized pentamidine with a secondary prophylaxis of *Pneumocystis carinii* pneumonia, June 1, 1991; 114:11:948–53.

National Institute of Allergy and Infectious Diseases, unpublished data, as presented in *ACC,* Oct. 1991; 3:10:80.

Neilsen, T., et al. Sulfamethoxazole-trimethoprim as secondary prophylaxis against PCP, abstract Th.B.412, Sixth International AIDS Conference, San Francisco, 1990.

Phair, J., et al. The risk of *Pneumocystis carinii* among men infected with the human immunodeficiency virus type I. *NEJM,* Jan. 18, 1990; 322:3:161–65.

Pierone, G., et al. Trimethoprim-sulfamethoxazole prophylaxis for *Pneumocystis carinii* pneumonia in AIDS, abstract TBO.6, Fifth International AIDS Conference, Montreal, 1989.

Ruskin, J., et al. Low-dose co-trimoxale for prevention of *Pneumocystis carinii* pneumonia in human immunodeficiency virus disease. *Lancet,* Feb. 23, 1991; 337:468–71.

Stein, D., et al. Thrice-weekly dosing of trimethoprim-sulfa for primary and secondary prophylaxis of *P. carinii* pneumonia [abstract]. Programs and Abstracts of the 30th Interscience Conference on Antimicrobial Agents and Chemotherapy, Atlanta, 1990; 854.

Wheat, L. Histoplasmosis in AIDS. *ACC,* Jan. 1992; 14:1:1–4.

CHAPTER 6—GENERAL HEALTH CARE

Blanche, S., et al. A prospective study of infants born to woman seropositive for human immunodeficiency virus type I. *NEJM,* June 22, 1989; 320:25:1643–48.

CDC. Condoms for prevention of sexually transmitted diseases. MMWR, March 11, 1988: 37:9:133–37.

Conant, M., et al. Condoms prevent transmission of AIDS-associated retrovirus. *JAMA,* 1986; 255:1706.

Des Jarlais, D., et al. Development of AIDS, HIV seroconversion, and co-factors for T4 cell loss in a cohort of intravenous drug users. *AIDS: An International Bimonthly,* 1987; 1:105–11.

Francis, D., et al. The prevention of acquired immunodeficiency syndrome in the United States. *JAMA,* 1987; 257:1360.

Friedland, G., and Klein, R. Transmission of the human immunodeficiency virus. *NEJM,* Oct. 10, 1987; 317:18:1125–35.

Fultz, P. Components of saliva inactivate human immunodeficiency virus. *Lancet,* 1986; 2:1215.

Hahn, R., et al. Prevalence of HIV infection among intravenous drug users in the United States. *JAMA,* May 12, 1989; 261:18:2677–84.

Hecht, F. Immunizations in HIV-infected persons, *ACC,* May, 1991; 3:5:36–37.

Hicks, D., et al. Inactivation of LAV/HTLV-III infected cultures of normal human lymphocytes by nonoxynol-9 in vitro. *Lancet* 1985; 2:1422.

Institute of Medicine, National Academy of Sciences. *Confronting AIDS,* 1986; 112.

Kaplan, L., et al. Treatment of patients with acquired immunodeficiency syndrome and associated manifestations. *JAMA,* March 13, 1987; 257:10:1367–74.

Katz, S., et al. Human immunodeficiency virus infection of newborns. *NEJM,* June 22, 1989; 320:25:1687–89.

Kotler, D. Studies of Nutritional Status in Patients with AIDS. In Kotler, D., ed. *Gastrointestinal and Nutritional Manifestations of the Acquired Immunodeficiency Syndrome.* Raven Press, Ltd., New York, 1991.

La Montagne, J. Immunization programs and human immunodeficiency virus. *Rev Inf Dis,* May–June, 1989; II:3:S639–S643.

Lifson, A., et al. The natural history of human immunodeficiency virus infection. *J Inf Dis,* Dec. 1988; 158:6:1364.

Minkoff, H. Care of pregnant women infected with human immunodeficiency virus. *JAMA,* Nov. 20, 1987; 258:19:2714–17.

Newman, C. Practical Dietary Recommendations in HIV Infection. In Kotler, D., ed. *Gastrointestinal and Nutritional Manifestations of the Acquired Immunodeficiency Syndrome.* Raven Press, Ltd., New York, 1991.

Sources

Padian, N. Male to female transmission of human immunodeficiency virus. *JAMA,* Aug. 14, 1987; 258:6:788–90.

Quinn, T., et al. Human immunodeficiency virus infection among patients attending clinics for sexually transmitted diseases. *NEJM,* Jan. 28, 1988: 318:4:197–203.

Recommendations of the Immunization Practices Advisory Committee (ACIP):

- Cholera Vaccine, *MMWR,* Oct. 14, 1988; 617–624.
- General Recommendations on Immunization, *MMWR,* Apr. 7, 1989, vol. 38:13:205–14, 219–27.
- Immunization of Persons with Altered Immunocompetence, Draft, revision 1, June 3, 1991.
- Protection Against Viral Hepatitis, *MMWR,* Feb. 9, 1990; 39:RR2:1–26.
- Smallpox Vaccine, *MMWR,* June 14, 1985; 34:23:341–42.
- Typhoid Immunization, *MMWR,* July 13, 1990; 39:RR-10:1–5.
- Use of BCG Vaccines in the Control of Tuberculosis, *MMWR,* Nov. 4, 1988; 37:43:663–64, 669–75.
- Varicella-Zoster Immune Globulin for the prevention of Chicken Pox, *MMWR,* Feb. 24, 1984; 33:7, 84–90, 95–100.
- Yellow Fever Vaccine, *MMWR,* May 4, 1990; 39:RR-6:1–6.

Riejtmeijer, C., et al. Condoms as physical and chemical barriers against human immunodeficiency virus. *JAMA,* March 25, 1988; 259:12:1851–53.

Schechter, M., et al. Can HTLV-III be transmitted orally? *Lancet,* 1985; 1:379.

Schmalz, J. Addicts to get needles in plan to curb AIDS. *The New York Times,* Jan. 31, 1988; 1.

Spurrett, B., et al. Cervical dysplasia and HIV infection. *Lancet,* Jan. 30, 1988; vol. 1 for 1988, 8579:237–39.

Stamm, W., et al. The association between genital ulcer disease and acquisition of HIV infection in homosexual men. *JAMA,* Sept. 9, 1988; 260:10:1429–33.

Tiollais, P., and Buendia, M. A. Hepatitis B virus. *Scientific American,* Apr. 1991; 264:4:116ff.

U.S. Public Health Service. Protection Against Viral Hepatitis. *MMWR,* Feb. 8, 1990; 39:RR-2:1–26.

Wilson, M., et al. Infections in HIV-infected travelers: risks and prevention. *AIM,* Apr. 1, 1991; 114:7:582–92.

Winick, M., et al. Guidelines for nutrition support in AIDS. *ACC,* Oct. 1989, 49–51.

Winkelstein, W., et al. Sexual practices and risk of infection by the human immunodeficiency virus. *JAMA,* Jan. 16, 1987; 257:3:321–25.

Sources

CHAPTER 7—YOUR STATE OF MIND

American Psychiatric Association: Diagnostic and Statistical Manual of Mental Disorders, third edition, revised (DSM-III-R). Washington, DC, American Psychiatric Association, 1987.

Hyman, S. *Handbook of Psychiatric Drugs.* Little Brown & Co., Boston/ Toronto, 1987.

CHAPTER 8—SEX, AGE, RACE, AND ETHNICITY

CDC. Acquired immunodeficiency syndrome (AIDS) among blacks and Hispanics—United States. *MMWR,* Oct. 24, 1986; 35:42:656–658, 663–666.

_____. AIDS in Women. *MMWR,* 1990; 39:845–46.

_____. *MMWR,* March 15, 1991; 40:RR–2.

_____. Risk for cervical disease in HIV-infected women—New York City. *MMWR,* 1990; 346–49.

Connor, E. Advances in the early detection of HIV infection. *JAMA,* Dec. 25, 1991; 266:24:3474–75.

Dowdle, W. AIDS Coordinator, U.S. Public Health Service. Cited in Houston-Hamilton A. A constant increase: AIDS in ethnic communities. *Focus,* Oct. 1986; 1:11:1–2.

Easterbrook, P., et al. Racial and ethnic differences in outcome in zidovudine-treated patients with advanced HIV disease. *JAMA,* Nov. 20, 1991; 266:19:2712–13.

Feingold, A. Cervical cytologic abnormalities and papillomavirus in women infected with human immunodeficiency virus. *J of AIDS,* 1990; 3:9:896–903.

Grubman, S. HIV Infection in Infants, Children, and Adolescents. To be published in *AIDS and Other Manifestations of HIV Infection,* ed. Wormser, Raven Press, 1992.

Lagakos, S., et al. Effects of zidovudine therapy in minority and other subpopulations with early HIV infection. *JAMA,* Nov. 20, 1991; 266:19:2709–12.

Lopez-Anaya, A. Pharmacokinetics of zidovudine (azidothymidine). III. Effects of pregnancy. *J of AIDS,* 1991; 4:1:64–68.

Minkoff, H., and Dehovitz, J. Care of infected women with the human immunodeficiency virus. *JAMA,* Oct. 23, 1991; 266:16: 2253–58.

_____. HIV Infection in women. *ACC,* May 1991; 3:5:33–35.

Minkoff, H. Care of pregnant women infected with human immunodeficiency virus. *JAMA,* Nov. 20, 1987; 258:19:2714–17.

Pomerantz, R. Human immunodeficiency virus (HIV) infection of the uterine cervix. *AIM,* March 1988; 108:3321–27.

Scott, G. HIV infection in children: clinical features and management. *J of AIDS,* 1991; 4:2:109–15.

Smith, M. Editorial: Zidovudine—does it work for everyone? *JAMA,* Nov. 20, 1991; 266:19:2750–51.

CHAPTER 9—LEARNING ABOUT EXPERIMENTAL TREATMENTS

No sources.

CHAPTER 10—ORGAN SYSTEM COMPLICATIONS

Cockerell, C. Cutaneous signs of AIDS other than Kaposi's sarcoma. In Friedman-Kien A. *Color Atlas of AIDS.* W. B. Saunders, Philadelphia, PA, 1989.

Chan, M. Management of AIDS-related diarrhea. *AIDS Patient Care,* Aug. 1991: 5:4:175–77.

Cotton, P. AIDS Giving Rise to Cardiac Problems. *JAMA,* Apr. 25, 1990; 263:16:2149.

Dalakas, M., et al. Mitochondrial myopathy caused by long-term zidovudine therapy. *NEJM,* Apr. 19, 1990; 322:16:1098–1105.

Grant, I., et al. Evidence for early central nervous system involvement in the acquired immunodeficiency syndrome (AIDS) and other human immunodeficiency virus (HIV) infections. *AIM,* 1987; 107:828–36.

Ho, D., moderator. The acquired immunodeficiency syndrome (AIDS) dementia complex, *AIM,* Sept. 1, 1989; 111:5:400–10.

Johanson, J., et al. Efficient management of diarrhea in the acquired immunodeficiency syndrome. *AIM,* 1990; 112:942–48.

Koralnik, I. A controlled study of early neurological abnormalities in men with asymptomatic human immunodeficiency virus infection. *NEJM,* Sept. 27, 1990; 323:13:864–70.

Perry, S. Organic mental disorders caused by HIV: update on early diagnosis and treatment. *American J Of Psychiatry,* June 1990: 147:6:696–710.

Price, R., et al. The AIDS dementia complex. *J Inf Dis,* Nov. 1988; 158:5:1079–83.

———. The brain in AIDS: central nervous system HIV-1 infection and AIDS dementia complex. *Science,* Feb. 5, 1988; 239:586–92.

Rosenblum, M., et al. *AIDS and the Nervous System.* Raven Press, 1988.

Schmitt, F., et al. Neuropsychological outcome of zidovudine (AZT) treatment of patients with AIDS and AIDS-related complex. *NEJM,* Dec. 15, 1988; 319:24:1573–78.

Schoenfeld, P. HIV Infection and Renal Disease. *ACC,* Feb. 1991; 3:29–11.

So, Y. Neurological manifestations of AIDS. *ACC,* Sept. 1989; 1:5:37–40.

Wilson, M., et al. Infections in HIV-infected travelers: risks and prevention. *AIM,* Apr. 1, 1991; 114:7:582–92.

▲ Cytomegalovirus (CMV)

Byne, W. Cytomegalovirus. *GMHC Treatment Issues Compilation.* Gay Men's Health Crisis, New York, Nov. 1987–Mar. 1989; 57.

Causey, D. Concomitant ganciclovir and zidovudine treatment for cytomegalovirus retinitis in patients with HIV infection: an approach to treatment. *J of AIDS,* 1991; 4:S1.

DeArmond, L. Future directions in the management of cytomegalovirus infections. *J of AIDS,* 1991; 4:S1.

Deiterich, D. Ganciclovir treatment of gastrointestinal infection caused by cytomegalovirus in patients with AIDS. *Rev Inf Dis,* July–Aug. 1988; 10:S3:532–37.

———. Cytomegalovirus colitis in AIDS: presentation in 44 patients and a review of the literature. *J of AIDS,* 1991; 4:S1.

Drew, L. Clinical use of ganciclovir for cytomegalovirus infection and the development of drug resistance. *J of AIDS,* 1991; 4:S1.

———. Cytomegalovirus infection in patients with AIDS. *J Inf Dis,* Aug. 1988;158:2:449–55.

———. Cytomegalovirus. *ACC,* Aug. 1990; 2:8:65–68.

Erice, A. Progressive disease due to ganciclovir-resistant cytomegalovirus in immunocompromised patients. *NEJM,* Feb. 2, 1989; 320:5:289–92.

Gilquin, J. "Genital and oral erosions induced by foscarnet" (letter). *Lancet,* Feb. 3, 1990; 35:287.

Hardy, D. Combined ganciclovir and recombinant human granulocyte-macrophage colony-stimulating factor in the treatment of cytomegalovirus retinitis in AIDS patients. *J of AIDS,* 1991; 4:S1.

Henderly, D. Diagnosis and treatment of cytomegalovirus retinitis. *J of AIDS,* 1991; 4:S1.

Hirsch, M. The treatment of cytomegalovirus in AIDS—more than meets the eye. *NEJM,* Jan. 23, 1992; 326:4:264–65.

Hochster, H. Toxicity of combined ganciclovir and zidovudine for cytomegalovirus disease associated with AIDS. *AIM,* July 15, 1990; 113:2:111–17.

Jacobson, M. Approaches in the treatment of cytomegalovirus retinitis: ganciclovir and foscarnet. *J of AIDS,* 1991; 4:S1.

Jacobson, M. Effect of foscarnet therapy on infection with human immunodeficiency virus in patients with AIDS. *J. Inf Dis,* Oct. 1988; 158:4:862–65.

Kotler, D. Cytomegalovirus colitis and wasting. *J of AIDS,* 1991; 4:S1.

Mills, J. Treatment of cytomegalovirus retinitis in patients with AIDS. *Rev Inf Dis,* July–Aug. 1988; 10:S3:S522–S531.

O'Donnell, Z. Cytomegalovirus. *ACC,* July 1989.

Schooley, R. Cytomegalovirus in the setting of the human immunodeficiency virus. *Rev Inf Dis,* Sept.–Oct. 1990; 12:S7:S811–S819.

Sources

Studies of Ocular Complications of AIDS Research Group, in collaboration with the AIDS Clinical Trials Group. Mortality in patients with the acquired immunodeficiency syndrome treated with either foscarnet or ganciclovir for cytomegalovirus retinitis. *NEJM,* Jan. 23, 1992: 326:4:213–20.

Van Der Pijl, J. "Foscarnet and penile ulceration" (letter), *Lancet,* Feb. 3, 1990; 35:286.

▲ Herpes Simplex Virus

Chatis, P. Successful treatment with foscarnet of an acyclovir-resistant mucocutaneous infection with herpes simplex virus in a patient with the acquired immunodeficiency syndrome. *NEJM,* 1989; 320:293–96.

▲ Hepatitis B Virus

Tiollais, P., and Buendia, M. A. Hepatitis B virus. *Scientific American,* Apr. 1991; 264:4:116ff.

U.S. Public Health Service. Protection against viral hepatitis. *MMWR,* Feb. 8, 1990; 39:RR-2:1–26.

▲ Progressive Multifocal Leukoencephalopathy

Chaisson, R. Progressive multifocal leukencephalopathy in AIDS, *JAMA,* July 4, 1990; 264:1:79–81.

Rosenblum, M. *AIDS and the Nervous System,* Raven Press, 1988.

▲ *Pneumocystis Carinii* Pneumonia (PCP)

Hoo, G. Inhaled or intravenous pentamidine therapy for *Pneumocystis carinii* pneumonia in AIDS. *AIM,* Aug. 1, 1990; 113:3:195–202.

Jules-Elysee, K. Aerosolized pentamidine: effect on diagnosis and presentation of *Pneumocystis carinii* pneumonia. *AIM,* 1990; 112:750–57.

Masur, H. Pneumocystis pneumonia: from bench to clinic. *AIM,* Nov. 15, 1989; 11:10:813–26.

Medina, I. Oral therapy for *Pneumocystis carinii* pneumonia in the acquired immunodeficiency syndrome. *NEJM,* Sept. 20, 1990; 323:12:776–82.

Sattler, F. Trimethoprim-sulfamethoxazole compared with pentamidine for the treatment of *Pneumocystis carinii* pneumonia in the acquired immunodeficiency syndrome—a prospective, non-crossover study. *AIM,* 1988; 109:280–87.

Telzak, E. Extrapulmonary *Pneumocystis carinii* infections. *Rev Inf Dis,* May–June 1990; 12:3:380–86.

▲ *Toxoplasma Gondii*

Dannemann, B. Treatment of toxoplasmic encephalitis in patients with AIDS. *AIM,* Jan. 1, 1992: 116:1:33–43.

Sources

DeGans, J. Pyrimethamine alone as maintenance therapy for central nervous system toxoplasmosis in 38 patients with AIDS. *J of AIDS,* Feb. 1991; 5:2:137–43.

Levy, R. Neurological manifestations of the acquired immune deficiency syndrome: experience at UCSF and review of the literature. *J of Neurosurgery,* 1985; 62:475–95.

Nott, V. Toxoplasmosis prophylaxis. GMHC Treatment Issues; 1:1:3. Gay Men's Health Crisis, New York.

———. Toxoplasmosis. GMHC Treatment Issues Compilation, Gay Men's Health Crisis, New York, Nov. 1987–March 1989: 69.

▲ *Histoplasma Capsulatum*

Graybill, J. Histoplasmosis and AIDS. *J Inf Dis,* Sept. 1988; 158:3:623.

Wheat, L. Histoplasmosis in AIDS. *ACC,* Jan. 1992; 4:1.

▲ **Cryptosporidium and** *Isospora Belli*

Kotler, D., ed. *Gastrointestinal and Nutritional Manifestations of the Acquired Immunodeficiency Syndrome.* Raven Press, 1991.

McMeeking, A. A controlled trial of bovine dialyzable leukocyte extract for cryptosporidiosis in patients with AIDS. *J Inf Dis,* Jan. 1990, 161: 108–12.

Pape, J. Treatment and prophylaxis of *Isospora belli* infection in patients with the acquired immunodeficiency syndrome. *NEJM,* Apr. 20, 1989; 320:16:1044–47.

Soave, R. Cryptosporidium and *Isospora belli* infections. *J Inf Dis,* Feb. 1988; 157:2:225–29.

▲ **Gastrointestinal Parasites**

Benenson, A., ed. *Control of Communicable Diseases in Man,* 15th edition. American Public Health Association, Washington, D.C., 1990.

Kassler, J. *Gay Men's Health,* Harper and Row, 1983.

Perlman, D. *Campylobacter jejuni* infections in patients infected with human immunodeficiency virus (HIV). *AIM,* Apr. 1988; 108:4:540–46.

▲ **Mycobacteria**

Agins, B. Effect of combined therapy with ansamycin, clofazamine, ethambutol, and isoniazid for Mycobacterium avium infections in patients with AIDS. *J Inf Dis,* Apr. 1989; 159:4:784–87.

Barnes, P. Tuberculosis in patients human immunodeficiency virus infection. *NEJM,* June 6, 1991; 324:23:1644–50.

Chiu, J. Treatment of disseminated mycobacterium avium complex infection in AIDS with amikacin, ethambutol, rifampin, and ciprofloxacin. *AIM,* Sept. 1, 1990: 113:5:359–61.

Sources

Countdown 18 Months. Position paper published by ACT UP, New York, 212-564-2437, 1991.

Horsburgh, R. Mycobacterium avium complex infection in the acquired immunodeficiency syndrome, *NEJM,* May 9, 1991; 324:1: 1332–38.

New York Statewide Professional Standards Review Council. *Criteria Manual for the Treatment of AIDS: AIDS Intervention Management System.* Draft, 1990.

Roth, J. Mycobacterial infections. GMHC Treatment Issues Compilation, Gay Men's Health Crisis, New York, Nov. 1987–March 1989: 76.

Small, P. Mycobacterium avium complex. *ACC,* Oct. 1990; 2:10:89.

Snyder, D., et al. The new tuberculosis. *NEJM,* March 5, 1992; 326:10:703–05.

Young, L. Mycobacterium avium complex infection. *J Inf Dis,* May, 1988; 152:5:863–67.

▲ Syphilis

Bolan, G. Syphilis in HIV-infected persons. *ACC,* Feb. 1990; 2:2:9–12.

Hook, E. Syphilis and HIV infection. *J Inf Dis,* Sept. 1989; 160:3:530–34.

Musher, D. Effect of human immunodeficiency virus (HIV) infection on the course of syphilis and on the response to treatment. *AIM,* Dec. 1, 1990; 113:11:872–81.

Zenker, P. Treatment of Syphilis, 1989. *Rev Inf Dis,* July–Aug. 1990; 12:S6:S590–S609.

▲ Cryptococcus Neoformans

Clark, R. Spectrum of *Cryptococcus neoformans* in 68 patients infected with human immunodeficiency virus. *Rev Inf Dis,* Sept.–Oct. 1990; 12:5:768–77.

Larsen, R. Azoles and AIDS, *J Inf Dis,* Sept. 1990; 162:727–30.

Powderly, W., et al. A controlled trial of fluconazole or amphotericin-B to prevent relapse of cryptococcal meningitis in patients with the acquired immunodeficiency syndrome. *NEJM,* March 19, 1992; 326:12:793–98.

Saag, M. Comparison of amphotericin-B with fluconazole in the treatment of acute AIDS-associated cryptococcal meningitis. *NEJM,* Jan. 9, 1992: 326:2:83–89.

Sugar, A., et al., Overview: Treatment of Cryptococcal Meningitis, *Rev Inf Dis,* March–Apr. 1990; 12:S3:S338–S348.

▲ Candida Albicans

DeWit, S. Comparison of fluconazole and ketoconazole for oropharyngeal candidasis in AIDS. *Lancet,* Apr. 8, 1989; 746–48.

Sources
CHAPTER 12—CANCERS

Beral, V. AIDS-associated non-Hodgkin's lymphoma. *Lancet,* Apr. 6, 1991; 337:8745:805-09.

Beral, V. Kaposi's sarcoma among persons with AIDS: a sexually transmitted infection? *Lancet,* Jan. 20, 1990; 335:8682:123.

Levine, A. Therapeutic approaches to neoplasms in AIDS. *Rev Inf Dis,* Sept.-Oct. 1990; 12:5:938-43.

Marx, J. Kaposi's sarcoma puzzle begins to yield. *Science,* Apr. 27, 1990; 248:4954:442-43.

Moore, R. Non-Hodgkin's lymphoma in patients with advanced HIV infection treated with zidovudine. *JAMA,* May 1, 1991; 265:17:2208-11.

Nakamura, S. Kaposi's sarcoma cells: long-term culture with growth factor from retrovirus-infected CD4 T cells. *Science,* 1988; 242:426-30.

Ziegler, J. Kaposi's sarcoma: introduction and overview. *J of AIDS,* 1990; 3:S1:S1-S3.

CHAPTER 13—PROCEDURES AND TESTS

Grubman, S. Blood tests: monitoring your immune system. Treatment Issues, Gay Men's Health Crisis, New York; 3:7:4-7.

Hecht, F. Laboratory tests for monitoring HIV infection. *ACC,* Feb. 1991; 3:2:12-13.

Skoutelis, A., et al. Indwelling central venous catheter infections in patients with acquired immune deficiency syndrome. *J of AIDS,* 1990; 3(4):335-42.

Sox, H., ed. *Common Diagnostic Tests,* 2nd edition, 1990, American College of Physicians.

CHAPTER 14—THE EXPERIENCE OF HOSPITALIZATION

No sources.

CHAPTER 15—DETAILS OF TESTING FOR HIV INFECTION

Groopman, J., et al. Antibody seronegative human T-lymphotropic virus type III (HTLV-III)-infected patients with acquired immunodeficiency syndrome or related disorders. *Blood,* 1985; 66:742-44.

_____. Lack of evidence of prolonged human immunodeficiency virus infection before antibody seroconversion. *Blood,* 1988; 71:1752-54.

Horsburgh, R., et al; Pan, L. Z., et al. Correspondence on "Imagawa, D. et al.: Human immunodeficiency virus type 1 infection in homosexual men who remain seronegative for prolonged periods." *NEJM,* Dec. 14, 1989; 321:24:1678-81.

Sources

Imagawa, D., et al. Human immunodeficiency virus type 1 infection in homosexual men who remain seronegative for prolonged periods. *NEJM,* June 1, 1989; 320:22:1458. *Later retracted by the author as irreproducible.*

Phair, J., et al. Diagnosis of infection with the human immunodeficiency virus. *J Inf Dis,* Feb. 1989; 159:2:320–23.

Ranki, A. Long latency precedes overt seroconversion in sexually-transmitted human-immunodeficiency-virus infection. *Lancet,* Sept. 12, 1987; 8559:589–93.

Wolinsky, S., et al. Human immunodeficiency virus type 1 (HIV-1) infection of a median of 18 months before a diagnostic Western blot. *AIM,* Dec. 15, 1989; 111:12:961–72.

CHAPTER 16—IMMUNOLOGY, PATHOGENESIS, AND ETIOLOGY

Broder, S., moderator. Antiretroviral therapy in AIDS. *AIM,* Oct. 1990; 113:8:604–18.

DeVita, V. *AIDS.* J. B. Lippincott, Philadelphia, 1985.

Fauci, A., moderator, Immunopathogenic mechanisms in human immunodeficiency virus HIV infection. *AIM,* Apr. 1991; 114:8:678–93.

Gallo, R. Human retroviruses: a decade of discovery and link with human disease. *J Inf Dis,* 1991; 164:235–43.

Haseltine, W. Development of antiviral drugs for the treatment of AIDS: strategies and prospects. *J of AIDS,* 1989; 2:311–34.

Merigan, T., and Katzenstein, D. Relation of the pathogenesis of human immunodeficiency virus to various strategies for its control. *Rev Inf Dis,* March–Apr. 1991; 13:292–302.

Rapoza, N., ed. *HIV infection and disease. AMA,* 1989.

Schindler, L. *Understanding the immune system.* National Institutes of Health, pub. no. 88-529, July 1988.

CHAPTER 17—HIV: VIROLOGY AND THERAPEUTIC STRATEGIES

Crowe, S., et al. Anti-HIV drug therapy. *ACC,* March 1990; 2:3:17–20.

DeClercq, E. Basic approaches to antiretroviral treatment. *J of AIDS,* 1991; 4:207–18.

Hirsch, M. Chemotherapy of human immunodeficiency virus infections: current practice and future prospects. *J Inf Dis,* 1990; 161:845–57.

Myers, M. New antiretroviral agents in the clinic. *Rev Inf Dis,* Sept.–Oct. 1990; 12:5:944–50.

Berzofsky, J. Approaches and issues in the development of vaccines against HIV. *J of AIDS,* 1991; 4:451–59.

CHAPTER 18—BLOOD AND BLOOD CELLS

General sources.

Sources

CHAPTER 19—UNDERSTANDING CLINICAL TRIALS

McGowan, J., and Hoth, D. AIDS drug discovery and development. *J of AIDS,* 1989; 2:335–43.

CHAPTER 20—MEDICAL INSURANCE

McCormack, T. *The AIDS Benefits Handbook,* Yale University Press, 1990.

CHAPTER 21—MONEY TO LIVE ON

McCormack, T. *The AIDS Benefits Handbook,* Yale University Press, 1990.
Petersen, D. *Personal Finances and HIV Disease,* Multi-Tasking Systems, 636 6th Avenue, Suite 3D, New York, NY 10011.

CHAPTER 22—SOME LEGAL MATTERS

Duckett, M., et al. AIDS-related migration and travel policies and restrictions—a global survey. *AIDS,* 1989; 3:supplement 1:S2231–S2252.
Gilmore, N., et al. International travel and AIDS. *AIDS,* 1989; 3: supplement 1:S2229.
Gostin, L. The AIDS litigation project—part I. *JAMA,* Apr. 11, 1990; 263:14.
_____. The AIDS litigation project—part II. *JAMA,* Apr. 18, 1990; 263:15:2086–93.
HIV reporting in the states. The George Washington University Intergovernmental AIDS Reports, Nov.–Dec. 1989: 2:5:1–3.
Leonard, A. Employment discrimination. In Rubenfeld A, ed. *AIDS Legal Guide,* second edition. Lambda Legal Defense and Education Fund, Inc., 1988. Tel.: 212-995-8585.

Appendices

What follows is a very brief list of some sources of information and services related to HIV disease. Start by locating your nearest AIDS organization and learning about the services available to you. If you have special needs or questions, your local AIDS organization or the National AIDS Clearing House mentioned immediately below may be able to provide specific referrals.

NATIONAL AIDS CLEARING HOUSE

The National AIDS Clearing House is a hotline run by the Centers for Disease Control that will give you information about AIDS service organizations in your area. Call 800-342-AIDS or 800-342-2437. The Clearing House can answer many types of questions and provide many types of referrals.

HIV ANTIBODY TESTING SITES

▲ Antibody Testing Sites

The following sites offer HIV antibody testing (ELISA confirmed by Western blot) and pre- and post-test counseling at a low fee or for free. You should be tested anonymously or at least use a false name. Most sites ask that you call during business hours for an appointment. There may be a waiting list for appointments. You must wait six months after your last possible exposure before testing is completely meaningful. If no site listed here is near your area, call the AIDS organization in the nearest large city or the National AIDS Clearing House (800-342-2437) and ask them to help you find a testing site nearby.

ANTIBODY TESTING SITES

State	City	Testing Site	Telephone
CA	Los Angeles	Edelman Health Center	(213) 464-7276
CA	San Francisco	Health Center #1	(415) 621-4858
DC	Washington	Whitman Walker Clinic	(202) 332-3926
FL	Fort Lauderdale	Broward Co. Health Dept.	(305) 467-4893
FL	Miami	Dade Co. Health Dept.	(305) 325-1234

(con't. on next page)

State	City	Testing Site	Telephone
GA	Atlanta	Atlanta Gay Center	(404) 876-5372
IL	Chicago	Health Dept.	(312) 744-4312
MA	Boston	Alternative Testing Site	(617) 727-6971
NJ	Jersey City	Jersey City Medical Center CTS	(201) 915-2545
NJ	Newark	St. Michael's Hospital	(201) 877-5525 (800) 877-5526
NY	Nassau County	HIV Hotline	(516) 535-2004
NY	New York City	Health Dept.	(212) 447-8200
NY	Suffolk County	HIV Hotline	(516) 853-2999
PA	Philadelphia	Alternate Test Site	(215) 735-1911
PR	San Juan	CLETS	(809) 754-8118
TX	Dallas	Dallas Co. Health Dept.	(214) 920-7916
TX	Houston	Montrose Clinic	(713) 528-5531

▲ Testing for HIV-2

If you have a history of transfusion, needle sharing, or unprotected sexual contact in a West African nation (including Guinea Bissau, Ivory Coast, Senegal, Burkina Faso, Cape Verde Island), you should be tested not only for antibodies to HIV-1 but for antibodies to HIV-2, a variant of HIV that is prevalent in West Africa. For anonymous HIV-2 testing, have your physician contact:

CDC, AIDS Program, Laboratory   (404) 639-3174.
   Investigation Branch

SOME SELF-EMPOWERMENT ORGANIZATIONS

In addition to direct services, some of these organizations have newsletters that may be of interest.

National Association   (202) 898-0414
  of People With
  AIDS (NAPWA),
  Washington, DC

People With AIDS   Office (212) 532-0290,
  Coalition (PWAC),   Hotline (212) 532-0568, 800-828-3280
  NYC

Body Positive, NYC   (212) 633-1782

410

Appendices

SOME LOCAL AIDS SERVICE ORGANIZATIONS

To find the AIDS organization nearest you, call the National AIDS Clearing House at 800-342-2437, or consult the following list.

State	City	Organization	Telephone No.
AZ	Phoenix	Arizona AIDS Project	(602) 420-9396
AZ	Tucson	Tucson AIDS Project	(602) 326-2437 Hotline
CA	Los Angeles	AIDS Project/L.A.	(213) 876-AIDS
CA	Los Angeles	AIDS Project/L.A. (So. Cal.)	(800) 922-AIDS from So. Cal.
CA	San Francisco	San Francisco AIDS Foundation	(415) 863-AIDS
CA	San Francisco	San Francisco AIDS Foundation	(800) FOR-AIDS
CO	Denver	Colorado AIDS Project	(303) 830-2437
CO	Denver	Colorado AIDS Project (nationwide)	(800) 333-2437
DC	Washington	Whitman Walker AIDS Program	(202) 332-AIDS (800) 342-AIDS
FL	Ft. Lauderdale	AIDS Center One	(305) 485-7175
FL	Miami	Health Crisis Network	(305) 634-4636 Spanish (305) 324-5148
GA	Atlanta	AIDS Atlanta	(404) 876-9944 AIDS Info. Line
GA	Atlanta	AIDS Atlanta (nationwide)	(800) 551-2728
IL	Chicago	AIDS Foundation of Chicago	(312) 642-5454
LA	New Orleans	New Orleans AIDS Task Force	(504) 944-2437
LA	New Orleans	New Orleans AIDS Task Force (LA)	(800) 992-4379
MA	Boston	AIDS Action Comm. of Mass.	(617) 536-7733
MD	Baltimore	HERO AIDS Hotline	(410) 945-AIDS
MI	Royal Oak	Michigan AIDS Hotline (MI)	(800) 872-AIDS
MI	Royal Oak	Michigan AIDS Hotline	(313) 547-9040
MN	Minneapolis	Minnesota AIDS Project	(612) 870-7773
MO	St. Louis	St. Louis Effort for AIDS	(314) 367-8400

(con't. on next page)

State	City	Organization	Telephone No.
NJ	New Jersey	Hyacinth Foundation Hotline	(800) 433-0254 Hyacinth Hotline
NJ	New Jersey	New Jersey AIDS Foundation	(908) 246-0204 Hyacinth Office
NY	New York City	Gay Men's Health Crisis	(212) 807-6655
NY	New York City	People With AIDS Coalition	(212) 532-0290 office (212) 532-0568 (800) 828-3280 Hotlines
OH	Columbus	Columbus AIDS Task Force	Office (614) 488-2437 Hotline (800) 332-2437
PA	Philadelphia	Philadelphia AIDS Task Force	(215) 732-AIDS (215) 985-AIDS PA (800) 662-6080
PR	San Juan	Puerto Rico AIDS Foundation	(809) 782-9600
TX	Dallas	Oaklawn AIDS Project Infoline	(214) 351-4335
TX	Houston	AIDS Foundation Houston Hotline	(713) 524-AIDS
WA	Seattle	Northwest AIDS Foundation	(206) 329-6923
WI	Milwaukee	Milwaukee AIDS Project (WI)	(800) 334-AIDS Wisconsin AIDS Line
WI	Milwaukee	Milwaukee AIDS Project	(414) 273-AIDS

AIDS COALITION TO UNLEASH POWER (ACT UP)

The AIDS Coalition to Unleash Power (ACT UP) is devoted to political activity around the issue of the HIV epidemic. There are ACT UP chapters throughout the country and internationally. You can get contact information for an ACT UP group near you by calling the New York chapter of ACT UP.

New York, NY	(212) 564–2437
San Francisco, CA	(415) 563–0742
Los Angeles, CA	(213) 669–7301

OTHER GROUPS THAT PROVIDE HIV-RELATED SERVICES

▲ Sexual Minorities (Gay Men and Lesbians)

Lambda Legal Defense and Education Fund   (212) 995–8585

National Gay and Lesbian Task Force (NGLTF)	(202) 332-6483
ACT UP/SF	(415) 563-0724
Human Rights Campaign Fund (HRCF)	(202) 628-4160
ACT UP/NY	(212) 564-2437
NY Lesbian & Gay Anti-Violence Project, AIDS-Related Crime Hotline	(212) 807-0197
NY Gay & Lesbian Community Center	(212) 620-7310
LA Gay & Lesbian Community Center	(213) 464-7400
Int'l Lesbian & Gay Association	(011-4471) 278-1496
Int'l 24-hour Lesbian & Gay Switchboard	(011-4471) 837-7324

▲ Women

Women's AIDS Network (SF AIDS Fdn)	(415) 864-5855, ext. 2007
National Organization for Women (NOW)	(212) 807-0721 NY
	(202) 331-0066 DC
	(415) 861-8880 SF
Planned Parenthood	NY (212) 541-7800
	SF (415) 441-7858

▲ Ethnic and Racial Minorities

National Minority AIDS Council	(202) 544-1076
IMPACT	(202) 546-7228
National Council La Raza—AIDS Project	(202) 289-1380
Midwest Hispanic AIDS Coalition	(312) 772-8195
COSSMHO (Hispanic health group)	(202) 387-5000
People of Color Against AIDS Network (Washington state)	(206) 322-7061
American Indian Health Care Association (Minnesota)	(612) 293-0233

▲ Hemophiliacs

National Hemophilia Foundation	(212) 219-8180

▲ Substance Users (Narcotics, Alcohol, etc.)

Alcoholics Anonymous Intergroup	(212) 683-3900 NY
	(415) 661-1828 SF
	(213) 387-8316 LA

▲ Children/Parents

National Pediatric HIV Center	(800) 362-0071
Pediatric AIDS Foundation	(310) 395-9051

▲ Teenagers

Hetrick-Martin Institute for Protection of Lesbian and Gay Youth	(212) 741-0451
AIDS and Adolescents Network of NY	(212) 925-6675

▲ More AIDS Information

AIDS Information Sourcebook, 1991–92   (800) 279–6799
   Oryx Publishing Co., $39.95
   4041 N. Central Ave., Suite 700
   Phoenix, AZ 85012

TREATMENT INFORMATION

To get information about clinical trials in your area that are open for enrollment, call 800-TRIALS-A (800-854-2572). Call Monday to Friday, 9:00 A.M. to 7:00 P.M. EST. This is an information service sponsored by the Centers for Disease Control (CDC). Information is available in both Spanish and English. You will get to speak to someone in person who will give you information about government-approved clinical trials and also about specific drugs, both antivirals and those for opportunistic infections. They will do computer searches for you. Services are free.

TREATMENT INFORMATION

Publication	Publisher	Subscription information
Treatment Issues	Gay Men's Health Crisis, NYC	(212) 337-1950
Notes from the Underground	People with AIDS (PWA) Health Group, NYC	(212) 255-0520
PI Perspectives and Briefing Papers	Project Inform, San Francisco	(800) 822-7422 outside California (800) 334-7422 inside California (415) 558-9051 inside San Francisco
BETA (Bulletin of Experimental Treatments for AIDS)	San Francisco AIDS Fdn.	(415) 863-AIDS
AIDS Treatment News	John James, San Francisco	(415) 255-0588
AmFAR Directory of Clinical Trials	American Foundation for AIDS Research	(212) 682-7440

Two reliable buyer's clubs (groups that supply "underground" AIDS drugs) are:

People With AIDS Health Group
150 W. 26th Street
New York, NY
Tel. (212) 255–0520

Healing Alternatives Foundation
1748 Market St., Suite 204
San Francisco, CA 94102
Tel. (415) 626-2316

Call these two clubs for information about the reliability of buyer's clubs in your area.

INFORMATION ON MAKEUP FOR KS LESIONS

Contact your local AIDS organization to find support groups and advice on how to cover KS lesions. A professional makeup artist has also volunteered to advise people with KS:

Debra Provenzano
7119 Shore Road
Brooklyn, NY 11209
(718) 680–6224

MONEY MATTERS

A book called *The AIDS Benefits Handbook,* by T. P. McCormack (Yale University Press, 1990), contains excellent and detailed information about a large variety of benefits programs.

An excellent resource that is constantly up-dated is *Personal Finances and HIV Disease* by David Petersen. It is available from Multi-Tasking Systems, 636 Avenue of the Americas, #3D, New York, NY 10011.

Information on the AIDS Drug Reimbursement Program is generally available by calling the Department of Health in your county. Some direct sources of information are:

U.S. Health Resources and Services Agency	(301) 443–9086
AIDS Drug Reimbursement Program	
N.Y. State AIDS Drug Assistance Program	(800) 542–2437
(ADAP)	
CA State Office of AIDS	(916) 324–8429

LEGAL MATTERS

For information and help regarding discrimination, contact your state and local Human Rights Commissions. A good collection of legal information available in bookstores is *AIDS and the Law,* edited by H. Dalton, S. Burris, and the Yale AIDS Law Project, Yale University Press, 1987. Contact Lambda Legal Defense to get its pamphlet *Living with AIDS* and its *AIDS Legal Guide,* a more detailed technical work. The National Lawyers' Guild AIDS Network publishes an *AIDS Practice Manual* for lawyers, as well as *The Exchange,* a newsletter on legal and political issues around AIDS. The Intergovernmental Health Policy Project has published *AIDS: A Public Health Challenge,* which contains information on state and federal legislation, plus broad discussions of AIDS policy issues. You may also wish to contact the following national organizations:

American Civil Liberties Union—AIDS Project	(212) 944–9800, Ext. 545
National Lawyers' Guild AIDS Network	(415) 285–5066
Intergovernmental Health Policy Project—AIDS Policy Center (George Washington University)	(202) 872–1445

If you are diagnosed with HIV disease while you are in the military, get legal help *immediately.* Some sources of help:

Military Law Task Force (National Military Project on AIDS)	(619) 233–1701
Citizen Soldier	(212) 777–3470
Midwest Committee for Military Counseling	(312) 939–3349
CCCO	(415) 474–3002, (215) 545–4626

INFORMATION RESOURCES FOR TRAVELERS

Call the Centers for Disease Control (CDC) International Travelers Hotline at 404-332-4555 for up-to-date information on health concerns for travelers, including current areas of infectious disease and current vaccination requirements for travel to various countries.

A booklet is also available from the CDC, entitled "Health Information for International Travel" ($5.00). Call 202-783-3238.

NUTRITION INFORMATION LITERATURE

There are a number of books that you can consult; one standard available in many bookstores is *Jane Brody's Nutrition Book* (Bantam Books).

In addition, there have been a number of pamphlets available to the public that provide up-to-date information specially tailored to people with HIV disease. You can get these pamphlets by calling The National AIDS Information Clearinghouse (phone 800-458-5231).

The Cutting Edge, P.O. Box 392, Fremont, CA 94537 (415-797-9768), can provide referrals to HIV-knowledgeable nutritionists and a database of available articles and pamphlets on nutrition and food safety in HIV disease.

Table of Therapeutic Substances Mentioned in the Text

(For current information, consult the AIDS/HIV Treatment Directory of the American Foundation for AIDS Research, 212-682-7440.)

Chem. name(s) & Formula	Brand name(s)	Category	Mfr.(s) & Availability
Acetominophen	Various including Tylenol	Analgesic	Various including McNeil OTC
Acyclovir	Zovirax	Antiviral	Burroughs-Wellcome Rx
AGM-1470	—	Antivaso-proliferative	Taketa Exp
AL721 Active lipids in a 7:2:1 ratio	Various brands	Antiretroviral	Various mfrs. OTC
Alpha interferon, low-dose	Kemron and others	Cytokine	Various mfrs. Exp
Alprazolam	Xanax	Psychoactive Benzodiazepine antianxiety	Upjohn Rx
Alumina and magnesia preparations	Mylanta Maalox	Antacid	J&J•Merck Consumer Rhône-Poulenc OTC
Amikacin	Amikin	Antibacterial Antitubercular	Apothecon Rx
Amitriptyline	Elavil	Psychoactive Cyclic antidepressant	Stuart Rx
Amoxapine	Asendin	Psychoactive Cyclic antidepressant	Lederle Rx

(con't. on next page)

KEY

OTC	=	Available over the counter (without a prescription)
Rx	=	Available by prescription
Exp	=	Experimental, may be available through clinical trials
Und	=	Available through underground sources such as buyer's clubs

Table of Therapeutic Substances Mentioned in the Text

Chem. name(s) & Formula	Brand name(s)	Category	Mfr.(s) & Availability
Amphetamine	Dexedrine	Psychoactive Stimulant anti-depressant	SmithKline Beecham Rx
Amphotericin-B	Fungizone	Antifungal	Squibb Rx
Ampicillin	Generic	Antibiotic	Rx
Ampligen	—	Antiretroviral	HEM Research Exp
Antisense oligomers	—	Antiretroviral	—
Aspirin Acetylsalicylic acid (ASA)	Various	Analgesic	Various OTC
Azidothymidine (AZT) Zidovudine 2',3'-azidothymidine	Retrovir	Antiretroviral	Burroughs-Wellcome Rx
Azithromycin	Zithromax	Antibiotic Macrolide	Pfizer Rx
Benzodiazepines (class of drugs)	—	Psychoactive	Rx
Benzoyl peroxide	Various brands	Mild antibacterial	Various Mfrs. Rx
BI-RG-587	—	Antiretroviral	Boehringer-Ingelheim Exp
Bismuth subsalicylate	Pepto-Bismol	Antidiarrheal	Procter & Gamble OTC
Bleomycin	Blenoxane	Chemotherapy	Bristol-Myers Oncology Rx
Bupropion	Wellbutrin	Psychoactive	Burroughs-Wellcome Rx
Buspirone	BuSpar	Psychoactive	Mead Johnson Rx

KEY

OTC = Available over the counter (without a prescription)

Rx = Available by prescription

Exp = Experimental, may be available through clinical trials

Und = Available through underground sources such as buyer's clubs

418

Table of Therapeutic Substances Mentioned in the Text

Chem. name(s) & Formula	Brand name(s)	Category	Mfr.(s) & Availability
BW566C80 Hydroxynaptho-quinone	—	Antiprotozoal	Burroughs-Wellcome Expanded access 800-755-2020
Carbamazepine	Tegretol	Psychoactive	Basel Rx
Castanospermine	—	Antiretroviral	NCI Exp
Cefaclor	Ceclor	Antibiotic Cephalosporin	Lilly Rx
Cephalosporin, a class of antibiotics	—	Antibiotics	Rx
Chloramphenicol	Chloromycetin	Antibiotic	Parke-Davis Rx
Chlordiazeapoxide	Librium	Psychoactive Benzodiazepine antianxiety	Roche Rx
Chlorhexidine	Hibiclens	Antimicrobial, topical	Stuart Rx
Chlorhexidine gluconate	Peridex	Antimicrobial oral rinse	Procter & Gamble Rx
Cimetidine	Tagamet	Antiulcer medication H2-receptor antagonist	SmithKline Beecham Rx
Ciprofloxacin	Cipro	Antibiotic	Miles Rx
Clarithromycin	Biaxin	Antibiotic Macrolide	Abbot Labs Rx
Clindamycin	Cleocin and others	Antiprotozoal	Upjohn Exp
Clindamycin and primaquine	—	Antibiotic Antiprotozoal	Exp, Und
Clofazimine	Lamprene	Antibiotic used against MAC	Geigy Rx

(con't. on next page)

KEY

OTC   =   Available over the counter (without a prescription)

Rx   =   Available by prescription

Exp   =   Experimental, may be available through clinical trials

Und   =   Available through underground sources such as buyer's clubs

419

Table of Therapeutic Substances Mentioned in the Text

Chem. name(s) & Formula	Brand name(s)	Category	Mfr.(s) & Availability
Clonazapam	Klonopin	Psychoactive Benzodiazepine	Roche Rx
Clotrimazole	Mycelex Lotrimin Gyne-Lotrimin (topical cream)	Antifungal	Miles Rx
Compound Q Tricosanthin GLQ223	—	Antiretroviral	GeneLabs Exp, Und
Cromolyn	Nasalcrom Opticrom	Antiallergic	Fisons Rx
Dapsone and trimethoprim	Dapsone	Antibiotic	Jacobus Rx
ddC 2',3'- dideoxycytidine Zalcitabine	Hivid	Antiretroviral	Hoffman-LaRoche Conditionally approved for Rx
ddI Dideoxyinosine Didanosine	Videx	Antiretroviral	Bristol-Myers FDA approved in 1991 for Rx
Desipramine	Norpramin	Psychoactive	Marion Merrell Dow Rx
Dexmethasone	Decadron	Corticosteroid anti-inflammatory	Merck Sharp & Dohme Rx
Dextran sulfate	—	Antiretroviral	Ueno Exp, Und
DHEA	—	Immunotherapy	ELAN Exp
Diazepam	Valium	Psychoactive Benzodiazepine antianxiety	Roche Rx
Diclazuril	—	Antiparasitic	Janssen Withdrawn

KEY

OTC = Available over the counter (without a prescription)

Rx = Available by prescription

Exp = Experimental, may be available through clinical trials

Und = Available through underground sources such as buyer's clubs

Table of Therapeutic Substances Mentioned in the Text

Chem. name(s) & Formula	Brand name(s)	Category	Mfr.(s) & Availability
Dicloxacillin	Various brands	Antibiotic	Various mfrs. Rx
Diethyl toluamide DEET	Skin-So-Soft	Insect repellent	Various OTC
Difluoromethyl- ornithine (DFMO)	—	Antiprotozoal	— Exp
Diphenhydramine	Benadryl	Antihistamine	OTC, Rx
Diphenoxylate with atropine sulfate	Lomotil	Antidiarrheal (opiate and anticholinegric)	Searle Rx
Disulfiram	Antabuse	Treatment of alcoholism	Wyeth-Ayerst Rx
Ditocarb sodium Sodium diethyl dithio- carbamate DTC	Imuthiol	Immunotherapy	Institut Mérieux Withdrawn from development
Doxepin	Sinequan	Pshychoactive Cyclic antidepressant	Roerig Rx
Doxorubicin	Adriamycin	Chemotherapy	Adria Rx
Doxycycline	Various brands (Doryx)	Antibiotic	Various mfrs. Rx
Erythromycin	Generic	Antibiotic	Rx
Erythropoietin EPO	Epogen Procrit	Cytokine Antianemic	Amgen Ortho Rx
Ethambutol	Myambutol	Antibiotic	Lederle Rx
Etoposide VP-16	VePesid	Chemotherapy	Bristol-Myers Oncology Exp

(con't. on next page)

KEY

OTC = Available over the counter (without a prescription)

Rx = Available by prescription

Exp = Experimental, may be available through clinical trials

Und = Available through underground sources such as
buyer's clubs

Table of Therapeutic Substances Mentioned in the Text

Chem. name(s) & Formula	Brand name(s)	Category	Mfr.(s) & Availability
Famotidine	Pepcid	Antiulcer medication H2-receptor antagonist	Merck Sharp & Dohme Rx
Fluconazole	Diflucan	Antifungal	Roerig Rx
Flucytosine 5-fluorcytosine (5FC)	Ancobon	Antifungal	Roche Rx
Fluocinonide	Lidex	Topical steroid	Syntex Rx
Fluoxetine	Prozac	Psychoactive Antidepressant	Dista Rx
Fluphenazine	Prolixin	Psychoactive	Princeton Rx
Flurozepam	Dalmane	Psychoactive	Roche Rx
Foscarnet Trisodium phosphonoformate	Foscavir	Antiviral	Adria Rx
Furazolidone	Furoxone	Antibiotic	Roberts Rx
Gancyclovir	Cytovene	Antiviral	Syntex Rx
Granulocyte colony stimulating factor G-CSF Filgastrin	Neupogen	Cytokine Antineutropenic	Amgen Rx
Granulocyte-monocyte colony stimulating factor GM-CSF Sagramostin	Leukine Prokine	Cytokine Antineutropenic	Hoechst-Roussel Rx
Haloperidol	Haldol	Psychoactive Antipsychotic	McNeil Rx
Hydrocortisone	Various	Steroidal anti-inflammatory	OTC, Rx

KEY

OTC = Available over the counter (without a prescription)

Rx = Available by prescription

Exp = Experimental, may be available through clinical trials

Und = Available through underground sources such as buyer's clubs

Table of Therapeutic Substances Mentioned in the Text

Chem. name(s) & Formula	Brand name(s)	Category	Mfr.(s) & Availability
Hydroxyzine	Vistaril	Antihistamine Psychoactive Antianxiety	Pfizer Rx
Hypericin St. John's Wort	—	Immunotherapy	Exp, Und
Ibuprofen	Various, including Advil, Motrin	Analagesic	Various, OTC
Imidazoles, a class of antifungal drugs	—	Antifungal	Rx
Imipramine	Tofranil	Psychoactive Cyclic antidepressant	Geigy Rx
Interferon alpha α-INF	Roferon-A Intron A	Cytokine	Roche Schering Rx
Isocarboxazid	Marplan	Psychoactive MAOI anti- depressant	Roche Rx
Isoniazid	INH	Antibiotic	CIBA Rx
Itraconazole	Sporanex	Antifungal	Janssen Rx
Kaolin-pectin suspension	Kaopectate	Antidiarrheal	Upjohn OTC
Ketoconazole	Nizoral	Antifungal	Janssen Rx
L-compounds	—	Antiretroviral	Merck Sharp & Dohme Exp
Letrazuril	—	Antiparasitic	Janssen Rx
Leucovorin calcium Folinic acid (not folic acid)	Leucovorin Wellcovorin	Adjunctive therapy for folic acid anatogonists	Lederle Burroughs-Wellcome Rx

(con't. on next page)

KEY

OTC = Available over the counter (without a prescription)

Rx = Available by prescription

Exp = Experimental, may be available through clinical trials

Und = Available through underground sources such as buyer's clubs

Table of Therapeutic Substances Mentioned in the Text

Chem. name(s) & Formula	Brand name(s)	Category	Mfr.(s) & Availability
Lithium carbonate	Various	Psychoactive Antimania	Various Rx
Loperamide	Imodium Imodium A-D	Antidiarrheal	Janssen, Rx McNeil, OTC
Lorazepam	Ativan	Psychoactive Benzodiazepine antianxiety	Wyeth-Ayerst Rx
Maprotiline	Ludiomil	Psychoactive Cyclic antidepressant	CIBA Rx
Megestrol acetate	Megace	Appetite stimulant	Bristol-Myers Co. Rx
Meperidine	Demerol	Narcotic Barbiturate	Sanofi Winthrop, Rx
Methionine enkephalin (MEK)	—	Immunotherapy	Sygma Exp
Methylphenidate	Ritalin	Psychoactive	CIBA Rx
Metoclopramide	Reglan	GI ulcer medicine	A. H. Robins Rx
Metronidazole	Flagyl	Antiprotozoal Antibacterial	Searle Rx
Miconazole	Monistat (topical cream)	Antifungal	Janssen OTC
Morphine	Various	Narcotic	Various Rx
N-acetylcysteine (NAC)	—	Immunotherapy	Zambon Und
N-butyl-DNJ Dexoynojirimycin	—	Antiretroviral	— Exp
Nortriptyline	Pamelor, Aventyl	Psychoactive Cyclic antidepressant	Sandoz Rx

KEY

OTC = Available over the counter (without a prescription)

Rx = Available by prescription

Exp = Experimental, may be available through clinical trials

Und = Available through underground sources such as buyer's clubs

Table of Therapeutic Substances Mentioned in the Text

Chem. name(s) & Formula	Brand name(s)	Category	Mfr.(s) & Availability
Nystatin	Mycostatin Mycolog	Antifungal	Various Rx
Octreotide acetate	Sandostatin	Synthetic hormone	Sandoz Rx
Opium (deodorized tincture)	—	Antidiarrheal	Rx
Oxazepam	Serax	Psychoactive Benzodiazepine antianxiety	Wyeth-Ayerst Rx
Paromycin Paromomycin sulfate	Humatin	Antibiotic	Parke-Davis Rx
Penicillins, a class of related antibiotics	Various	Antibiotics	Various Rx
Pentamidine isethionate Aerosolized pentamidine (AP)	Pentam NebuPent	Antiprotozoal	Fujisawa Rx
Pentoxyfiline	—	Immunotherapy	Hoechst-Roussel Exp
Peptide T	—	Antiretroviral	Bristol-Myers Exp, Und
Perphenazine	Trilafon	Psychoactive Antipsychotic	Schering Rx
Phenelzine	Nardil	Psychoactive MAOI anti-depressant	Parke-Davis Rx
Phenobarbitol	Various brands	Antiseizure	Various Rx
Phenylephrine and phenylpropanol-amine and guaifenesin	Entex	Decongestant Expectorant	Norwich Eaton Rx

(con't. on next page)

KEY

OTC = Available over the counter (without a prescription)

Rx = Available by prescription

Exp = Experimental, may be available through clinical trials

Und = Available through underground sources such as buyer's clubs

Table of Therapeutic Substances Mentioned in the Text

Chem. name(s) & Formula	Brand name(s)	Category	Mfr.(s) & Availability
Phenytoin	Dilantin	Antiseizure	Parke-Davis Rx
Piritrexim	—	Antiprotozoal Folate antagonist	Burroughs-Wellcome Exp
Povidone-iodine	Betadine	Antimicrobial, topical	Purdue Frederick Rx
Prednisone	Various brands (Deltasone)	Steroid	Various (Upjohn) Rx
Probenecid	Benemid	Adjunctive therapy with penicillin	Merck Sharp & Dohme Rx
Prochlorperazine	Compazine	Psychoactive Antipsychotic Antinausea	SmithKline Beecham Rx
Promethazine	Phenergan		Wyeth-Ayerst Rx
Protease inhibitors RO-31-8959 (Hoffman)	—	Antiretroviral	Hoffman-LaRoche Upjohn Not available
Protriptyline	Vivactil	Psychoactive Cyclic antidepressant	Merck Sharp & Dohme Rx
Pyrazinamide	PZA	Antitubercular	Lederle Rx
Pyrimethamine	Daraprim	Antiprotozoal	Burroughs-Wellcome Rx
Pyrimethamine and sulfadoxine	Fansidar	Antiprotozoal Sulfa drug	Roche Rx
Quinacrine	Atabrine	Antiparasitic	Sanofi Winthrop Rx
Ranitidine	Zantac	Antiulcer medication H2-receptor antagonist	Glaxo Rx

KEY

OTC = Available over the counter (without a prescription)

Rx = Available by prescription

Exp = Experimental, may be available through clinical trials

Und = Available through underground sources such as buyer's clubs

Table of Therapeutic Substances Mentioned in the Text

Chem. name(s) & Formula	Brand name(s)	Category	Mfr.(s) & Availability
Recombinant gp160 rgp160	—	Immunotherapy	VaxSyn BIOCINE Bristol-Myers Immuno-US MicroGeneSys Exp
Recombinant soluble CD4 (rsCD4)	—	Antiretroviral	Genentech Exp
Ribavirin	Virazole	Antiretroviral	ICN Pharm. Exp, Und
Rifabutin	Ansamycin	Antibiotic	Adria Exp
Rifampin	RIF Various brands	Antibiotic	Various Rx
SCH39304	—	Antibiotic Antifungal	Schering Exp
Secobarbitol	Seconal	Psychoactive	Lilly Rx
SP-PG	—	Antivaso-proliferative	Daiichi Exp
Spiramycin	—	Antibiotic	Rhone-Poulenc Exp
Sucralfate	Carafate	Antiulcer medication	Merrell Dow
Sulfa drugs, a class of related antibiotics	—	Antibiotics	Rx
Sulfadiazine	Microsulfon	Bacteriostatic	Consolidated Midland Rx
Tacrine	—	Immunotherapy	— Exp
tat inhibitor RO-24-7429	—	Antiretroviral	Hoffman-LaRoche Exp
Temazapam	Restoril	Psychoactive Benzodiazepine antianxiety	Sandoz Rx

(con't. on next page)

KEY

OTC = Available over the counter (without a prescription)

Rx = Available by prescription

Exp = Experimental, may be available through clinical trials

Und = Available through underground sources such as buyer's clubs

Table of Therapeutic Substances Mentioned in the Text

Chem. name(s) & Formula	Brand name(s)	Category	Mfr.(s) & Availability
Terfenadine	Seldane	Antihistamine	Marion Merrell Dow Rx
Tetracycline	Various brands	Antibotic	Various Rx
Thioridazine	Mellaril	Psychoactive Antipsychotic	Sandoz Rx
Thymotrinin (TP3)	—	Immunotherapy	Ortho Exp
TIBO compounds e.g. R82913	—	Antiretroviral	Janssen Exp
Tinidazole	—	Antiparasitic	Rx
Tranylcypromine	Parnate	Psychoactive MAOI anti-depressant	SmithKline Beecham Rx
Trazodone	Desyrel	Psychoactive Cyclic antidepressant	Mead Johnson Rx
Tretinoin	Retin-A	Uncategorized	Ortho Rx
Triazolam	Halcion	Psychoactive Benzodiazepine antianxiety	Upjohn Rx
Triazoles, a novel class of antifungal drugs	—	Antifungal	Rx, Exp
Trifluoperazine	Stelazine	Psychoactive Antipsychotic	SmithKline Beecham Rx
Trimethoprim sulfamethoxazole (TMP-SMX)	Bactrim Septra	Antibiotic Sulfa drug	Roche Burroughs-Wellcome Rx
Trimetrexate	—	Antiprotozoal Folate antagonist	Warner Lambert Exp

KEY

OTC = Available over the counter (without a prescription)

Rx = Available by prescription

Exp = Experimental, may be available through clinical trials

Und = Available through underground sources such as buyer's clubs

Table of Therapeutic Substances Mentioned in the Text

Chem. name(s) & Formula	Brand name(s)	Category	Mfr.(s) & Availability
Trimipramine	Surmontil	Psychoactive Cyclic antidepressant	Wyeth-Ayerst Rx
Valproate	Depakote	Psychoactive	Abbott
Vinblastine	Velban	Chemotherapy	Lilly Rx
Vincristine	Oncovin	Chemotherapy	Lilly Rx

KEY

OTC	=	Available over the counter (without a prescription)
Rx	=	Available by prescription
Exp	=	Experimental, may be available through clinical trials
Und	=	Available through underground sources such as buyer's clubs

INDEX

B cell defects, 337
B cells, 332–33, 334, 358
B lymphocytes, 232, 237, 296–97, 328, 332
Bacille Calmette Guerin (BCG) vaccine, 264
Bacteremia, 269, 357
Bacteria, 191, 212–13, 299, 330
  drug-resistant, 113
  encapsulated, 338
  intestinal, 114
Bacterial infections, 185–86, 197, 257–72, 357
  in children, 167, 172
Bacterial pneumonias, 79, 271–72
Bactrim (trimethoprim/sulfamethoxazole; Septra), 55, 79–82, 84, 85, 86, 113, 114, 209, 247, 248, 268, 269, 357
  allergic reaction to, 188
  clinical trials, 363
  intravenous, 73
  in treatment of *Isospora belli*, 254
  in treatment of PCP, 241–42, 243
  use during pregnancy, 165
  used with other drugs, 243–44
Basophils, 296, 328, 335, 357, 358
Benadryl (diphenhydramine), 81, 188, 189
Benefits, 376–77
Benzodiazepines, 149, 154–55, 305
BETA (Bulletin of Experimental Treatments for AIDS), 177
Beta-2 Microglobulin (B2M) (test), 40, 45–46
Betadine, 186
Biofeedback, 144
Biliary tract, 226
Biopsy(ies), 163, 185, 192, 197, 232, 233, 291, 303, 305
  bone marrow, 306
  brain, 206, 207, 237, 247, 306–07
  CMV, 222
  CMV colitis, 225
  esophagitis, 224, 225
  lung, 304
  open-lung, 241
  skin, 284
  tissue, 259–60
  transbronchial, 241
Bird droppings, 249, 272
Birth control, 106
Bismuth subsalicylate (Pepto-Bismol), 225
Blame(ing), 131, 132, 134, 135, 138
Bleeding
  with procedures/tests, 293–94, 305, 306
Bleomycin, 286
Blinding (clinical trials), 362–63
Blindness, 223
Blood, 9, 13, 14, 103, 104, 321, 355–58
  donated, 7, 8
  infection from, 166, 217
Blood-brain barrier, 72, 230, 247, 361
Blood cell suppression, 248
Blood cells, 260
  development of, 355–56
  types and functions of, 356–58
Blood chemistry, 295, 297
Blood cultures, 268
Blood disorders, 243, 355
Blood pressure, 28, 149, 150
Blood products, 13, 166
Blood sugar, 205

Blood supply
  screening, 166, 235
Blood tests, ix, x–xi, 29, 40, 41, 54, 211, 276–77, 295–96
  for anemia, 54
  for CMV, 222
  in fever evaluation, 208
  for hepatitis B, 98, 234, 236
  with in-dwelling catheter, 308
  for kidney function, 210, 230
  monitoring AZT use, 55
  for non-Hodgkin's lymphomas, 291
  for syphilis, 271
  for toxoplasmosis, 86, 246, 247
Bodily fluids, 103–04, 106, 110
Body
  changes in, 123–24
Body Positive (org.), 176
Bone marrow, 228, 249, 260, 266, 290, 328–29, 332, 355, 357, 358
Bone marrow biopsy, 306
Bone-marrow suppression toxicity, 56, 228, 229, 286
Brain, 199, 237, 245, 361
  HIV infection of, 201, 202
Brain biopsy, 206, 207, 237, 247, 306–07
Brain CT scans, 301
Breast feeding, 99, 165
Breathing problems, 196–97
  see also Shortness of breath
Bristol-Myers, 67
Bronchoalveolar lavage (BAL), 197, 240–41, 304
Bronchodilators, 84
Bronchoscopy, 226, 240–41, 304
Budding (HIV), 343, 350
Bullous impetigo, 185, 186
Bupropion (Wellbutrin), 150
Burroughs-Wellcome company, 59, 60–61, 55, 85, 221
Buspirone (Buspar), 154, 155
Buyer's clubs, 177, 178, 179, 261, 414–15
BW566C80 (hydroxynaphthoquinone), 85

Calcium, 230, 231, 297
Campylobacter, 102, 113
Campylobacter jejuni, 191, 257, 269
Campylobacter pylorides, 225, 251
Cancer, x, 55, 68, 71, 168, 187, 194, 213, 278–92, 357, 358
  cervix, 162, 163
  in children, 168
  effect on immune system, 335
  with HIV disease, 338–39
  liver, 235
  lung, 301
  mouth, 185
  nervous system, 205
  skin, 185, 190
Candida albicans (thrush), 43, 87, 88, 92, 161–62, 184, 186, 250, 272, 275–77
  in esophagitis, 224
Candidiasis, 28, 78, 194, 205, 275–77
  cause of esophagitis, 224
  prevention of, 86, 88
Carbamazepine (Tegretol), 152
Carcinogens, 279, 281–82
Carcinomas, 279

433

Computerized tomography (CT) scans, 201,
202, 203, 204, 205, 206, 237, 247, 273,
291, 300, 301–02, 305, 306, 307
Concorde 1 trial, 64
Condom use, 89, 103, 104, 105, 106–07, 108,
109, 110, 218
and incidence of KS, 281
Condoms, 3, 6, 9, 12, 14, 27, 58, 115, 124,
163, 164, 220, 232, 235
Condyloma acuminata, 29, 163
Confidentiality, 3–4, 15, 141
and medical insurance, 373–74
Confirmatory testing, HIV antibody, 5, 7, 8, 14
Constipation, 149, 150
Constitutional symptoms, 92, 208, 239
Contagious diseases, 217, 218
TB, 262, 263
Controlled trials, 362–63
Corticosteroids, 81, 169, 211, 243–44
Cosmetic treatment
KS, 284, 285, 286, 288–89, 415
Costs
AZT, 49, 50–51
drugs, 275
procedures and tests, 208, 293
psychotherapy, 139–40
Cotton-wool spots, 223
Cough(ing), 28, 79, 196, 239, 301
Counselors, counseling, 4, 11, 12, 14, 17,
130, 135, 176
Course of illness
in children, 166, 167–68
and corresponding interventions, 217–19
differences between women and men in,
160
drug use and, 110
CPK (creatinine phosphokinase), 55
Cranial imaging, 291
Cranial irradiation, 291–92
Cranium, 200
Creatine kinase (CK), 208
Creatinine clearance, 230
Creatinine levels, 229, 242
Cross-resistance, 57
Cryosurgery, 163, 283
Cryotherapy (freezing therapy), 187, 285–86
Cryptococcal disease, 168
meningitis, 200, 203, 205, 206, 246
cryptococcosis, 44, 78, 211, 272–75, 307
prevention, 85, 87–88
cryptococcus neoformans, 200, 204, 206,
209, 250, 272–75
Cryptosporidiosis, 43, 113, 168, 194, 252–53
Cryptosporidium, 191, 225, 237, 244, 251–54
Cultures, 233, 268, 299
blood, 208
in diagnosis of TB, 266
with histoplasmosis, 250
for MAC, 259–60
sputum, 264
stool, 269
Cunnilingus, 14, 104–05
Cytokines, 329–30, 345
Cytology, 303
Cytomegalovirus (CMV), 44, 78, 79, 85, 88,
165, 181, 191, 193, 196, 197, 205, 206,
209, 211, 219, 220–26, 241, 253
avoiding infection, 220

in children, 168
as co-factor, 231–32, 281–82
colitis, 305
diagnosis, 193, 221–22
disease, 44
in the eye, 222–23, 307
in the gut, 223–26
mononucleosis, 221
pneumonia, 301, 304
prevention of, 22, 85, 88
primary infection, 220, 221
tests for, 298
transmission of, 220
treatment of, 227–32

Daiichi Pharmaceuticals (co.), 288
Dapsone, 68, 84, 85, 86, 247, 267
in prevention of PCP, 79, 82–83
in treatment of cryptosporidiosis, 253
Dapsone/trimethoprim, 243
ddC, 57, 66, 68, 70–75, 172, 207, 229, 344,
346, 347
benefits of, 71
combined with other drugs, 73–75
as sole antiviral therapy, 66–67, 72–73
ddI, 50, 57, 66, 67–70, 72, 73, 207, 229, 343,
346, 347, 373
and alcohol use, 115
benefits of, 68, 69–70
combined with dapsone, 83
dosage, 68, 69
side effects, 67–69
use in children, 172
Death, 122, 137
as clinical end point, 365
from hepatitis B, 234, 235
from toxoplasmosis, 245
Deaths from AIDS, x, 159, 160, 166, 259
cancers in, 278
PCP, 76
Decadron (steroid), 185, 248, 349
DEET (diethyltoluamide), 189
Defenses, 135–37, 330
Degenerative brain disease (encophalopathy),
168
Dehydration, 114, 191, 193, 210, 230
Delirium, 200
Dementia, 53, 200–05, 237, 339
Demerol, 157
Demyelination, 237
Dendritic cells, 334
Denial, 135–37, 138
Dental care, 89, 99–100, 184
Deoxyribonucleic acid (DNA), 213, 331,
341–42, 345, 346, 348
proviral, 347
replication, 325–26
Deoxyribonucleic acid (DNA) amplification
testing, 8, 10–11, 324, 325–26
Deoxyribonucleic acid (DNA) polymerase, 54,
345–46
Dependency, 122, 130–31
Depression, 2, 4, 34, 121, 137, 146, 156, 175,
203, 204
in cognitive therapy, 143
criteria for, 147–48
professional help with, 138

434

435

Emotional aspects
  functioning, 2, 27
  issues, xi, xiii, 11, 59
  physician and, 34, 35
  psychoactive medications in treatment of
    distress, 144–58
  reactions to starting treatment, 58–59
  reactions to testing positive, 15–16
  responses, 132
  support, 11–12, 16–17, 142
Employer-based insurance, 370
Encapsulated bacteria (bacterial pneumonia),
    257, 271–72
Encephalitis, 200–01, 205–06, 226–27, 245, 272
Encephalopathy, 167, 200, 204
Endocarditis, 27, 173
Endocrine problems, 210–11
Endoscope, 226, 304, 305
Endoscopy, 193, 224, 233, 277, 304–05
  CMV colitis, 255
  esophagitis, 224–25
Enemas, 107–8
Entamoeba histolytica (amoebas), 191, 225,
    237, 251, 254–56
Enteral nutrition, 195
Enteric infections, 112–14
Entitlements, 376, 377–80
Enzyme-linked immunosorbent assay
    see ELISA test
Enzymes, 278, 342, 350
Eosinophilic pustular folliculitis, 190
Eosinophils, 295, 328, 357, 358
Epidemics, 112, 215
Epidemiology, 214–16
  cryptococcosis, 272
  histoplasma capsulatum, 249
  KS, 281
  TB, 262–63
  Toxoplasma gondii, 245
Epithelium, 251, 338
Epstein-Barr virus (EBV), 221, 231, 290
Erythema multifome, 188
Erythematous candidiasis, 276
Erythrocytes, 357
Erythromycin, 253, 269
Erythropoiesis, 54, 356
Erythropoietin (EPO, Epogen), 54, 356
Escherichia coli, 113, 191
Esophageal candidiasis, 44, 160, 168, 193,
    275, 276, 277, 304
Esophageal problems, 193
Esophagitis
  CMV, 224
Esophagus, 223, 224
  herpes simplex of, 232, 233
Ethambutol (Myambutol), 87, 260–62, 267
Ethnicity, 166, 172–74
  and AZT efficacy, 63
Etiology, 339–40
Etoposide (VP-16, Vepesid), 288
Europe, 77, 112, 245
Evolution
  in immune system, 330, 331, 334
Exchange, The (newsletter), 385
Excision, 303
Expanded access programs, 67–68, 359, 362,
    365
Experimental drugs/treatments, 20, 248, 261,

343–44
  access to, 359, 362
  candidiasis, 277
  CMV, 231
  histoplasmosis, 250
  insurance reimbursement for, 373
  learning about, 175–79, 236
  in treatment of cryptococcal meningitis, 274
  in treatment of KS, 288
  in treatment of PCP, 243
Extrapulmonary pneumocystosis (PCP), 82,
  84
Extrapulmonary TB, 266
Eye(s), 28, 181
  CMV in, 222–23
  exam, 222

Failure to thrive, 168
False negatives, 4, 10, 222, 255, 326
False positives, 4–5, 7, 8, 325
Family, 129–32, 134, 169
Family/couple therapy, 130, 142–43
Famotidine (Pepcid), 225
Fansidar, 84–85, 86, 188, 248, 254
Fatigue, 40, 62, 92, 238
Fecal-oral transmission, 112, 114, 251, 253,
    255, 268
Feces contamination, 112–13
Federal employment, 384
Feelings
  age-inappropriate, 122–23
  about being sick, 119, 121–24
  about body change, 123–24
  unhelpful, 119, 132–38
Fellatio, 14, 104, 105
Fetus, 99, 217, 244, 302, 303
  risks to, 164, 165
Fever, 40, 51, 71, 92, 114, 208, 219, 239, 249
  in children, 167
  diagnosis, 306
Fingernails/toenails, 53, 186
566C80 (hydroxynapthaquinone), 243
Fluconazole (Diflucan), 87–88, 162, 224, 250,
    273, 274, 275, 277
Flucytosine (Ancobon), 274
Fluid testing, 295–99
Fluoxetine (Prozac), 150
Flurazepam (Dalmane), 154, 156
Focal neurological disorders, 200–01, 204,
    205, 206
Follicles, 185
Folliculitis, 185–86
Food and Drug Administration (FDA), 49, 60,
    66, 67, 70, 287, 373
  and drug development process, 359–60,
    362
Food safety, 89, 100–03, 112, 113
Food stamps, 318, 380
Formed elements (blood), 295, 355
Foscarnet (Foscavir), 88, 210, 223, 224, 225,
    227, 230–31, 233
Fraud, 178
Free virions, 350
Friends, 17, 20, 22, 25, 31, 125–26, 130
  HIV-positive, 176
Functional psychiatric disorders, 199
Fumagillin, 288
Fungal diseases, 85, 87–88

Histoplasma capsulatum, 26, 237, 249–50
Histoplasmosis, 77, 86, 88, 211, 249–50
HIV (human immunodeficiency virus), ix, 1,
  217, 218, 231, 251
  AZT-resistant strains of, 56, 57, 58, 64, 72
  as cause of AIDS, 215, 216, 339–40
  causing disease, 282, 336–39
  ddl resistant, 69
  drug strategies to disrupt reproductive
    cycle of, 343–51
  hepatitis B and, 236
  immunologic therapeutic strategies against,
    352–54
  as medical specialty, 19–20, 21
  physical structure of, 342–43
  repeat exposure to, 103
  therapeutic strategies, 343–54
  virology, 341–43
  wild-type, 56
HIV antibody testing, ix, 1, 3–17, 41, 120,
    137, 159, 298
  accuracy of results, 8
  arranging for, 14
  and discrimination, 14–15, 383–84
  initial and confirming, 7
  mandatory, 383–85
  psychological preparation for, 11–12
  reaction to testing positive, 15–17
  reasons against, 3–4
  reasons for, 4–5
  risk self-assessment, 12–14
  significance of results of, 9
HIV antibody testing sites, 409–10
HIV culture, 166
HIV disease, ix–xiii, 121–22, 123, 216
  experience of, 119
  manifestations in children, 166–68
  measuring immune deficiency, 41, 42–44
  opportunistic complications of, 76–85
  organ system complications in later stages
    of, 183–211
  progression of, 49, 51, 64
  science of, 321
  unfairness, randomness of, 135
  and weight loss, 194
HIV genetic material, 56
HIV-induced (idiopathic) thrombocytopenia
    purpura, 53
HIV infection, ix, xi, 9, 86, 181, 201
  acute/primary, 219–20
  CMV infection with, 232
  testing for, 321, 323–26
HIV-2, 8
HIV-related services, 412–14
Hives, 188
Hoffman-LaRoche (co.), 70, 348, 349
Holistic remedies, 150
Home health care, 309, 318, 373
Homophobia, 27, 140, 142, 314
Homosexuality, 120, 131, 133, 134, 142, 144
Hopelessness, 147
Hospital(s), 20, 24
  with AIDS units, 21, 314
  choosing, 313–14
  personnel, 315–18
  physician affiliation, 21
  routine, 319–20
  teaching, 23, 313–14, 375

Hospitalization, 112, 137, 181, 186, 271
  and applying for benefits, 378
  experience of, 313–21
  insurance reimbursed, 372
  pain medication, 157–58
Hotlines, 176, 177
Housing, 382, 384
H2-receptor antagonists, 225
Human papilloma virus (HPV), 163
  infection, 187–88
  lesions, 183, 184
Human Rights Commissions, 382
Humatin (paromycin), 193, 195
Hydrocortisone, 115, 189, 274
Hydroxynaphthoquinones, 243
Hygiene, 251
Hyperrcin, 354
Hyperkalemia, 211, 243
Hypersensitivity (skin), 185, 188–89
Hypnosis, 158
Hypocalcemia, 230
Hypoglycemia, 242
Hypomania, 151–52
Hyponatremia, 211, 230, 242
Hypoxemia, 168, 169, 226

Ibuprofen (Advil, Motrin), 157, 169, 274
IFA (test), 7, 14
Illness
  as punishment, 134, 135
Imaging techniques, 201, 206, 240, 299–303
Imidazole, topical, 186, 187, 190
Imipramine (Tofranil), 149, 154
Immigration, 385
Immune complex, 47, 331, 332, 333
Immune deficiency, 221, 336
  illnesses at stages of, 181
  and TB, 264, 265
Immune function, 272, 321
Immune globulins, 113, 166, 171–72, 231,
    331–32, 335
  specific ("adaptive") immunity, 331–33
Immune modulators, 354
Immune processes
  causing tissue damage, 334–35
Immune response, 330, 333, 334, 348, 350
  failure of, 337
  to HIV, 338, 352
  suppression of, 335
  to vaccines, 353
Immune status
  pregnancy and, 164
Immune suppression, 41
  through chemotherapy, 284, 292
  and CMV, 221
  and cryptosporidiosis, 252
  and dementia, 202
  and herpes, 232, 233
  and KS, 280, 281
  and opportunistic infections, 76–77
Immune surveillance system (hypothesis), 281
Immune system, 6, 29, 45, 206, 218, 321, 335
  distributed activity, 329–30
  HIV eluding, 347
  impaired, ix, 238, 245, 249–50, 276
  monitoring, x–xi, 1, 40–47
  natural (nonspecific), 338
  parts of, 327–29

438

positive thinking and, 137–38
self-nonself distinction, 333–34, 335, 337
Immunity, 6, 236
  nonspecific ("native"), 330–31, 338
  specific ("adaptive"), 331–33
Immunizations, 89, 93–97, 113, 218, 264
  for children, 171–72
  hepatitis B, 114, 234, 235–37
  routine adult, 95
Immunodeficiency disorders, 290
Immunoglobulins, 13, 94, 166
Immunologic therapeutic strategies, 352–54
Immunology, 327–36, 353
Immunosuppression
  JC virus, 237
  and response to vaccines, 93–94
Imodium, 114, 193, 195, 199
Impetigo, 167
Imuthiol, 354
Inactivated (killed) vaccines, 94
Income, 376, 377
Incubation period, 219
Independence, 122, 130
Induced sputum test, 240, 241
Infants
  hepatitis B transmitted to, 235
  herpes transmitted to, 233
  HIV-infected, 9, 11, 164, 165, 166, 325
Infections, x, 212–77
  basic information about, 212–19
  skin, 185–88
Infectious diseases, 111, 112, 160, 213, 217, 218
Inflammation, 334
Inflammatory neuropathy, 207
Influenza vaccinations, 92, 94, 95, 114, 171
Information, xi–xiii, 13, 25–26
  friends as source of, 20
  about treatment, 175–77
Informed consent, 361
Infusaport, 224
Infusions, 307, 308, 309
Infusion pump, 230
Inhalation, 79, 82, 84, 196, 209
Injection practices, 137
Insect bite reactions, 188, 189
Insertive partner in sexual intercourse, 14, 104
Insomnia, 69, 150, 156–57
Institutional review board (IRB), 361
Insurance industry, 25, 369, 371
  open enrollment, 371–72, 375
Integrase, 345, 350
Intercourse, 13, 14, 56, 105, 109, 115, 217
  sexually transmitted diseases in, 162–64
  unprotected, 6, 9, 13, 14, 27, 104, 108, 134, 159
  see also Condoms
Interferons, 286, 345, 348
Internal organs, 282, 303
International Certificates of Vaccination, 96
Interns (hospital staff), 316
Interstitial pneumonia, 226
Interventions
  in course of illness, 217–19
  see also Early intervention
Intestinal parasites, 105
Intracranial disorders, 200, 205–07

Intravenous (IV) drug use, 9, 14, 45, 110–11, 123
  and AZT, 63
  and kidney problems, 210
Intravenous feeding, 195, 307
Intravenous immune globulins (IVIG), 172
Intravenous therapy
  ganciclovir, 228–29
  pentamidine, 209
Invasive procedures, 137, 279, 293, 303–09
Investigational new drug (IND), application, 361
Irresponsibility, 133–34
Isocarboxazid (Marplan), 150
Isoniazid (INH), 207, 262, 265, 266
Isospora belli, 191, 237, 244, 251, 252, 253–54
Isosporiasis, 194
ITP (idiopathic thrombocytopenia purpura), 49
Itraconazole (Sporanex), 88, 162, 179, 250, 274, 277

Jane Brody's Nutrition Book, 101
JC virus, 204, 219, 237
Jock itch, 187
Joints, 29

Kaolin-pectin suspension (Kaopectate), 253
Kaposi's sarcoma (KS), 64, 190, 193, 197, 211, 252, 278–79, 289–90, 301, 303, 339
  alpha-interferon, 348
  AZT and, 28, 49, 51
  cause of, 232
  cause or co-factors, 281–82
  in children, 168
  common sites of, 282–83
  costs/benefits of treatment, 284, 285
  course of illness, 282
  definitive diagnosis of, 284
  diagnosis, 283–84
  patterns of illness, 280
  rare among women, 160
  symptoms in mouth, 185
  T4 count and, 43
  treatment, 284–89
Karnofsky scores, 53
Ketoconazole (Nizoral), 88, 162, 186, 187, 190, 193, 211, 224, 250, 266, 276–77
Kidney problems, 168, 209–10, 230, 242, 247–48, 297
Kidneys, 229, 230, 299, 355
Killer T8 cells, 44, 333, 334, 336, 338
Kissing, 14, 106
Kupffer cells, 328, 330, 332

Laboratory tests, 40–41
  see Tests/procedures; and under specific type, e.g., Blood tests
Lactate dehydrogenase (LDH) elevation, 240, 291
Lambda Legal Defense, 385
Laser surgery, 163, 185, 283, 285
Latency (monitoring and prophylaxis), 218, 219, 265, 269
Latent infections, 231, 338
  CMV, 221, 227
  histoplasmosis, 249
  PCP, 238
  toxoplasmosis, 248

439

multiple, 77–78
paradox of, 123–24
psychoactive, 138, 144–58
unproven, 177–79
see also Drugs
Meditation, 158
Megace (megesterol acetate), 195
Megakaryocytes, 358
Mellaril, 152
Membranes, 329, 334
viral, 341, 342
Memory B lymphocytes, 352
Memory cells, 333
Memory impairment, 90, 157, 203, 246
Men who have sex with men, 109–10, 220, 258, 268, 269
and hepatitis B, 235, 236
Meninges, 200, 206, 272, 290
Meningitis, 87, 200, 201, 204, 205, 206, 272
cryptococcal, 273–75
Meningo-encephalitis, 272
Menstrual blood, 104, 105
Menstruation, 105
Mental disorders, 198, 199
Mental life, 119, 136
Mental state, 33–34
changes in, 203, 230, 246
Meperidine (Demerol), 274
Messenger RNA, 349
Metabolic dysfunctions, 149, 195, 196, 205
Metastasis, 279
Methadone, 110, 171, 267
Metheglobinemia, 243
Methionine enkephalin (MEK), 354
Methylphenidate (Ritalin), 151
Metronidazole (Flagyl), 192, 254, 255–56
Microbiology, 295, 299
Miconazole (Monistat), 186
Microconidia, 249
Microorganisms, 76, 225
blood examined for, 299
categories of, 214
causing infections, 212–14
drug-resistant strains of, 78
Microsporidiosis, 251
Microsporidium, 191
Middle East, 96, 112, 235, 236
Minerals, 100, 102, 355
Minorities, 2, 173, 174
see also African-Americans; Latinos
Mississippi River valley, 249
Molecular weight, 325
Molluscum contagiosum, 187
Money matters, 367, 376–81, 415
Monistat, 162
Monitoring, 76–77
cryptococcosis, 273
histoplasmosis, 249
HIV-infected children, 169
MAC, 260–61
side effects of AZT, 55
strategies/psychologies in, 41
toxoplasmosis, 246–47
Monoamine oxidase inhibitors (MAOI), 150, 154
Monoclonal antibodies, 231
Monocytes, 231, 296, 328, 329, 334, 336, 357, 358

Monokines, 329
Moral issues/systems, 124, 133–34, 135, 137
Morphine, 157, 171
Motor coordination, 237, 246
Motor dysfunction, 203–04
Mouth, 28, 92, 100, 108, 235
inflammation of (stomatitis), 71
KS of, 283
problems, 183–85
semen in, 104, 105
Movement disorders, 156
MRC/INSERM, 64
Mucormycosis, 205
Mucous membranes, 9, 103–04, 105, 217, 232, 235, 275, 303, 330
Multicenter AIDS Cohort Study (MACS), 61
Multiple myeloma, 335
Multiple sclerosis, 335
Muscle disease, 207–8
Muscles, 29
Myalgia (muscle pain), 53–54, 55, 207–8
Myasthenia gravis, 335
Mycobacteria, 241, 257–67, 338
Mycobacterium avium, 225, 257
Mycobacterium avium complex (MAC), 44, 78, 168, 191, 194, 197, 209, 211, 251, 258–62, 301
diagnosis, 193, 259–60, 304
monitoring and prevention, 85–87, 260–61
outside AIDS, 258
signs and symptoms, 260
treatment, 259, 261–62
Mycobacterium avium-intracellulare, 196, 209
Mycobacterium hemophilum, 257–58
Mycobacterium intracellulare, 257, 258
Mycobacterium kansaii, 257
Mycobacterium tuberculosis, 197, 257, 262–67
Mycoplasma, 197, 212, 214
Myelopathy, 53, 199, 201
Myelosuppression, 286, 287
Myopathy (muscle disease), 53–54, 55, 61, 64, 207–08

N-acetylcysteine (NAC), 354
N-butyl-DNJ (deoxynojirimycin), 350
Nail pigmentation, 188
Narcotics, 157
Narcotics Anonymous (NA), 118
Nasogastric feeding, 195
National Academy of Sciences, 110
Food and Nutrition Board, 102
National AIDS Clearing House, 176, 409
National AIDS Information Clearinghouse, 101
National Association of People with AIDS (NAPWA), 176
National Lawyers' Guild AIDS Network, 385
"Native" immune system, 330–31
Natural killer cells (NK cells), 231, 328, 330, 331, 332, 336
dysfunction in, 338
Nausea, 59, 64, 71, 90, 193–94, 219, 252–53
Nebulizer, 84
Needle cleaning, 89, 110–11, 220
Needle sharing, 3, 6, 8, 12, 45, 110–11, 117, 123, 131, 258
and cardiac problems, 209
and clinical trials, 364
and CMV, 220

441

Reglan, 194
Regulatory genes (HIV), 347–48
Rejection, 108, 124, 134
Relapse, 250
Relations with other people, 119, 122, 124–32
Relaxation, 144, 158, 294–95
Renal failure/insufficiency, 210, 229
Renal test, 55
Research subjects, 51
Residents, 316, 318
Resistance, 66, 114, 219
  acyclovir, 233
  AZT, 49, 56–58
  ddC, 72
  ddI, 69
  ganciclovir, 228
  microorganisms, 78
  mycobacteria, 257
  reverse transcriptase inhibitors, 347
Respiratory problems/symptoms, 79, 114,
  196–97, 249, 301
Response to treatment
  differences between men and women, 160
  race/ethnicity and, 173–74
Restless leg syndrome, 156
Reticulocyte count, 297, 357
Reticuloendothelial system, 258
Retina, 222, 223, 250
Retinal detachment, 223
Retinitis, 245
  CMV, 221, 222–23, 226, 227, 228
Retroviruses, 212, 213, 321, 341–42, 345
Reverse transcriptase (RT), 48, 56, 67, 70,
  213, 342, 345
Reverse transcriptase inhibitors
  experimental nonnucleoside, 347
  nucleoside-analog, 346
Reverse transcriptase (RT) inhibitors, 48–49,
  51, 54, 345–47
Reverse transcription (HIV), 343, 345–47
Reversible vascular hyperplasia, 281
Ribavirin, 56, 349
Ribonuclease II, 345, 346
Ribosomes, 341, 342, 348, 349
Richman, 60
Rifabutin (Ansamycin), 87, 260, 261
Rifampin (RIF), 211, 261, 262, 265, 266–67
Rimming. See Oral-anal contact (rimming)
RIPA (test) (radio-immunoprecipative assay), 7
Risk factors
  non-Hodgkin's lymphomas, 290
Risk for HIV infection, 3, 4, 5, 8, 11
  drug use as, 111
  levels of, 12–13
  in schools, 172
  for women, 159
Risk pools, 372
Risk reduction, 3, 4, 12, 14, 103, 108–10
Risk self-assessment, 12–14
RNA, 213, 342, 345, 346, 348, 349, 350
RNA polymerase, 348
RO-31-8959, 349

Safer sex, 3, 5, 103–10, 137, 220
Safety (drug), 177–78, 344, 359
  clinical trials, 361–62
  postexposure vaccination, 352
Saliva, 104, 106

Salmonella, 102, 167, 191, 225, 251, 257,
  267–68
Salmonellosis, 113, 194, 267–68
San Francisco, 117, 176, 189, 375
San Francisco AIDS Foundation, 20, 177
Sarcomas, 279
Scaly skin (papulosquamous disorders), 185,
  189–90
Scapegoating, 131, 133
SCH39304, 88
SCID-HU mouse, 361
Scraping, 303
Seborrhea, 92
Seborrheic dermatitis, 189–90
Secobarbitol (Seconal), 155–56
Secondary prophylaxis, 78, 219
Secondary syphilis, 269, 271
Sedative effect of drugs, 148, 149–50
Sedatives, 117
Seizures, 149, 150, 168, 200, 206–07, 230,
  246, 248
Self-destructive behavior, 132–33, 136, 143
Self-education, 25
Self-esteem, 124
Semen, 9, 14, 103, 104, 105, 108, 220
Sepsis, 250
Septra. See Bactrim
Septra Suspension, 81
Seroconversion, 8
Serology, 295, 298
Serum, 324
Serum creatinine, 231
Serum fasting triglyceride levels, 69
Serum osmolality, 297
Serum neopterin, 45, 46
Serum sodium concentrate, 297
Sex
  between patient and therapist, 141
  risk from, 13, 14, 217
  unsafe, 8, 58
  see also Intercourse, unprotected; Safer sex
Sex toys, 107–08
Sexism, 160
Sexual behavior
  balance in, 109
  risk categories, 103–09
Sexual history, 27
Sexual partners, 13, 14, 309
  disclosing HIV status to, 108–09, 124–25
Sexual practices, 125
Sexual side effects
  of psychoactive drugs, 151
Sexuality, 133, 134
Sexually transmitted diseases, 5, 27, 29, 103,
  106, 108, 160, 164, 217
  genital warts, 187
  KS, 281
  in women, 162–63
Shame, 132–35, 138
Shigella, 82, 102, 191, 225, 251, 257, 268–69
Shigellosis, 113, 194
Shingles (herpes zoster), 43
Shortness of breath, 28, 79, 90, 196, 209,
  239, 301
Side effects, 77, 114, 123–24, 158, 177, 224,
  257, 348
  alpha-interferon, 348
  AZT, 49–50, 52, 53–54, 55, 59, 60, 62,

445

447

448